Gut and Psychology Syndrome

Natural treatment for

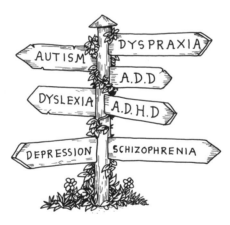

Dr. Natasha Campbell-McBride MD,
MMedSci (neurology), MMedSci (nutrition)

© Natasha Campbell-Mcbride, 2010

Gut and Psychology Syndrome

ISBN 13: 978-0-9548520–2–3

First published in the United Kingdom in September 2004 by
Medinform Publishing
10 Adelaide Close
Soham
Cambridge CB7 5FJ

Revised and expanded edition published November 2010
Seventh reprint February 2012

Typeset by Cambrian Typesetters, Frimley, Surrey
Printed by Maple-Vail Book Manufacturing, York, Pennsylvania

To my sons, Nicholas and Matthew, and to my husband, Peter, without whose support and encouragement this book would never have been written.

Reviews

Dr. Natasha Campbell-McBride is to be congratulated on putting together such a well-researched and provocative book. From the overuse of antibiotics to the promotion of breast-feeding and healthier diets, Dr. Campbell-McBride writes with the authority of a practising doctor and with the warmth and feeling of a mother of a child with autism. Every parent with a child who has autism, attention-deficit hyperactivity disorder, dyslexia or dyspraxia will find much to value in this book, which in turn delights and shocks the reader. I warmly recommend it.

Dr Basant K Puri, MA, PhD, MB, BChir, BSc MathSci, MRCPsych, DipStat, MMath, Head of the Lipid Neuroscience Group, MRI Unit, Hammersmith Hospital, Imperial College, London; and author of the books The Natural Way to Beat Depression; Chronic Fatigue Syndrome; and Natural Energy.

Dr. Natasha Campbell-McBride has done an excellent job of summarising the nutritional biochemical connections with pyschiatric and neurological disorders and gastrointestianl function. She has done an admirable job in relating specific digestive disorders in conditions such as schizophrenia, autism, attention deficit disorder and other problems of child development. The book is full of valuable and interesting facts that can be used by people to optimise the health of themselves and their children.

Dr. William Shaw, PhD., Great Plains Laboratories, Kansas, USA

Dr. Campbell-McBride's book provides important information and great insight into the understanding and treatment of gastrointestinal disorders in those with developmental disabilities and other disorders. The book contains basic information for the beginner as well as in-depth information for those at an advance level. Thank you Dr. Campbell-McBride for writing this book.

Dr. Stephen M. Edelson, Ph.D., Center for the Study of Autism, Oregon USA.

This book is fantastic and will become a classic. Every medic should have one. . . No, every household should have one!

An invaluable resource for patients with 'syndrome diseases' and so-called 'mental health problems'. The medicine of the future already in practice.

Martina Watts BA(Hons) DipION MBANT,
practising nutritionist and journalist

This book presents the case for investigating the nutritional aspects, how the gut works and how poor gut function seriously impacts not only physical health but also brain function, for all children with learning and behaviour difficulties.

Countless parents seeking help from The Hyperactive Children's Support Group find their children benefit greatly from dietary and nutritional interventions. Vitamin, mineral and essential fatty acid deficiencies are all too frequently discovered.

This book offers an insight to how the digestive system affects the brain.

Sally Bunday, Founder Director,
The Hyperactive Children's Support Group,UK

Wicken Fen

The old wooden gates swinging wide open
leaving room for a path of wood stretching out in front of you.
The heavenly scent of the clean fresh air.
The whistling sound of the grass and the trees
swaying left and right in the breeze.
At night you stare at the wonderful sight.

The path leading over the moist soft grass.
You walk on the bridge over a gently flowing river.
The hill reaching so high, almost touching the sky.
The windmill still stands as you walk the stairs
which have been there for years.

The buzzing of the bees busy in their hive.
All the sounds surround you.
The warm feeling of welcome is quick to arrive.
The sun shining bright on the grass
as green as the leaves in summer.

The way forward getting thinner leaving the feeling that lasts.
The adventure is over.
Feeling warm inside.
Farewell until next time.

Nicholas Campbell-McBride, 11 years old,
Cambridge, UK

Contents

To the Parents of Autistic Children
– an Open Letter

Not many people would choose to become parents of an autistic child. Yet it is happening to more and more of us in our modern world. There is an unmistakable epidemic of autism going on across the globe. If this can possibly be of any comfort for a parent, then I would say that you are certainly not alone!

Autism used to be a rare disorder, so that the majority of doctors never saw it in their practice and most people had never heard of it. About twenty years ago in Western countries the incidence of autism used to be on average one child in 10,000. Now according to the UK Department of Health 1 in 150 children in Great Britain are diagnosed with autism. According to the USA Centers for Disease Control (CDC) around 1 out of 150 American children are diagnosed with autistic spectrum disorders now and the numbers are growing every day. Similar numbers are reported by the Autism Canada Foundation. A Finnish study published in the *European Journal of Child and Adolescent Psychiatry* (2001, volume 9) reported an incidence rate of 1 child in 483 diagnosed autistic in Finland. In Sweden a rate of 1 child in 141 was reported.

So, what is happening? Why do we have such a dramatic increase in the numbers of children falling prey to this terrible disorder, deemed incurable by orthodox medicine?

Is the reason for this epidemic genetic? The truth is – we don't know! However, what we do know, is that genetic disorders do not show such a sudden increase in incidence. Genetics just don't work that way. This kind of increase in new diagnosis of autism cannot be explained by genetics. On the contrary, it provides a strong argument to support the statement that genetics may not play an important part in the development of autism after all.

Is this epidemic due to better diagnosis? That is what some very well-established British medical experts are trying to tell us. So, in effect, are they saying that 15 years ago doctors in the UK were so bad at recognising and diagnosing autism that they were missing one child in 150? If that is the case, where are all these children today? They would by now be teenagers with autism, because we know that this disorder does not disappear with age. We clearly do not have 1 in 150 teenagers in the UK with autism. So, this argument does not convince anybody. Something else is going on. Something that cannot simply be explained away and something that cannot be fixed with a pill.

Most parents of autistic children can clearly recall that traumatic moment when the diagnosis of "Autism" was announced to them by a doctor, followed by the statement "There is nothing that can be done." Well, being a doctor myself, I have to say that your doctor is wrong, there is a lot that can be done! I would even go further, depending on your commitment and certain circumstances, you have a good chance of bringing your child as close as possible to normality! Hundreds of autistic children across the globe, appropriately treated and educated become almost indistinguishable from their typically developing (normal) peers. The sooner the treatment starts, the better the results, because the younger the child is, the less damage there is to undo and also because they have less catching up to do in their development with normal children of their age. Thankfully, the medical profession-als, though often unhelpful as far as treatment is concerned, are much better nowadays at diagnosing autism. The majority of children get diagnosed by the age of three, which was not the case 15–20 years ago. Receiving the diagnosis so early gives the parents a chance to start acting early, which gives the child a better chance of recovery.

In the Western world there is a general tendency to delegate respon-sibility for our health to the medical profession. If you are ill you go to the doctor. When it comes to autism, after establishing the diagnosis, official medicine has virtually nothing to offer the child. It is a big shock for parents to suddenly find themselves facing this monster called "Autism" on their own. Most of the parents I have met are intel-ligent and often well-educated people. The first thing they do is to learn as much as possible. Today there is a whole world of information available on the subject of autism, including solid scientific research. Looking at the amount of research done in other areas of medicine in the last 15 years, it is often less than what has been achieved in the field of autism. I believe the reason is that research in autism is almost entirely driven by the most motivated people on Earth – the parents of autistic children. Among them are doctors, biochemists, biologists and simply intelligent people looking for solutions to their child's problem. There is a network of parent organisations across the world keen to share information and help each other. I know a lot of parents who would spend hours on the phone to comfort and help another parent in the same situation. Treating autism is not an easy task. It takes years of continuous effort and commitment. But, being a parent of a recovered child myself, I can tell you that it is one of the most rewarding experiences on Earth! In this book I would like to share with you what I strongly believe to be the appropriate treatment for an autistic child.

Information on nutrition is not included in the curriculum of Western medical schools and consequently doctors have very little idea about the value of nutrition in the treatment of disease. Yet appropriate nutrition is a corner-stone of any successful treatment for any chronic disease. Autism and other learning disabilities are no exception. There are many popular misconceptions in this area, which have to be clarified.

Autism used to be a diagnosis considered hopeless. With all the knowledge we have today it is very far from that. And we are still learning every day. Children diagnosed today are much more fortunate than children diagnosed 15 years ago (if the word fortunate can be used at all), because their parents have so much more information available to them to start helping their child immediately. Fifteen years ago we did not know half of what we know today. Parents of newly diagnosed children now have no time to despair – there is too much learning to do! I think that is very positive. The learning roller coaster your child will take you through will change your life forever. Who knows, it may open new horizons and opportunities for you, as it has done for so many people.

So, let's keep learning!

Introduction

This book has evolved over a period of three years when I worked with hundreds of children in my clinic. Initially the book was planned to be about autism as the majority of children who came to see me were indeed autistic. However, the more children I saw, the more it became clear that we have other epidemics emerging. Attention deficit disorder with hyperactivity and without it (ADHD/ADD), dyspraxia, dyslexia, various behavioural and learning problems, allergies, asthma, eczema all have reached epidemic proportions. But more than that, these seemingly unrelated conditions overlap with each other. After years of working with the children in my clinic I hardly met one child who presented with just one of the above conditions. Every child has two, three or more of these health problems at once. For example, a child would present with allergies; at the same time the parents would describe a couple of asthmatic episodes and eczema and then would talk about their child's extreme clumsiness (dyspraxia) and learning problems. A large percentage of allergic and asthmatic children are dyspraxic and hyperactive to various degrees. Many of them have problems with concentration and attention span, which affect their learning ability. There is an approximate 50% overlap between dyslexia and dyspraxia and a 30–50% overlap between ADHD and dyslexia. Children who suffer severe eczema in infancy quite often develop autistic features later in life. Autism and ADHD overlap with every one of the above-mentioned conditions. Apart from being hyperactive many autistic children have severe allergies, asthma, eczema, dyspraxia and dyslexia.

As we can see, modern medicine has created all these separate diagnostic boxes to fit our children in. But the modern child does not fit into any one of them; the modern child fits into this rather lumpy picture.

Why are all these conditions related? What underlying problem are we missing in our children which makes them susceptible to asthma, eczema, allergies, dyspraxia, dyslexia, behavioural problems, ADHD and autism in different combinations? Why, when they become teenagers, do many of these children fall prey to substance abuse? Why

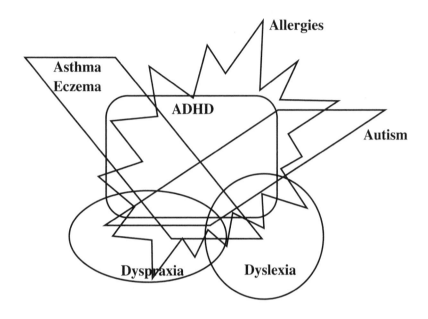

THE OVERLAPPING PICTURE

do many of these children grow up to become diagnosed with schizo-phrenia, depression, bipolar disorder and other psychological and psychiatric problems?

To answer all these questions we have to look at one factor, which unites all these patients in a clinical setting. This factor is the state of their digestive system. I have yet to meet a child with autism, ADHD/ADD, asthma, eczema, allergies, dyspraxia or dyslexia, who has not got digestive abnormalities. In many cases they are severe enough for the parents to start talking about them first. In some cases the parents may not mention their child's digestive system, yet when asked direct questions would describe a plethora of gut problems. But what have digestive abnormalities got to do with autism, hyperactiv-ity, inability to learn, mood and behaviour problems? According to recent research and clinical experience – a lot! In fact it appears that the child's digestive system holds the key to the child's mental devel-opment. The underlying disorder, which can manifest itself in different children with different combinations of symptoms, resides in the gut! Rather than trying to fit a child with autistic tendencies, asthma, eczema and hyperactivity or a child with dyspraxia, dyslexia and allergies into any particular diagnostic box we need to have a name for the underlying disorder, which originates in the gut and manifests itself as any combination of the above conditions.

Here I propose a name: **Gut And Psychology Syndrome** or **GAP Syndrome**. Children with GAP Syndrome often fall into the gap – the gap in our medical knowledge. As a result they do not receive appropriate treatment. In the following chapters we are going to talk in detail about what the GAP Syndrome means, how it develops and how to treat it.

Apart from childhood learning disabilities: autism, ADHD/ADD, dyslexia, dyspraxia and various learning and behavioural problems, there is another group of conditions which fit into the GAP Syndrome. These conditions are schizophrenia, depression, eating disorders, manic depression or bipolar disorder and obsessive compulsive disorder. The father of modern psychiatry French psychiatrist Phillipe Pinel (1745–1828), after working with mental patients for many years, concluded in 1807: "The primary seat of insanity generally is in the region of the stomach and intestines." And yet, the last thing a modern psychiatrist would pay attention to is the patient's digestive system! We will discuss the scientific and clinical evidence pointing in the direction of gut–brain connection in schizophrenic patients.

It is beyond the scope of this book to look at other psychiatric conditions. Hopefully, future clinical experience and research will shed light on how many of them may belong to Gut And Psychology Syndrome. Here we will concentrate on the conditions which receive the diagnostic labels of Autistic Spectrum Disorder, ADHD/ADD, Dyslexia, Dyspraxia and Schizophrenia. This book may also be useful for patients who are diagnosed with allergies, including asthma and eczema.

Part One: WHAT IS GOING ON?

1. All Diseases Begin in the Gut

Hippocrates, 460–370 BC

GAPS children and adults have digestive problems, sometimes quite severe. Colic, bloating, flatulence, diarrhoea, constipation, feeding difficulties and malnourishment, all to various degrees, are a typical part of autism, schizophrenia and other GAPS conditions. Doctors often explain these symptoms as a result of patients' "funny" feeding habits and are not inclined to investigate them.

Whether we look at a child or an adult with GAPS, in the majority of cases digestive problems start at weaning time or times when breast milk gets replaced with formula milk and other foods get introduced. In many cases parents clearly remember that the diarrhoea or constipation started in the second year, but thinking back would recall that their child had colic, vomiting (reflux) or other digestive symptoms in the first year as well. In cases of GAPS adults it is important to speak to the parents of the patient (if possible) in order to collect a detailed medical history starting from birth. In those cases where an adult did not have a history of gut problems from childhood the digestive problems would start later in life due to some health-damaging event.

The second year of life is the time when many GAPS children start developing fussy eating habits, refusing a whole lot of foodstuffs and limiting their diet to a handful of foods, usually starchy and sweet: breakfast cereals, crisps, chips, popcorn, cakes, biscuits, sweets, bananas, bread, rice, sweet yoghurts. Most of these children would refuse to have vegetables, fruit (apart from bananas), meats, fish and eggs. About 60–70% of the autistic children I have seen in my clinic would have an extremely limited diet, consisting sometimes of two or three items. It is quite rare to meet an autistic child who is not fussy with food. Other GAPS children may not be as extreme as autistic children but the majority of them also limit their diets in the same typical fashion.

It is also very rare for parents of GAPS children to describe their child's stool as normal. The picture is particularly striking in autistic children. Diarrhoea and constipation would often alternate and, in many cases, undigested food is clearly visible in the stool. Very often the stool would have an extremely strong, unpleasant smell and at other times it would be so liquid and frothy that the child cannot hold it. Sometimes the stool would be very acid and burn the child's skin in the nappy area. In many cases the stool has a pale whitish colour and floats on the surface of the water, indicating that the child is unable to digest fats. Often the child would have such severe constipation, that he or she would not open the bowel for 5–7 or more days, which then would result in an extremely large and painful stool. This sort of experience makes children fearful of passing stool, so they hold on for as long as they can, making the whole problem even worse. In some cases parents do not notice anything wrong with the stool, but when asked would acknowledge that their child has pronounced flatulence and bloating. In many of these cases the child would wake up at night screaming, when the parents do not know what is wrong. As the excessive gas gets released or simply moves to a different place in the bowel the pain would disappear and the child would settle down.

In the case of autism all these symptoms undoubtedly cause children a lot of discomfort and pain. But unfortunately, due to their inability to communicate, most autistic children cannot tell their parents about it, so they express their feelings in other ways: self-stimulation, self-destruction, tantrums, refusing to eat, etc. Many children would assume strange postures and positions in order to relieve abdominal discomfort, usually pressing their tummies on hard parts of furniture. Children with other GAPS conditions who do not have communication problems often complain of tummy aches and feeling nauseous.

In most cases these children are not tested or investigated by gastro-enterologists. In a few published cases when autistic children have been investigated, an X-ray of their digestive tract almost invariably showed a condition called "faecal compaction with an over-spill syndrome". What does it mean? It means that large amounts of old, compacted faeces are literally glued to the walls of the digestive tract, where they can stay for many months, providing a fertile rotting environment for all sorts of parasites, bacteria, fungi and viruses to breed and thrive, constantly producing a lot of toxic substances which are absorbed into the bloodstream of the child. In this condition new food, eaten by the child, seeps through a narrow channel between these compacted faecal masses. So, whatever stool comes out of these children is an over-spill, which does not empty the bowel, hence the name – an over-spill syndrome.

Until the last few years, apart from a few anecdotal reports in medical literature on an over-spill syndrome in autistic children, there was virtually no research done in this area. Then in 1998 Dr Andrew Wakefield, a consultant gastro-enterologist at the Royal Free Hospital in London, and his team published their research, suggesting a connection between chronic inflammatory bowel disease and autism. They performed endoscopy and biopsy on a group of autistic children, who were referred to them with gastrointestinal symptoms. Endoscopy is a procedure where a special pipe is inserted into the digestive tract of a patient, through which an investigator can see what is going on there. While an endoscopy is being performed, a small bit of the gut wall can be obtained using a special biting instrument to be later examined under the microscope. This is called taking a biopsy.

As a result of their research, Dr Wakefield and his team have identified a condition in the bowel of these children, which they named *Ileal – Lymphoid – Nodular Hyperplasia and Non-Specific Colitis*. Let us see what it all means.

First we will look at the *Ileal – Lymphoid – Nodular Hyperplasia*. Ileum is a name given to the last three-fifths of the small intestine. The ileum is approximately 3.5 m long in adults and at its end connects to the bowel. The major function of the small intestine in general is food absorption. However, not much food absorption happens in the ileum. The walls of this part of the small intestine are packed with large numbers of lymph nodes, called Peyer's patches, which are small, round or bean shaped structures, ranging in size from 1 to 25 mm. These lymph nodes are a very important part of our immune system. We know of two major functions that they fulfil.

1. The first function is filtering the lymph (tissue liquid) coming from the ileum and removing bacteria, viruses, fungi, dead cells (including cancer cells) and various toxins from it. It is a good place to look at what particular infectious agents might be lurking in your

intestine because the lymph nodes are like a prison for these viruses, bacteria, dead cells and fungi – if they cannot destroy them, they imprison them. So, when gastro-enterologists perform endoscopies, they always try to get a sample of these lymph nodes to be examined under the microscope. This is what Dr Wakefield's team has done.

2. A second function of lymph nodes is production of lymphocytes – a large group of immune system cells, a major function of which is fighting infections. In fact lymph nodes themselves are made primarily of lymphocytes, together with some other cells. So, when the lymph nodes are faced with an infection, they start producing a lot of lymphocytes to fight the infection, which makes the lymph nodes large and inflamed, sometimes painful. This enlargement of the lymph nodes is called lymphoid nodular hyperplasia and this is what Dr Wakefield has found in the ileum of autistic children.

Because many of the children from his study have developed autistic features after MMR vaccine, this is the direction Dr Wakefield pursued when looking at what particular infection may have caused this enlargement of the lymph nodes. Suspecting that it might be the measles virus, he involved in his research a well-known virologist Dr John O'Leary, a professor of pathology from Dublin. Sure enough, Dr O'Leary has found the same measles virus used in the MMR vaccine in the ileal lymph nodes of the autistic children. This particular part of Dr Wakefield's research, concerning the measles virus and MMR vaccine, caused a lot of controversy and vigorous resistance from government and the medical establishment which distracted attention from the main issue. The main issue is: autistic children have enlarged and inflamed lymph nodes in their gut wall, which is a clear sign of a fight with some infection going on there.

Let us now look at the second part of the condition which Dr Wakefield described in his group of autistic children, the *Non-Specific Colitis*. The term Colitis means an inflammation of the colon. Doing the endoscopies, Dr Wakefield's team has found various stages of chronic inflammation in the gut of these children, erosions of the mucous membranes of the colon and intestines, abscesses filled with pus, ulcers and plenty of faecal compaction. In some places the gut wall was so inflamed with such enlargement of the lymph nodes, that it almost obstructed the lumen of the gut. In some ways this inflammation resembled ulcerative colitis, in some – Crohn's disease, when some features were completely unique to these autistic children. That is why this colitis was named non-specific, because it could not be assigned to any existing diagnosis. Dr Wakefield's team called it AUTISTIC ENTEROCOLITIS. This term is yet to be accepted into the official medical vocabulary, but for those who work with autistic children it is a very good term to use.

The findings of Dr Andrew Wakefield and his team, who have examined hundreds of autistic children, have been independently supported by a number of other researchers in the world (Buie *at al.*, Uhlmann *et al.*, Furlano *et al.*, Morris *et al.*). Apart from published research, there are number of practising doctors around the world whose clinical observations support the fact that autistic children have a digestive disorder, the severity of which may differ in different children. Based on my clinical experience I would strongly add my voice to theirs: in fact I have yet to meet an autistic child without digestive problems.

So far we have been talking mostly about autism. What about the rest of GAPS patients? There has been a substantial amount of research linking schizophrenia with digestive abnormalities similar to coeliac disease. C. Dohan, R. Cade, K. Rachelt, A. Hoffer, C. Pfeiffer and other doctors and scientists have established a hypothesis of gut–brain connection in schizophrenia and backed it by very serious scientific findings, which we will discuss in detail in the following chapters. Clinical experience shows that the majority of schizophrenic patients suffer from digestive problems. In most cases these problems start in early childhood.

Apart from autism and schizophrenia there is much less published scientific data on gut problems in ADHD, dyslexia, dyspraxia, asthma, allergy, eczema and other GAPS conditions. However, when it comes to clinical observations almost all children and adults with GAPS have digestive problems to various degrees. Many patients have typical symptoms of IBS (Irritable Bowel Syndrome): abdominal pain, bloating, stool abnormalities and flatulence. A small percentage of patients may have normal stools, but would suffer from malnutrition, reflux, "heartburn", abdominal pains and flatulence. In the case of GAPS children most of them limit their diets in the typical GAPS fashion, preferring processed carbohydrates to the exclusion of everything else. Many GAPS adults also have similar fussy attitudes to food. I had a number of patients who did not complain of any particular digestive problems. However, when put on a GAPS treatment programme they have improved dramatically.

The question is: why do GAPS children and adults have their digestive systems in such a condition? What has it got to do with their mental state? To understand that we need to look at some very important fundamental aspects of the human gut.

2. The Roots of a Tree

A human body is like a planet inhabited by huge numbers of various micro-creatures. The diversity and richness of this life on every one of us is probably as amazing as the life on Earth itself! Our digestive system, skin, eyes, respiratory and excretory organs are happily co-existing with trillions of invisible lodgers, making one ecosystem of macro- and micro-life, living together in harmony. It is a symbiotic relationship, where neither party can live without the other. Let me repeat this: we, humans, cannot live without these tiny micro-organisms, which we carry on and in our bodies everywhere.

The largest colonies of microbes live in our digestive system. A healthy adult, on average, carries 1.5–2 kg of bacteria in the gut. All these bacteria are not just a chaotic microbial mass, but a highly organised micro-world with certain species predominating and controlling others. The number of functions they fulfil in our bodies are so vital to us, that if our gut got sterilised, we would probably not survive. In a healthy body this microbial world is fairly stable and adaptable to changes in their environment. Let's look at who is who in there?

Gut micro-flora can be divided into three groups:

1. **Essential or beneficial flora** This is the most important group and the most numerous in a healthy individual. These bacteria are often referred to as our indigenous friendly bacteria. The main members of this group are: *Bifidobacteria, Lactobacteria, Propionobacteria,* physiological strains of *E.coli, Peptostreptococci* and *Enterococci*. We are going to look in detail at what good work they do in our bodies.
2. **Opportunistic flora** This is a large group of various microbes, the number and combinations of which can be quite individual. These are: *Bacteroids, Peptococci, Staphylococci, Streptococci, Bacilli, Clostridia,* Yeasts, *Enterobacteria* (*Proteus, Clebsielli, Citrobacteria,* etc.), *Fuzobacteria, Eubacteria, Catenobacteria* and many others. There are around 500 various species of microbes known to science so far which can be found in the human gut. In a healthy person their numbers are normally limited and are tightly controlled by

the beneficial flora. Each of these microbes is capable of causing various health problems if they get out of control.

3. **Transitional flora** These are various microbes which we daily swallow with food and drink, usually non-fermenting gram-negative bacilli from the environment. When the gut is well protected by beneficial bacteria, this group of microbes goes through our digestive tract without doing any harm. But if the population of the beneficial flora is damaged and not functioning well this group of microbes can cause disease.

So, what are all these microbes doing there and why do we need them?

Health and integrity of the gut

A human digestive tract is a long tube open to the outside world at its start and at its end. Whatever harmful things there are in the outside world, our digestive system is a perfect entrance for them into our bodies. We eat and drink plenty of micro-organisms, chemicals and toxins every day. How do we survive?

One of the major reasons is the fact that the whole length of the digestive tract is coated with a bacterial layer, much like a thick layer of turf on the surface of the gut epithelium, providing a natural barrier against invaders, undigested food, toxins and parasites. And, just like a soil unprotected by turf becomes eroded, the gut wall suffers if its protective bacterial "turf" gets damaged. How do our indigenous bacteria protect the gut wall?

Apart from providing a physical barrier, they work against invasive pathogenic micro-organisms by producing antibiotic-like substances, anti-fungal volatiles, anti-viral substances, including interferon, lizocym and surfactins, that dissolve membranes of viruses and bacteria; they engage the immune system to respond appropriately to invaders. In addition, by producing organic acids, the beneficial bacteria reduce pH near the wall of the gut to 4.0–5.0, making a very uncomfortable acidic environment for growth and activity of pathogenic "bad" microbes, which require more alkaline surroundings.

Pathogenic microbes produce a lot of very potent toxins, not to mention all the toxic substances that we ingest with food and drink.

Our healthy indigenous gut flora has a good ability to neutralise nitrates, indoles, phenols, skatol, ksenobiotics and a lot of other toxic substances, inactivate histamine and chelate heavy metals and other poisons. The cell walls of beneficial bacteria absorb many carcinogenic substances, making them inactive. They also suppress hyperplastic processes in the gut, which is the basis of all cancer formation.

So, if the beneficial bacteria in the gut are damaged and are not functioning as they should, then the "walls of the city" are not protected very well, which is a typical situation in a GAPS gut. Without protection the gut wall is open to invasion by anything that comes along: a virus from vaccination or the environment, a ubiquitous fungus such as *Candida albicans*, various bacteria and parasites and toxic substances, all of which are very capable of damaging our digestive system and causing a chronic inflammation in its walls. And we must not forget about the opportunistic flora, which normally lives in the gut, tightly controlled by the beneficial bacteria. They are always there and ready to cause trouble, if their guardians, the good bacteria, are weakened. Studies with microscopic examination of a biopsy of the gut wall show that in healthy individuals there is a thick bacterial band attached to gut mucosa, keeping it intact and healthy. In inflammatory bowel disease different pathogenic bacteria are found in the mucosa, even inside the gut cells, which means that the protective bacterial band has been broken and allowed the pathogens to reach the sacred gut wall.

To make the situation even worse, without well-functioning gut flora the gut wall not only becomes unprotected, but also malnourished. Normal gut flora provides a major source of energy and nourishment for the cells which are lining the digestive tract. The beneficial bacteria living on the gut epithelium digest the food which comes along, converting it into nourishing substances for the gut lining. In fact it is estimated that gut epithelium derives 60–70% of its energy from bacterial activity. When the gut flora is compromised, the lack of nourishment it would produce adds to the damage of the digestive wall. This sets up a chain of degenerative changes in the digestive wall structure, which would further impair its ability to digest and absorb nutrients.

To understand what exactly happens in the gut of your child, let us have a look at some anatomy and physiology of the gut lining. The absorptive surface of intestines has a wonderful structure of finger-like protrusions, called villi, and deep crypts between them. The epithelial cells called enterocytes, which coat the villi, are the very cells which complete the digestive process and absorb the nutrients from food. These cells work very hard, so they have to be always young and in good shape to do their job efficiently. As usual, Mother Nature organised it in the most marvellous way. These enterocytes are constantly born in the depth of the crypts. Then they slowly travel to the top of the villi, doing their job of digestion and absorption and getting more and more mature on the way. As they reach the top of the villi, they get shed off. This way the epithelium of intestines gets constantly renewed to ensure its ability to do its work well. (Fig 1)

Animal experiments with sterilisation of the gut found that when the beneficial bacteria living on the intestinal epithelium are removed, this process of cell renewal gets completely out of order. The time of cell travel from the crypts to the top of the villi becomes a few times longer, which upsets the maturation process of enterocytes and often turns them cancerous. The mitotic activity in the crypts gets significantly suppressed, which means that much less cells will be born there and much less of them will be born healthy and able to do their job properly. The state of the cells themselves becomes abnormal. All because their housekeepers, the healthy gut bacteria, are not there to take care of them. (Fig 2)

That is what happens in a laboratory animal with a sterilised gut. In a human body the absence of good bacteria always coincides with bad bacteria getting out of control, which makes the whole situation much worse. Without the care of beneficial bacteria while under attack from pathogenic flora, the whole structure of gut epithelium changes, starting a process of pathology or disease developing. The villi degenerate and become unable to digest and absorb food properly, leading to malabsorption, nutritional deficiencies and food intolerances.

Gut flora is the housekeeper of the digestive system. The state of the house and its ability to fulfil its purposes directly depends on how good the housekeeper is. Anatomical integrity of our digestive tract, its functionality, ability to adapt and regenerate, ability to defend itself and many other functions are directly dependent on the state of its

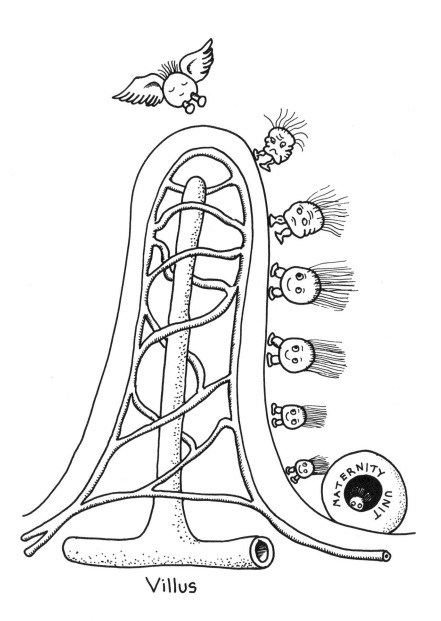

Villus

FIG 1   The life-cycle of an enterocyte

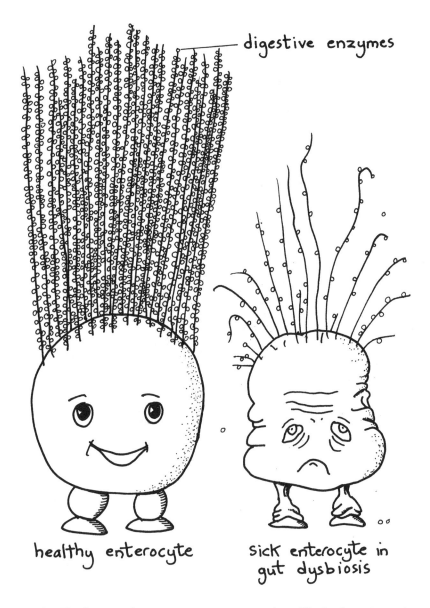

digestive enzymes

healthy enterocyte

sick enterocyte in gut dysbiosis

FIG. 2 The hair on the enterocytes represent microvilli. As the enterocytes cover the surface of the villi their hair (microvilli) make a so-called brush-border, where the last steps in digestion of food happen

microscopic housekeepers – our gut flora. As we will see later, GAPS children and adults have a very abnormal gut flora, which results in digestive abnormalities.

Nourishment of the body

Everybody knows that the main purpose of having a digestive system is to be able to digest and absorb food. Scientific and clinical experience shows that without healthy gut flora the digestive system cannot fulfil these functions efficiently. A good example is the digestion of milk and wheat proteins, which happens in two stages. The first stage occurs in the stomach where, under the influence of digestive juices produced by the stomach walls, milk and wheat proteins get split into peptides, some of which have morphine-like structures called casomorphines and gluteomorphines (or gliadinomorphines). It is a normal process and happens in all of us. Then these peptides move to the small intestine where the next stage of their digestion happens. They get subjected to pancreatic juices and then reach the intestinal wall where they are broken down by enzymes, called peptidases, on the microvilli of enterocytes. This is the stage which is missing in people with abnormal gut flora because of the poor state of their enterocytes. As a result casomorphines and gluteomorphines get absorbed into the bloodstream unchanged and cause problems in the body, in particular interference with brain function and immune system function. There has been a considerable amount of research in this area in patients with autism, schizophrenia, ADHD, psychosis, depression and auto-immunity, who show high levels of casomorphines and gluteomorphines in their bodies, which means that their gut wall is in no fit state to complete appropriate digestion of these substances. Clinical experience shows that when the gut flora is restored, many GAPS patients can digest casein and gluten in moderate amounts without their symptoms returning.

Apart from keeping the gut wall in good shape, the healthy gut flora populating this wall has been designed to take an active part in the very process of digestion and absorption. So much so, that the normal digestion and absorption of food is probably impossible without well-balanced gut flora. It has an ability to digest proteins, ferment carbohydrates and break down lipids and fibre. By-products of bacterial activity in the gut are very important in transporting minerals, vitamins, water, gases and many other nutrients through the gut wall into the bloodstream. If the gut flora is damaged, the best foods and supplements in the world may not have a good chance of being broken down and absorbed.

Certain ingredients in our foods cannot be digested by a human gut at all without the help of beneficial bacteria. A good example is dietary fibre. In a gut with healthy gut flora the fibre gets partially broken down to oligosaccharides, amino-acids, minerals, organic acids and other useful nutrients to feed the gut wall and the rest of the body. Most of us are aware that dietary fibre is good for us. Fresh fruit and vegetables, whole grains, nuts and seeds, beans and pulses are all good sources of fibre. Supplemental fibre in the form of sachets, capsules or drinks is often prescribed to people by doctors to lower their blood cholesterol levels, to remedy constipation and many other digestive problems, to help bile metabolism, to prevent bowel cancer, to improve glucose tolerance in diabetics, etc., etc. There is a long list of benefits from regular consumption of dietary fibre. Well, fibre is one of the natural habitats for beneficial bacteria in the gut. They feed on it, producing a whole host of good nutrition for the gut wall and the whole body, they engage it in absorbing toxins, they activate it to take part in water and electrolytes metabolism, to recycle bile acids and cholesterol, etc., etc. It is the bacterial action on dietary fibre that allows it to fulfil all those good functions in the body. And when these good bacteria are damaged and are not able to "work" the fibre, dietary fibre itself can become dangerous for the digestive system, providing a good habitat for the bad pathogenic bacteria and aggravating the inflammation in the gut wall. This is when gastroenterologists have to recommend their patients have a low-fibre diet. Consequently, dietary fibre alone without the beneficial bacteria present in the gut can end up not being all that good for us. And indeed GAPS children and adults who are prone to diarrhoea or loose stools have to have low fibre in their diet until the diarrhoea clears.

Apart from fibre there is another substance which most of us would not be able to digest without our good bacteria in the gut. This substance is milk sugar, called Lactose. It is a well-known fact that a lot of people are Lactose intolerant, which means that they can't digest milk. Most GAPS children and adults are among these people. The explanation offered by science so far is that many of us lack an enzyme called Lactase to digest Lactose. If we are not meant to digest Lactose, then why do some people seem to manage it perfectly well? The answer is that these people have the right bacteria in their gut. One of the major Lactose-digesting bacteria in the human gut is *E.coli*. It comes as a surprise to many people that physiological strains of *E.coli* are essential inhabitants of a healthy digestive tract. They appear in the gut of a healthy baby from the first days after birth in huge numbers: 10^7–10^9 CFU/g and stay in these same numbers throughout life, providing that they do not get destroyed by antibiotics and other environmental influences. Apart from digesting Lactose, physiological strains of *E.coli* produce vitamin K2, vitamins B1, B2, B6, B12, produce antibiotic-like substances, called colicins, and control other members of their own family which can cause disease. In fact having your gut populated by the physiological strains of *E.coli* is the best way to protect yourself from pathogenic species of *E.coli*. They also take a huge and complex part in appropriate functioning of the immune system, which we will talk about later.

Apart from *E.coli*, other beneficial bacteria in the healthy gut flora will not only ensure appropriate absorption of nutrients from food but also actively synthesise various nutrients: vitamin K2, pantothenic acid, folic acid, thiamin (vitamin B1), riboflavin (vitamin B2), niacin (vitamin B3), pyridoxine (vitamin B6), cyanocobalamin (vitamin B12), various amino acids and other active substances. In the process of evolution Nature made sure that when the food supply is sparse, we humans don't die from vitamin and amino acids deficiencies. Nature provided us with our own factory for making these substances – our healthy gut flora. And when this gut flora is damaged, despite adequate nutrition, we develop vitamin deficiencies. Why? Because many vitamins and other active substances have a fairly short life in the body. So, unless one is taking these vitamins every hour (providing that they can get absorbed at all without healthy gut flora), there will be periods during the day when the body would be deficient in these vitamins. That is what happens to people with damaged gut flora which is unable to provide a constant steady stream of vitamins and other active substances for the body to use. Every tested GAPS child or adult shows deficiencies in those very vitamins which their gut flora is supposed to produce. Restoring the beneficial bacteria in their gut is the best way to deal with those deficiencies.

Most people with abnormal gut flora have various stages of anaemia. It is not surprising. They not only can't absorb essential-for-blood vitamins and minerals from food, but their own production of these vitamins is damaged. On top of that, people with damaged gut flora often have a particular group of pathogenic bacteria growing in their gut, which are iron-loving bacteria (*Actinomyces spp.*, *Mycobacterium spp.*, pathogenic strains of *E.coli*, *Corynebacterium spp.* and many others). They consume whatever iron the person gets from the diet, leaving that person deficient in iron. Unfortunately, supplementing iron makes these bacteria grow stronger and does not remedy anaemia.

The majority of GAPS patients I have seen look pale and pasty and their blood tests often show changes typical for anaemia. Many of these patients have been prescribed iron tablets by their doctors. However, it takes much more to remedy anaemia than supplementing iron. To have healthy blood the body needs magnesium, copper, manganese, iodine, zinc and many other minerals, a whole host of vitamins: B1, B2, B3, B6, B12, C, A, D, folic acid, pantothenic acid and many amino acids. It has been shown in a large number of studies all over the world, that just supplementing iron does not do much for anaemia. It saddens me to see that doctors still prescribe it to anaemic patients giving them a lot of unpleasant digestive side effects due to encouraging growth of pathogenic iron-loving bacteria and direct negative effect on the cells of the gut lining, which are already inflamed and very sensitive in GAPS patients.

People with abnormal gut flora have multiple nutritional deficiencies due to all the factors described above. Every GAPS child and adult who has been tested shows a typical picture of nutritional deficiencies in many important minerals, vitamins, essential fats, many amino acids and other nutrients. The most common deficiencies are in magnesium, zinc, selenium, copper, calcium, manganese, sulphur, phosphorus, iron, potassium, sodium, vitamins B1, B2, B3, B6, B12, C, A, D, folic acid, pantothenic acid, omega-3, omega-6 and omega-9 fatty acids, taurine, alpha-ketoglutaric acid, glutathione and other nutrients. This usual list of nutritional deficiencies, commonly seen in GAPS patients, includes some of the most important known nutrients for normal functioning and development of the brain, immune system and the rest of the body. Despite the fact that some of GAPS children appear to grow very well, often being large for their age, they are malnourished in very important micronutrients. And knowing the state of their digestive system, it is not surprising. *A well-functioning gut with healthy gut flora holds the roots of our health. And, just as a tree with sick roots is not going to thrive, the rest of the body cannot thrive without a well-functioning digestive system.* The bacterial population of the gut – the gut flora – is the soil around these roots, giving them their habitat, protection, support and nourishment.

As we know, the roots of a tree, invisible, hidden deep under the ground, play a crucial role in the well-being of every branch, every twig, every little leaf of that tree, no matter how proudly high and far they may be from those roots. In the same way the diverse and multiple functions of gut flora reach in the body far beyond the gut itself. Let us look at one of the most important "branches" in the body – the immune system.

3. Immune System

People with GAP Syndrome have a compromised immune system. When we test their immune status, deficiencies in various immunoglobulins are found, while other immunoglobulins may be increased out of proportion. Deficiencies in complement, various cells, enzymes and other parts of the immune system are common. It appears that the whole of the immune system in GAPS children and adults is out of balance. But the most scary thing that happens is that their immune system starts to produce antibodies attacking the body's own tissues, including the brain and the rest of the nervous system. It is an immune system deeply upset and out of control, scavenging on its own body.

Why does this happen? Has it got anything to do with the state of these patients' digestive system? There is no doubt that it has!

The epithelial surface of the digestive system inhabited by huge numbers of bacteria can truly be described as the cradle of the immune system, both systemic and mucosal. A baby is born with an immature immune system. Population of the baby's digestive tract with healthy bacterial flora plays a crucial role in the appropriate maturation of its immune system. If establishment of balanced gut flora does not take place around the first 20 days of life, then the baby is left immune-compromised. The beneficial bacteria which take up residence on the epithelium of the gut wall play a major immunomodulating role in a number of ways. Let us look at some of them in detail.

Essential or beneficial bacteria in our digestive system engage a very important member of the immune system – the lymphoid tissue of the gut wall – and take part in the production of huge numbers of lymphocytes and immunoglobulins. For example, in the cell wall of *Bifidobacteria* (the good bacteria largely populating the human colon) there is a substance called Muramil Dipeptide which activates synthesis of one of the most important groups of immune system cells – lymphocytes. As a result, a healthy gut wall is literally infiltrated, jam-packed with lymphocytes, ready to protect the body from any invader. Scientific research shows that in people with damaged gut flora there are far fewer lymphocytes in the gut wall, which leaves it poorly protected. There are commercial companies trying to make supplements from Muramil Dipeptide to help the immune system. I believe that it is better to restore a healthy colony of *Bifidobacteria* in the gut, which will produce Muramil Dipeptide naturally, as well as many other useful substances which these bacteria normally supply.

Lymphocytes in the gut wall produce immunoglobulins. The most important one in the gut is Secretory Immunoglobulin A (IgA). Secretory IgA is a substance which is produced by lymphocytes in all mucous membranes in the body and excreted in body fluids. It is found in breathing passages, nose, throat, bladder, urethra, vagina, saliva, tears, sweat, colostrum, breast milk and, of course, the mucous membranes of the digestive system and its secretions. Its job is to protect mucous membranes by destroying and inactivating invading bacteria, viruses, fungi and parasites. It is one of the immune system's ways of dealing with the unwelcome invaders coming with food and drink into our digestive system. Microbiological science has established that when the healthy gut flora is compromised in humans and in laboratory animals the number of cells producing IgA falls dramatically and their ability to produce this important immunoglobulin is severely reduced. This, of course, would greatly lessen the ability of the gut to protect itself. In addition, quite soon after being excreted, the Immunoglobulin A naturally degrades. Apart from stimulating its production, the beneficial bacteria slow down its degradation through a very complex process, allowing the IgA more time to do its work. IgA is commonly deficient in GAPS children and adults due to their abnormal gut flora. As a result their gut wall has poor ability to defend itself from fungi, viruses from vaccinations or the environment, bacteria and parasites.

Lymphocytes are not the only immune cells which should be present in abundance in the digestive wall. When there is a deficiency of beneficial bacteria in the gut, other groups of immune cells, called neutrophils and macrophages cannot do their job properly either. These are the cells which gather in infected and inflamed tissues and clean them up by literally swallowing viruses, toxins and bacterial and cellular debris and destroying them. Approximately 126 billion neutrophils per day leave the blood and pass through the wall of the gastrointestinal tract. In people with abnormal gut flora these cells reduce their ability to tackle antigens; in other words they can't destroy invaders and their toxins efficiently, even when their phago-cytic (swallowing) ability may appear to be normal. We don't know yet how it happens. What we do know is that this will allow viruses, bacte-ria and other invaders to survive and persist inside of neutrophils and macrophages – the very cells which are supposed to destroy them.

Apart from ensuring the appropriate function of lymphocytes, IgA and phagocytes, healthy gut flora takes a very important part in the production of interferons, cytokines and many other active regulators of immune response, particularly in fighting viral infections. Millions of children and adults around the world are exposed to viruses from vaccines or the environment. If these people have well-functioning gut flora, then these viruses do them no harm, because their bodies are well equipped to deal with them. In GAPS people, due to the abnor-malities in their gut flora, viruses from vaccines or the environment have a good chance to survive and persist. A good example is the measles virus found in the gut wall and spinal fluid of autistic children. It is quite reasonable to suspect that this virus comes from the MMR (measles-mumps-rubella) vaccination.

Another fascinating way in which beneficial bacteria work with the immune system is a so-called "mimicking phenomenon". The bacteria on the surface of gut epithelium and the cells of this epithelium swap antigens, rather like children swapping their hats when playing hide and seek to fool the seeker. This swapping of antigens improves effi-ciency of a large number of various immune responses, particularly in local immunity. Unfortunately, in GAPS patients this swapping can work against them, as many pathogenic microbes can play this game as well. There is a debate in scientific literature about the measles virus using this mimicking phenomenon to fool the immune system into attacking its own tissues.

Gut flora's influence on the immune system reaches far beyond the gut itself. The research shows that when the gut flora is damaged, not only do the levels of IgA, lymphocytes, macrophages, interferons, cytokines, etc. in the digestive system drop but the whole immune system in the body gets out of balance. This process makes the person immune-compromised.

To understand all this, let's imagine a medieval fort with high stone

walls. The soldiers are on the walls defending them with guns, cata-
pults and other weapons appropriate for the job of fighting. Inside the
fort there are civilians, who grow crops, cook food for the defenders
and do all the civilian jobs. They have spades, cooking pots and other
tools for doing their jobs. When an enemy comes, it is the job of the
soldiers to fight them. Imagine that the soldiers fail and the enemy
starts getting inside the fort. Now the civilians are faced with the job
of the soldiers. The civilians do not have appropriate training or tools
for fighting so they are going to use whatever they have to hand – their
gardening tools, cooking pots, etc. These tools are not made for fighting so the civilians are not going to be as effective at defending the fort
as the soldiers with their weapons.

Something along these lines happens in the body when the gut flora
is compromised. There are two major armies in the immune system:
Th1 immunity (the soldiers on the walls of the fort) and Th2 immunity (the civilians inside the fort). The soldiers on the walls, Th1 immunity (T-cell helper type 1) promotes a so-called cell-mediated
immunity, which is located everywhere the body is in contact with the
outside world. Its role is to fight infections in the mucous membranes,
skin and inside cells. It is a first and very effective barrier to any invasion into the body. Secretory immunoglobulin A is assigned to this
system as well as Interleukin-2 (IL-2), Interleukin 12 (IL-12), gamma
interferon and some other substances. As we have seen, healthy gut
flora plays an extremely important role in keeping this part of immunity active and up to its job. When the bodily flora is damaged, then
this part of immunity becomes less efficient and starts letting
unwanted microbes and toxins through into the body. The body
responds by activating the second army in the immune system (the
civilians inside the fort) the Th2 immunity (T-cell helper type 2)
responsible for humoral immunity or immunity in the liquids of the
body. The main players in this system are Interleukins 4, 5, 6 and 10,
alpha interferon and IgE. Immunoglobulin E (IgE) is the master of
allergic reactions in the body; it is very active in people with asthma,
eczema, hay fever and other allergies. In a person with abnormal gut
flora this Th2 system becomes overactive, which predisposes the
person to atopic or allergic type reactions, chronic inflammation,
autoimmunity and many other undesirable effects. Like civilians in a

fort, armed with the wrong tools and not trained to fight, the Th2 system is not going to defend the fort in the right way.

We need both the Th1 and Th2 immunity in the body, but they have to be in the right balance. The imbalance between Th1 and Th2 immunity with underactive Th1 and overactive Th2 is a usual picture in chronic viral infections, allergies, chronic fatigue syndrome, candidiasis, asthma, eczema, autism and most other GAPS conditions. Why? Because all these conditions, though they look quite different, have one big thing in common – a gut dysbiosis or abnormal gut flora, which is the major balancing agent between Th1 and Th2 immunity. To carry on with the medieval fort analogy, it is the gut flora that keeps the soldiers on the walls in large numbers, alert, well trained and always ready to fight. When the gut flora is not functioning well, then the soldiers become relaxed and lazy; some of them go inside the fort to help the civilians with their jobs, so the number of soldiers on the walls becomes smaller, making the Th1 immunity weak and out of balance with the Th2 immunity.

On the whole it is hard to overestimate how important the state of our gut flora is in the appropriate functioning of our immune system. It has been estimated that around 80–85% of our immunity is located in the gut wall. The gut wall with its bacterial layer can be described as the right hand of the immune system. If the bacterial layer is damaged or, worse than that, abnormal, then the person's immune system is trying to function with its right hand tied behind its back.

In the previous chapter we covered in detail the various nutritional deficiencies which people with abnormal gut flora develop. An immune system cannot function without constant nourishment: it requires most known vitamins and minerals, amino acids and fats to be able to do its job. GAPS patients have a long list of nutritional deficiencies, due to abnormal digestion and absorption, so their immune system is not only unbalanced, but also malnourished.

But as if all that is not enough, an immune system in a body with abnormal bacterial flora is exposed to a whole host of extremely toxic substances, many of which have a direct damaging effect on immunity. These toxins come from all the opportunistic microbes which happily flourish in the gut and elsewhere in the body of a person with GAPS, thanks to the absence of beneficial flora's control.

We have already examined what happens to the digestive wall when the gut flora is abnormal: it becomes damaged and leaky. A constant stream of invaders and undigested food comes through the damaged epithelial barriers in the gut. The immune system has to deal with all that, while being malnourished, deficient, compromised, unbalanced and intoxicated.

So, should it come as a surprise to us that the immune system of GAPS children and adults is in such a poor state?

4. What Can Damage Gut Flora?

We have looked in detail at the different roles our indigenous gut flora plays in the body. We have seen how important it is for us to keep this microscopic world inside us healthy and active. However, in our modern world this task has become extremely difficult, if not impossible. Let us have a look at what dangers our gut flora has to face on a regular basis.

Antibiotics

We all have taken antibiotics in our lives. It is one of the most commonly prescribed medications in our modern world. Since the moment we are born we are likely to be exposed to this group of drugs on a regular basis, not only through prescription, but also through food. Farm animals and poultry are routinely given antibiotics, so all the products we get from them (meat, milk, eggs) will provide us with a constant supply of antibiotics and antibiotic-resistant bacteria, which these animals develop in their bodies as well as all the toxins which these bacteria produce. Farmed fish and shellfish have antibiotics routinely added to their tanks. A lot of fruit, vegetables, grains, legumes and nuts are sprayed with antibiotics to control disease. The way things are in our sophisticated modern world we simply cannot avoid exposure to antibiotics. It has become such a "normal" part of life that not many of us ask the question "What are they doing to us?" And as the production of antibiotics grew from hundreds of tons a year in the 1950s to tens of thousands of tons a year in the 1990s, so grew the evidence and worried research into the harmful effects of this group of drugs on human health. Let us see what this research shows:

- Antibiotics have a devastating effect on beneficial bacteria in the human body, not only in the gut but in other organs and tissues.
- Antibiotics change bacteria, viruses and fungi from benign to pathogenic, giving them an ability to invade tissues and cause disease.
- Antibiotics make bacteria resistant to antibiotics, so the industry has to work on more and more powerful new antibiotics to attack

these new changed bacteria. A good example is tuberculosis, where wide use of antibiotics has created new varieties of the Mycobacterium Tuberculosis resistant to all existing antibiotics.

- Antibiotics have a direct damaging effect on the immune system, making us more vulnerable to infections, which leads to a vicious cycle of more antibiotics and more infections.

Let us have a look at what different groups of antibiotics do to the gut flora.

Penicillins

In this group we have very widely used Amoxicillin, Ampicillin, Flucloxacillin and all other antibiotics with "-cillin" at the end of their name. These drugs have a damaging effect on two major groups of our beneficial resident bacteria: *Lactobacilli* and *Bifidobacteria*, while promoting growth of the pathogenic *Proteus* family, *Streptococci* and *Staphylococci*. This particular group of antibiotics allow bacteria normally found only in the bowel to move up to the intestines, which predisposes the person to development of IBS (Irritable Bowel Syndrome) and other digestive disorders.

Tetracyclines (Tetracycline, Doxycycline and other "-cyclines")

This group of drugs is routinely prescribed to teenagers for acne as a long course, lasting from three months to two years. Tetracyclines have a particular toxic effect on the gut wall by altering protein structure in the mucous membranes. This in turn does two things. First, it makes the gut wall anatomically vulnerable to invasion by pathogenic microbes; second, it alerts the immune system to attack these changed proteins, starting an auto-immune reaction in the body against its own gut. In parallel, tetracyclines stimulate growth of disease-causing *Candida* fungus, *Staphylococci* and *Clostridia* in the digestive tract.

Aminoglycosides (Gentamycin, Kanamycin), Macrolides (Erythromycin) and other "-mycins"

These drugs have a particular devastating effect on colonies of beneficial bacteria in the gut such as physiological *E.coli* and *Enterococci*. A prolonged course of treatment can completely eliminate these bacteria from the digestive system, leaving it open to invasion by pathogenic species of *E.coli* and other microbes.

Antifungal antibiotics (Nystatin, Amphotericin, etc.)

These drugs lead to selective stimulation of growth of the *Proteus* family and lactose-negative *E.coli* species, capable of causing serious disease.

Combinations of antibiotics have stronger damaging effects on the gut flora than single drugs. The damage is worse when antibiotics are administered orally and when the course of antibiotic is a lengthy one on a low dose, like the one prescribed for acne, chronic cystitis, chronic ear infection and other chronic infections. Medical personnel and workers in the pharmaceutical industry are at a particular risk of chronic exposure to low doses of antibiotics, and indeed gut dysbiosis is very common among these people.

When an antibiotic is prescribed in a high dose, it leaves the gut with a lot of empty niches to be populated by whatever bacteria, viruses or fungi get there first. This is a crucial time to administer a good probiotic to make sure that these niches get populated by friendly bacteria instead of pathogenic ones. Even when the course of antibiotic is short and the dose is low, it takes beneficial bacteria in the gut a long time to recover: physiological *E.coli* takes one to two weeks, *Bifidobacteria* and *Veillonelli* take two to three weeks, *Bacteroids* and *Peptostreptococci* take a month. If, in this period, the gut flora is subjected to another damaging factor(s), then gut dysbiosis may well start in earnest.

The majority of GAPS patients I have seen have been exposed to numerous courses of antibiotics during their life. The most common reasons in children are repeated ear infections, chest infections, impetigo and mastitis in the breast-feeding mother, when the baby would get antibiotics through the breast milk. Given that many of these children had little chance to develop a healthy gut flora from the beginning, these courses of antibiotics have a devastating effect on their fragile gut ecology.

Other drugs

Most drugs, particularly when prescribed for long periods of time or permanently, have a detrimental effect on gut flora.

Pain killers or analgesics (aspirin, ibuprofen, etc.) are often prescribed for long periods of time to people with chronic pain. These drugs stimulate growth of haemolytic forms of bacteria and *Campylobacter* in the gut, all of which are capable of causing disease.

Steroid drugs, like Prednisolone, Hydrocortisone, Betamethasone, Dexamethasone, etc., damage gut flora. In addition, they have a strong immunosuppressing ability, which makes the body vulnerable to all sorts of infection. For example, it is known that a course of steroids is almost invariably associated with fungal overgrowth in the body, particularly of *Candida* species.

Contraceptive pills, or The Pill, are something many women take for many years, often from a very young age. This group of drugs has a devastating effect on the gut flora. By the time a woman is ready to have children, she has been on these drugs for a long period of time and has an abnormal gut flora. A human baby is born with a sterile gut and acquires most of its gut flora from the mother. So if the mother has an abnormal gut flora, that is what she will pass to her child, predisposing this child to eczema, asthma and other allergies, and in severe cases to learning disabilities.

Many other groups of drugs, including sleeping pills, "heartburn" pills, neuroleptics, cholinolytic drugs, cytotoxic drugs, etc., etc., cause different damage to the gut flora, digestive system and immune system.

Drug-induced gut dysbiosis is usually the most severe and the most resistant to treatment. In the last 50 years we have seen a tremendous increase in drug use by the western population. It has almost become a normal part of life to take some sort of prescription or over-the-counter drug, something to talk about with your neighbours. Yet not many people think about what these drugs are doing to their bodies, let alone to their gut flora.

What other factors can have an effect on gut flora?

Diet

What we eat has a direct effect on the composition of the gut flora. A modern diet of convenience rather than nutrition, full of processed foods, has a serious detrimental effect on the gut flora.

Too many sugary foods and processed carbohydrates increase numbers of different fungi, *Candida* species in particular, *Streptococci*, *Staphylococci*, some *Clostridia* species, *Bacteroides* and some aerobic opportunistic bacteria. Processed and sugary carbohydrates (white bread, cakes, biscuits, pastries and pasta) also promote population of the gut with worms and other parasites.

A diet high in fibre from grains (bran and breakfast cereals in particular) has a profound negative effect on the gut flora, gut health and general body metabolism, predisposing the person to IBS, bowel cancer, nutritional deficiencies and many other problems. Fruit and vegetables provide a better quality fibre that is not as harsh for the digestive system.

Bottle-fed babies develop completely different gut flora to breastfed babies.

Breastfeeding is essential for appropriate population of the baby's gut with balanced, healthy gut flora. Babies are born with a sterile gut. Breastfeeding is the one and only opportunity we have in our lives to populate the entire surface of our gut with a healthy mixture of bacteria to lay the very basis of our future health. Bottled-fed babies have their gut populated by a combination of different bacteria, which predisposes them later to many health problems. We have a whole generation of people, mainly born in the 1960s and 1970s, who were not breastfed because it was not fashionable. A whole host of medical problems that arose from that fashion have made it obvious to the medical profession and the rest of us how important breastfeeding is. Thankfully, now, a majority of mothers do their best to breastfeed their newborn babies.

Prolonged fasting, starvation and overeating can seriously alter the composition of gut flora and start a chain of health problems, so supplementing beneficial bacteria in a form of probiotic would be a good idea in these situations.

Generally, when gut dysbiosis is caused exclusively by poor diet it is usually fairly mild and can be corrected by better eating habits. Unfortunately, in our modern world, it is rare not to be exposed to other factors which also damage your gut flora, antibiotics for example.

Disease

Different infectious diseases, like typhoid, cholera, dysentery, salmonella and some viral infections, can cause lasting damage to the gut flora. Repopulating the gut with beneficial bacteria has to be an important part of the treatment of patients with these serious infections.

Different chronic illnesses such as diabetes, autoimmune disease, endocrine disease, obesity and neurological conditions are accompanied by serious defects in gut flora. Such defects are a common after-effect of surgery, chemotherapy, hormone therapy and radiotherapy.

Stress

A short-term stress has a detrimental effect on the gut flora, but it usually recovers well after the stressful situation is over. However, a long-term physical or psychological stress can do permanent damage to the indigenous flora.

Other factors

Physical exertion, old age, alcoholism, pollution, exposure to toxic substances, seasonal factors, exposure to ionising radiation and extreme climates all have a profound effect on our friendly bacteria.

Every one of us carries a unique mixture of microbes in the gut. Under the influence of drugs and other factors, listed above, this gut flora will be changed in a unique way in every one of us, predisposing us to different health problems. It is a completely unpredictable process and science so far has not developed very reliable methods of testing for the full range of microbes in the gut, let alone treating any abnormalities. This damage gets passed from generation to generation as a newborn child gets its gut flora from the mother. And as the damage is passed through generations, it gets deeper and deeper. This process reflects in the severity of health problems related to abnormal gut flora seen in generations. For example, this is quite a common scenario, which I see in my clinic: a grandmother has mild digestive problems as a result of low-key gut dysbiosis. She passes moderately abnormal gut flora to her daughter. On top of that she decides not to breastfeed, because it is not fashionable. As a result, her daughter suffers from allergies, migraines, PMS and digestive problems. Then she takes contraceptive pills from the age of 16, which deepens the damage to her gut flora, not to mention a few courses of antibiotics along the way for various infections and a diet of fast foods. After 10 years of being "on the pill" she has children, to whom she passes her seriously abnormal gut flora. Her children develop digestive and immune problems, which then lead to eczema, asthma, autism and other learning problems.

Most of the factors described here are hard to escape in the modern world. Under the influence of these factors, the beneficial bacteria in the gut lose their ability to fulfil all the functions we have looked at in the previous chapters. They are unable to protect the digestive tract from opportunistic flora and transitional bacteria, viruses and fungi, which sets up a whole chain of pathology in the gut and the rest of the body. To gain more understanding of what happens in this situation, let us have a look at the opportunistic flora which lives in our digestive system.

5. The Opportunistic Flora

We talked in detail about the essential flora (the good bacteria) of the gut and its multiple functions. Let's now look at the second group of bacteria – the opportunistic flora. This is a large group of various microbes, the number and combinations of which can be quite unique. There are around 500 different species of them found in the human gut. These are the most common: *Bacteroids, Peptococci, Staphylococci, Streptococci, Bacilli, Clostridia, Yeasts, Enterobacteria* (*Proteus, Clebsielli, Citrobacteria,* etc.), *Fuzobacteria, Eubacteria, Spirochaetaceae, Spirillaceae, Catenobacteria,* different viruses and many others. Interestingly, many of these opportunistic bacteria, when in small numbers and under control, actually fulfil some beneficial functions in the gut, like taking part in the digestion of food, breaking down lipids and bile acids.

In a healthy gut their numbers are limited and tightly controlled by the beneficial flora. But when this beneficial flora is weakened and damaged, the opportunists get out of control. Each of these microbes is capable of causing various health problems. It is a fascinating area for future research, because it appears that it is the character of our individual opportunistic flora that may determine what disease we succumb to. Yes, we carry most of our future health problems in our own gut pretty much from birth. As long as we take good care of our defenders, the beneficial flora, those baddies may never show their ugly faces. Unfortunately, our modern life styles sooner or later damage our indigenous bodily flora, and whatever opportunists were waiting for their turn become active.

The best known is the fungus *Candida albicans*, which causes untold misery to millions of people. There is an abundance of literature published about candida infection, so we will not concentrate on it here. However, I have to say that a lot of what is described as Candida Syndrome is, in effect, a result of gut dysbiosis (abnormal gut flora), which include the activity of lots of other opportunistic and pathogenic microbes. *Candida albicans* is never alone in a human body. Its activity and ability to survive and cause disease depend on the state of trillions of its neighbours – different bacteria, viruses, protozoa, other yeasts and many other micro-creatures. In a healthy body *Candida* and many other disease-causing microbes are very well controlled by the beneficial flora. Unfortunately, the era of antibiotics gave *Candida albicans* a special opportunity. The usual broad-spectrum antibiotics kill a lot of different microbes in the body – the bad and the good. But they have no effect on *Candida*. So, after every course of antibiotics *Candida* is left without anything to control it, so it grows and thrives. At the dawn of the antibiotic era the medical profession recognised this phenomenon, so it used to be a rule to prescribe Nystatin (an anti-candida antibiotic) every time a broad-spectrum antibiotic was administered. However, for whatever reason, doctors stopped this practice decades ago, and now we are paying the price for it – candida infection has become extremely common. Apart from antibiotics, another factor in our modern world plays a major role in *Candida* overgrowth – our diet. *Candida* flourishes on sugar and processed carbohydrates and these are the foods which nowadays dominate our Western eating habits.

Some opportunists, listed above, when out of control, get through the gut wall barrier into the lymph and bloodstream and cause problems in various organs in the body. But of course, the first place to suffer will be the digestive system. Holding an abnormal bacterial mass, it is no surprise that the digestive system cannot function well. The most common result of gut dysbiosis is the infamous Irritable Bowel Syndrome (IBS), where a whole host of opportunistic bacteria populate the intestines, causing the unpleasant symptoms of IBS. More and more research is coming out linking Crohn's disease and ulcerative colitis with the activity of opportunistic gut flora getting out of control.

Certain opportunists, when not controlled by good bacteria, get access to the gut wall and damage its integrity, making it "leaky". For example, microbiologists have observed how common opportunistic gut bacteria from the families *Spirochaetaceae* and *Spirillaceae* have an ability, due to their spiral shape, to push apart intestinal cells, breaking down the integrity of the intestinal wall and allowing through substances which normally should not get through. *Candida albicans* has this ability as well. Its cells attach themselves to the gut lining, literally putting "roots" through it and making it "leaky". Partially digested foods get through this leaky gut wall into the blood stream, where the immune system recognises them as foreign and attacks them. This is how food allergies or intolerances develop. What is happening is that foods do not get a chance to be digested properly before they are absorbed through the damaged gut wall. In many cases, when the gut wall is healed food allergies disappear.

Opportunistic flora constantly produces toxic substances, which are the by-products of their metabolism. In a healthy situation many of these by-products can be physiological because in the process of evolution they got included in the normal functioning of the human body. For instance, a well-known group of toxins produced by gut bacteria are the amines – the metabolites of amino acids. Many of them have some important roles to play in the normal physiology of the body. A good example is histamine – an important neurotransmitter in the body. Certain cells in the body normally produce histamine. However, it is also produced by *Proteus* family, *E. coli* family, *Staphylococci* and many other bacteria in the gut. In a situation where these opportunistic bacteria overgrow, due to the lack of control from the beneficial flora, they start producing too much histamine. As histamine takes part in many different functions in the body, all these functions go wrong with the excess of histamine coming into the blood. These are the common symptoms of this condition: allergies, constantly low blood pressure, excessive production of body fluids, like saliva, dysfunction of the hypothalamus with hormonal changes (PMS is a common result), emotional instability, sleep abnormalities, addictions and many others. An excess of histamine in the body is called histadelia. This condition was found by Dr Carl Pfeiffer in many people with depression, schizophrenia, addictions and autism. Antihistamine drugs are used by psychiatrists to treat schizophrenia. Nobody has yet looked at correcting the gut flora in order to normalise histamine production in the body and remedy symptoms of histadelia.

Other well-studied amines, such as dimethylamine, piperidine, pyrrolidine, tyramine, octopamine, which are produced by bacterial activity in the gut from amino acids choline, lecithin, methylamine, lysine, arginine, ornithine and tyrosine, are also known to cause cerebral depression with symptoms of withdrawal, intellectual regression, behavioural and emotional abnormalities.

A group of chemicals called kryptopyrroles play a role in mental dysfunction. Kryptopyrroles are often found in the urine of GAPS people. This condition is called pyroluria and can produce irritability, anger, poor memory, impaired intellectual function, poor immunity and inability to deal with stress. So far pyroluria has been treated symptomatically by supplementing zinc, vitamin B6 and other nutrients, because medicine did not know where kryptopyrroles come from. Now there are studies indicating that they are produced by abnormal gut flora.

GAPS children and adults routinely show overgrowth of opportunistic microbes in their stool tests (the ones we can test for). The most commonly seen are *Candida albicans, Bacteroids, Clostridia spp., Proteus* family, *Streptococci* and *Staphylococci*. Invariably, this overgrowth is combined with either the absence or greatly reduced numbers of beneficial bacteria. Unfortunately, the stool testing so far available to us is quite primitive. There has not been a lot of money put into this research. There is a debate going on between professionals about the validity of stool analysis, as it only shows what microbes may be in the lumen of the bowel. It gives no information on the most important inhabitants of the gut – the ones that live on the gut wall, the mural bacteria. These are the bacteria which maintain gut integrity and its ability to digest and absorb food and which play such an important role in our immunity. There are limited studies done with biopsy of the gut wall and following microbiological analysis which show that the mural bacteria can be quite different from the ones which live in the lumen of the gut. Apart from that, stool analysis only reflects the microbial population of the bowel and does not reflect what lives higher in the intestines where the very important digestion and absorption happens. Unfortunately, we are still in the very early stages when it comes to testing for gut flora. Nevertheless, there is a large amount of information available now about what the bacterial population of a normal healthy person's stool should look like, and compared to that information GAPS people have very abnormal results.

A group of opportunistic gut bacteria, called **Bacteroids**, routinely found in GAPS stool analysis, deserves some attention. It is the most ubiquitous opportunistic bacteria in the gut of adult population in the

Western world, which may be explained by what these bacteria like to eat – sugar, starch, lactose – the backbone of the Western diet. There are in excess of 22 different members of this family identified so far in the human body, the most common being *Bacteroides fragilis* and *Bacteroides melaninogenicus*. These bacteria are almost always found in infected tissues of the digestive tract, abscesses, ulcers, urinary infections, lung infections, peritonitis, infected heart valves, blood infections, mouth infections, teeth and gum disease, gangrene and post-operative infections. They are opportunists always hanging around in every mucous membrane of the body waiting for their opportunity to cause trouble. However, they usually do not cause trouble alone but join some bigger bully on the playground, and in that company really show their ability to cause disease. For example, they are usually found in company with *Clostridia*. They appear to be good friends with the *Clostridia* family, which is considered to be more dangerous than Bacteroids. But *Bacteroids* seem to show their ability to cause disease better in the company of *Clostridia,* at the same time assisting *Clostridia* in its activity.

Members of **Clostridia family** are almost always detected in the stool analysis of autistic children and adults. There are about a hundred different *Clostridia* species known so far. Apart from autism they are also present in the stools of people with schizophrenia, psychosis, severe depression, muscle paralysis, muscle tonus abnormalities and some other neurological and psychiatric conditions. Many *Clostridia* species are normal inhabitants of a human gut. For example *Clostridium tetani* is routinely found in the gut of healthy humans and animals. Spores of this bacterium are passed through faeces into soils, where they can survive for years. Most soils in the world test positive for tetanus spores. Everybody knows that tetanus is a deadly disease, due to an extremely powerful neurotoxin *Clostridium tetani* produces. Anybody who gets a wound or even a scratch contaminated by soil is immediately advised to have a shot of anti-tetanus vaccine. But we contract tetanus only when the bacterium gets directly into our tissues or blood. *Clostridium tetani,* which lives in the gut, normally does not do us any harm because its toxin cannot get through the healthy gut wall. GAPS patients do not have a healthy gut wall, which allow toxins to get into the body.

Many other species of *Clostridia* (*perfringens*, *novyi*, *septicum*, *histolyticum*, *sordelli*, *aerofoetidum*, *tertium*, *sporogenes*, etc.) routinely found in the human gut, produce toxins similar to tetanus toxin as well as many other toxins. So how can we have these deadly bacteria in our gut and be healthy? Because they are controlled by our friendly bacteria, which will not allow them to flourish and, most importantly, does not allow their toxins through the gut lining into the blood-stream.

However, in the GAPS gut where the person hasn't got the benefi-cial bacteria to protect the gut wall and control *Clostridia*, neurotoxins have a good chance of getting into the bloodstream and into the brain and the rest of the nervous system, affecting its development and func-tioning. Sensitivity to light and noises is a typical symptom of tetanus infection and GAPS conditions like autism, schizophrenia, psychosis and dyslexia, so it seems plausible that the two may be connected. Most GAPS children and adults whom I see in my clinic have abnor-malities of muscle tonus similar to low exposure to tetanus neurotoxin. Typically extensor muscles have higher tonus than contractor muscles. Maybe that is the reason why autistic children and adults walk on tiptoes and often self-stimulate by stretching their arms, fingers and legs in odd positions. In these cases, where the patient's stool has been tested, almost without exception an overgrowth of *Clostridia spp.* is observed. Recent research at the University of Reading in the UK by a microbiological team led by Professor Glenn Gibson has found very high levels of *Clostridia* in the gut of 150 autistic children, and a second research programme found similarly high levels in the gut of another 60 autistic children, which were not present in their non-autistic siblings.

Just like *Candida albicans*, the *Clostridia* family was given a special opportunity by the era of antibiotics, because *Clostridia* are also resis-tant to them. So, every course of broad-spectrum antibiotics removes good bacteria, which leaves *Clostridia* uncontrolled and allows it to grow. Different species of *Clostridia* cause severe inflammation of the digestive system, for example *Clostridium difficile* causes a potentially fatal pseudo-membranous colitis. Some species of *Clostridia* have been linked to such debilitating digestive disorders as Crohn's disease and ulcerative colitis. I have no doubt that the *Clostridia* family plays an important role in the development of autistic enterocolitis as well. Future research will show whether this is the case. However, there are some facts already which support this idea. For example, William Shaw at Great Plains Laboratories reports a number of cases where a course of anti-clostridia drugs Metronidazole (Flagyl) and Vancomycin reduced autistic symptoms and improved digestion and the biochemical picture in autistic children. However, in almost all cases, as soon as the drug was stopped, all the symptoms and biochemical abnormalities returned. Unfortunately, anti-clostridia drugs are toxic, they have serious side effects, so we can not prescribe them for long periods of time to children or adults. *Clostridia* are spore-forming bacteria, which makes them impossible to eradicate. We can only control them, and the best way to do it is Nature's way – with beneficial bacteria.

Another large group of bacteria, which commonly overgrow in the gut dysbiosis situation are **sulphate-reducing bacteria**. There are many species of sulphate-reducing microbes. To mention just a few: *Proteobacteria, Thiobacilli, Chromatiaceae, Desufotomaculum spp.*, some gram-positive bacteria, some fungi and *Bacteroids*. These microbes metabolise sulphate from food into sulphites, many of which are toxic. Severe deficiency in sulphates has been found in 95% of autistic children. Undoubtedly, sulphate-reducing bacteria play an important role in causing this deficiency. Sulphates are needed in the body for many functions, some of which are detoxification and normal metabolism of brain neurotransmitters. An overgrowth of sulphate-reducing bacteria would make sulphur unavailable for the body to use, turning it into toxic substances like hydrogen sulphide, which is the gas with a rotten egg smell. Many parents of autistic children tell me that their child's stool and flatus has this characteristic smell.

Here we have looked at some pathogens found in the gut of GAPS patients. To their happy company we can add the **measles virus** found by Dr A. Wakefield's research group. This is only one virus, which received such detailed attention. There are some indications in literature that members of the **herpes virus** family are also very active in these patients. How many other viruses may there be in the GAPS gut which have never been studied? How many other pathogenic bacteria, fungi, protozoa and other microbes are there which we have no methods to detect or study yet? I have no doubt that sooner or later science will catch up with them and we will learn what they are and how to deal with them. In the meantime, what should we do to help our GAPS children and adults now? As always, Nature has a good answer – the beneficial flora. Having good bacteria in the gut is the best way to keep *Clostridia*, *Candida*, *Bacteroids*, viruses and many many other microbes under control. Well-functioning healthy gut flora would not only keep those pathogens down but would maintain the integrity of the gut wall so it does not let through the toxins from those pathogenic microbes. This is Nature's way of dealing with them, and the smart thing for us is to try and copy it.

Due to the absence or greatly reduced numbers of beneficial bacteria, the GAPS digestive system gets taken over by opportunistic and pathogenic microbial flora, constantly producing a river of toxicity flowing from the gut to the brain. This is the toxicity which is probably making these children and adults autistic, schizophrenic, hyperactive, dyspraxic, dyslexic, psychotic, depressed, obsessed, etc., etc.

We have already looked at some of these toxins. Let us have a look at a few more.

6. The Gut–Brain Connection

One only sees what one looks for,
one only looks for what one knows.
Goethe

Modern medicine has divided us, human beings, into different systems and areas: cardio-vascular system, digestive system, nervous system, etc. According to this division different medical specialities have been created, each concentrating on a particular bit of the human body: cardiology, gastro-enterology, gynaecology, neurology, psychiatry etc., etc. There is a reason for that. Medical science over the years has accumulated an enormous amount of knowledge. No doctor in the world can possibly know it all in detail, so specialising allows doctors to concentrate on a particular area of knowledge, to learn it thoroughly and to become an expert in that area.

However, from the early years of this specialisation many doctors have recognised a problem developing. A specialist in a particular area tends to pay attention to the organs which he or she knows best, ignoring the rest of the body. The fact that every organ in the body exists and works in contact with the rest gets forgotten. The body lives and functions as a whole, where every system, organ, tissue and even cell depend on each other, affect each other and communicate with each other. One should not look at, let alone treat, any organ without taking the rest of the body into account.

One area of medicine is particularly prone to look at its organ separately from the rest of the body. That area is psychiatry. Mental problems are examined from all sorts of angles: genetics, childhood experiences and psychological influences. The last thing that would be considered is looking at the patient's digestive system. Modern psychiatry just does not do that. And yet medical history has plenty of examples, where severe psychiatric conditions were cured by simply "cleaning out" the patient's gut. A renowned Japanese professor, Kazudzo Nishi, has estimated that at least one in ten psychiatric conditions is due to self-intoxication coming from the bowel.

The vast majority of psychiatric patients suffer from digestive problems, which are largely ignored by their doctors. The gut–brain connection is something which, for some reason, many modern doctors do not understand. As they give out millions of prescriptions for antidepressants, sleeping pills and other drugs, which the patients have to place into their digestive systems in order to affect their brains, they still fail to see the connection between the digestive system and the brain. Everybody knows what effect alcohol has on our brains. Where do we place alcoholic drinks? Into our digestive systems of course. However, we don't have to consume toxic substances to affect our brains. Having particular microbes in the digestive system can provide us with our own permanent source of toxicity.

As discussed in the previous chapters, a GAPS (Gut And Psychology Syndrome) person's digestive system becomes a major source of toxicity in the body. An unknown number of various neurotoxins are produced by abnormal flora in the gut of these children and adults, these are absorbed through the damaged gut wall into the blood and taken to the brain. The mixture of toxins can be very individual, and this is one of the reasons why all GAPS patients are so different. As I mentioned, the number of different toxins is unknown. However, we have accumulated a considerable knowledge of some of the neurotoxins commonly found in GAPS children and adults. These are the kind of toxins which can make anybody mentally ill. In the previous chapter we looked at some of them. Unfortunately, there are more to examine.

Ethanol and acetaldehyde

When thinking about autism, ADHD, schizophrenia, dyslexia, dyspraxia and other psychological problems, not many people would think about alcoholism. And yet there is a very serious connection. We know that due to various factors GAPS children and adults develop an overgrowth of pathological flora in their bodies. One group of these pathogens, almost without exception, are yeasts, including *Candida* species. Yeast requires glucose and other sugars as food. Sugars come from the digestion of carbohydrates. In healthy people dietary glucose gets converted into lactic acid, water and energy through a biochemical process called glycolysis. In people with yeast overgrowth *Candida* highjacks the glucose and digests it in a different way, called alcoholic fermentation. In this biochemical process *Candida* and other yeasts convert dietary glucose into alcohol (ethanol) and its by-product acetaldehyde. This phenomenon was first described in adults, who appeared to be drunk without consuming any alcohol. Later on it was found that these adults had an overgrowth of yeast in their gut, which produced alcohol and made them permanently "drunk". These people were particularly "drunk" after a carbohydrate meal, because carbohydrates are consumed by *Candida* with the production of alcohol. Despite the fact that these people did not consume alcohol, they developed some typical symptoms of alcoholism.

Alcohol and its by-products have a small molecular weight, which makes it very easy for them to cross any barrier in the body. They get absorbed into the blood very quickly and have a very good ability to get through the placenta to a developing foetus. Pregnancy is a natural state of immune suppression. If a woman already has *Candida* overgrowth in her body, pregnancy would make this problem worse. Overgrowing yeast in a pregnant woman would produce alcohol and its by-products, affecting the child's development. After the child is born it will continue to get alcohol and its by-products through breast milk, which usually contains the same amount as the woman's blood. Then because the child inherits the mother's bodily flora, overrun by yeast, the child starts producing its own alcohol and many other toxins. Alcohol consumption and yeast overgrowth in fathers also has an effect on the child's development, so fathers with yeast overgrowth contribute to the problem as well. Indeed, in my clinic more than 50% of fathers of autistic children suffer from abnormal gut flora and related health problems.

So what does alcohol and its by-products do to us? Everybody knows that alcohol is very toxic, particularly for a child. There is no part of the body that will not suffer from the constant supply of alcohol even in tiny amounts. Here are just a few results of chronic presence of alcohol in the body:

- Reduced ability of the stomach wall to produce stomach acid.
- Pancreas degeneration with reduced ability to produce pancreatic enzymes, which impairs digestion.

- Direct damage to gut lining, causing malabsorption.
- Nutritional deficiencies through malabsorption of most vitamins, minerals and amino acids. Deficiencies in B and A vitamins are particularly common.
- Damage to the immune system.
- Liver damage with reduced ability to detoxify drugs, pollutants and other toxins.
- Inability of the liver to dispose of old neurotransmitters, hormones and other by-products of normal metabolism. As a result, these substances accumulate in the body, causing behavioural abnormalities and many other problems.
- Brain damage with lack of self-control, impaired co-ordination, impaired speech development, aggression, mental retardation, loss of memory and stupor.
- Peripheral nerve damage with altered senses and muscle weakness.
- Direct muscle tissue damage with altered ability to contract and relax and muscle weakness.
- Alcohol has an ability to enhance toxicity of most common drugs, pollutants and other toxins.
- Alteration of metabolism of proteins, carbohydrates and lipids in the body.

Acetaldehyde is considered to be the most toxic of alcohol by-products. One of the most devastating influences of this chemical is its ability to alter the structure of proteins. We are largely made up of proteins; a myriad of various active substances from hormones to enzymes are proteins. When they are changed by acetaldehyde they cannot do their jobs properly. Acetaldehyde-altered proteins are thought to be responsible for many autoimmune reactions, which means that the immune system starts attacking its own body. Antibodies which the immune system makes to destroy these acetaldehyde-altered proteins may also attack the normal proteins in the body with a similar structure. GAPS patients are commonly found to have antibodies against their own tissues. One of the commonest is an antibody against a protein in a substance called myelin. Myelin is an integral part of the brain anatomy and the rest of the nervous system, coating brain cells and their branches, the nerve fibres. When myelin is damaged in adults it manifests itself as multiple sclerosis. There are some similarities in the neurological picture of autistic and dyspraxic children and patients with multiple sclerosis which may be due to acetaldehyde produced by the yeast overgrowth in these children.

Alcohol and acetaldehyde render a lot of essential nutrients useless in the body. For example, binding to proteins, acetaldehyde causes functional deficiency of vitamin B6, which is a co-factor in production of neurotransmitters, fatty acid metabolism and many other functions in the body. What is a functional deficiency? It means that the person may get plenty of vitamin B6 in the diet, but because acetaldehyde occupied the working sites of this vitamin on proteins, it cannot do its job. So, it floats around the body in a rather useless fashion and eventually gets excreted. This does not happen just to vitamin B6 but also to many other active substances in the body which have to bind to proteins in order to fulfil their purposes. Another common functional deficiency in GAPS patients is thyroid dysfunction. The thyroid gland may be producing plenty of hormones, but their working sites are occupied by acetaldehyde and other toxins. As a result the person develops typical symptoms of thyroid deficiency: depression, lethargy, fatigue, weight gain, poor body temperature control, poor immunity, etc.

So, we talked about alcoholism in connection with children and young adults. Shocking, isn't it?! What next?! Well, next we are going to talk about drug addiction.

Opiates from gluten and casein

Opiates are drugs, like opium, morphine and heroin, which are commonly used by drug addicts. What have they got to do with GAPS children and adults?

Gluten is a protein present in grains, mainly wheat, rye, oats and barley. Casein is a milk protein, present in cow, goat, sheep, human and all other milk and milk products. In the bodies of GAPS people these proteins do not get digested properly and turn into substances with similar chemical structures to opiates, such as morphine and heroin. There has been quite a substantial amount of research done in this area by Dohan, Reichelt, Shattock, Cade and others, where gluten and casein peptides, called **gluteomorphins** and **casomorphins**, were detected in the urine of patients with schizophrenia, autism, ADHD, post-partum psychosis, epilepsy, Downs syndrome, depression and some autoimmune problems, like rheumatoid arthritis. These opiates from grains and milk are thought to get through the blood–brain barrier and block certain areas of the brain, just as morphine or heroin would do.

Why does this happen? The explanation is undoubtedly hidden in the person's digestive system.

As we saw earlier, GAPS patients' digestive systems are in a poor state. The digestion of proteins starts in the stomach with the action of pepsin, a protein-digesting enzyme produced by the stomach wall. Stomach acid is essential for protein digestion, as it provides normal conditions for pepsin to do its work of breaking down proteins into shorter peptide chains. GAPS people commonly have low stomach acidity due to abnormal gut flora and overgrowth of pathogenic flora. For example, *Candida* alone can make toxins which have a strong suppressing ability on stomach acid production. These toxins would be excreted with breast milk in a mother with *Candida* overgrowth in her gut. It is possible that, while being breastfed, GAPS children receive these toxins from the mother through the breast milk, which impair production of stomach acid from the very beginning of the child's life. As the breast milk requires virtually no digestion the child does not need much stomach acid while exclusively breastfed. But when other foods get introduced, the child's low stomach acidity becomes a problem. By the time the breastfeeding stops the child's digestive system would probably have grown enough of its own *Candida* and other pathogens to produce toxins, which would carry on reducing the stomach acidity. The most usual weaning proteins first introduced to the child's digestive system are casein from formula milk and gluten from wheat. In a stomach with low acidity the first steps in the digestion of these and many other proteins would not go well. Then these maldigested proteins would be passed into the intestines, where pancreatic digestive enzymes are supposed to carry on breaking down proteins. Low stomach acidity would impair production of pancreatic enzymes, so the next step in protein digestion would also go askew. Next these maldigested proteins reach the final stage of their digestion

– the intestinal wall. The intestinal wall is lined by highly sophisticated cells, called enterocytes, which on their surface have a whole host of different digestive enzymes to complete the final steps in the digestion of various nutrients. As we have already discovered in the chapter on the gut flora, in GAPS people these cells are in poor shape due abnormal gut flora. They are not able to accomplish these final steps in the digestion of casein, gluten and many other nutrients. As Dr J. Robert Cade from the University of Florida said in his interview with *Health Science Centre* in March 1999, "We think that with autism and schizophrenia, the basic disorder is in the intestine, and these individuals are absorbing beta-casomorphin-7 that they normally should break down in the body as amino acids, rather than peptide chains up to 12 amino acids long".

There has been some research published on one of the protein-digesting enzymes which sit on the enterocytes. It is called dipeptidyl peptidase IV (DPP IV) and it is supposed to break down casomorphin and gliadomorphin into smaller peptides. GAPS children show deficiency in this enzyme. Interestingly, people who suffer from alcoholism, schizophrenia, depression or autoimmune disease also have low levels of this enzyme, due to the fact that in these conditions the patient's enterocytes are also damaged. Based on this research DPP IV is now added to some digestive enzyme formulations which can be supplemented to GAPS patients. The problem is that this is only one enzyme which we have studied and know something about. How many more enzymes are there on the surface of enterocytes which we know nothing or very little about at present? With the lack of beneficial bacteria, which normally live on these cells to feed them, look after them and protect them, these cells fall ill and become unable to function properly. As a result, maldigestion and malabsorption set the scene in the GAPS gut. At the same time, pathogenic bacteria, fungi and viruses damage the gut wall and allow maldigested proteins, like casomorphin and gliadomorphin, and other substances to be absorbed into the blood and carried to the person's brain.

There is another aspect to this problem. Normally proteins should be broken down into amino acids before they are absorbed in the gut. Apparently we all absorb some of our proteins in the form of peptides (partially broken down proteins) or even unchanged. These dietary peptides act as inhibitors of a special group of enzymes in the body, called peptidases, responsible for breaking down our neurotransmitters, hormones and many other active substances after they have performed their jobs. In GAPS patients these peptidases get severely suppressed by too many dietary peptides coming in, flooding the body with debris of our own inner peptides, which themselves can cause damage and psychological symptoms.

Based on the research into gluteomorphin and casomorphins, a gluten-and casein-free diet (GFCF diet) was developed. Some autistic children show dramatic improvement on this diet. However, many children do not. The reason for that is that there is much more to GAP Syndrome than gluteomorphins and casomorphins. So, for the majority of affected patients the diet has to take into account many other aspects of GAPS.

Other toxins

In the previous chapter we have talked about the *Clostridia* family and their toxins. *Clostridia* are difficult to study due to the fact that they are strict anaerobes. However, in his book Dr William Shaw describes in detail a number of autistic children who showed significant improvements in their development and biochemical tests while on anti-clostridia medication. Unfortunately, as soon as the medication was stopped the children slipped back into autism. As we have mentioned in the previous chapter, the best way to deal with *Clostridia* and many other pathogens in the gut is establishing proper healthy gut flora, as the beneficial bacteria are the natural way of controlling *Clostridia*.

Other frightening toxic substances have been found in autistic children by biochemist Dr Alan Friedman. These chemicals are called deltorphin and dermorphin. They were first found on the skin of poison dart frogs in South America where native people used to dip their darts into the mucus on these frogs in order to paralyse their enemy, because deltorphin and dermorphin are extremely potent neurotoxins. Dr Friedman believes that it is not the frog that produces these neurotoxins, but a fungus, which grows on their skin. It is possible that this fungus grows in the gut of autistic children. Hopefully, future research will elucidate this issue for us.

A number of other potent toxins have been identified and studied in GAPS people. To look at all of them is beyond the scope of this book. The important point is that GAPS children and adults are very toxic people. This toxicity comes from their digestive systems. So it is the person's digestive system we have to concentrate on first and foremost in order to treat the condition.

7. The Families

As the mother of a recovered autistic child, I am very familiar with the feeling of guilt, which so many parents experience. We feel that we have done or haven't done something which caused our child's condition. It is a perfectly natural feeling and, as parents, we have to learn to deal with it, as well as everything else our GAPS children bring into our lives. When we start reading and learning about what could have caused our child's condition on biochemical and physiological levels, we start feeling even guiltier. If only we could have avoided this and that and if only we could have done things differently, our child might have been different! In this chapter I am going to talk about the health of parents of GAPS children and how it could contribute to your child's condition. In no way do I want to make anybody feel guilty about it. We are what we are! Our children are physically made by us from whatever we are made of. Some of these things, like genetics, we are born with, and there is nothing we can do about them. Some were given to us by our parents, like our bodily microbial flora and our eating habits. Some were created by our life styles and choices. Some were imposed on us by our modern society and the world we live in. Most parents of GAPS children I have met, rather than concentrating on their feeling of guilt, find a way of learning as much as possible about their children's condition, and concentrating on what can be done about it.

So, let's carry on learning!

As far as science knows, an unborn baby is sterile. Its body has no bacteria, viruses or fungi living in it. When the time of birth comes, as the baby goes through the birth canal, it gets its first dose of microbes. Its skin, eyes and mucous membranes in the mouth and nose acquire their first micro-flora. Through swallowing liquids in the mother's vagina the baby's digestive system gets its first population of bacteria, viruses and fungi. So, whatever lives in the vagina of the mother is what the baby would get.

Now, let's have a look at what lives in a mother's vagina. A healthy woman has a very large population of microbes in her vagina, called vaginal flora. Normally it is dominated by *Lactobacillus* species, namely *Lactobacillus acidophilus*, *Lactobacillus casei*, *Lactobacillus fermentum* and others. These good bacteria keep the pH in the vagina quite acid, around 4.7, which does not allow other bacteria to take hold and grow. This normal flora in the vagina is absolutely vital for the woman's health. It protects her from infections, keeps the mucous membrane of the vagina and other organs in that area healthy and stimulates the production of large numbers of immune cells and immunoglobulins in the walls of the vagina to keep it well defended from any invaders. But when these good bacteria are damaged the problems start.

Let's see what can have a damaging effect on vaginal flora.

Antibiotics and other systemic antibacterial drugs have a direct effect on the composition of vaginal flora, because they destroy the beneficial bacteria in the vagina, as well as everywhere else in the body. If the beneficial bacteria in the vagina are not there then the coast is clear for any invading bacteria, fungus, virus or parasite to take hold and grow. The pH in the vagina goes up and various aerobic, anaerobic and micro-aerophilic species start populating the woman's vagina, such as *Gardnerella vaginalis*, *Prevotella spp.*, *Peptostreptococcus spp.*, *Mycoplasma hominis*, *Ureaplasma urealyticum and Mobilincus spp.*, causing inflammation with many very unpleasant symptoms. A well-known family of fungi, called *Candida albicans*, is a very common inhabitant of an unhealthy vagina, causing thrush. This fungus cannot live in a vagina with a good population of healthy bacteria.

The contraceptive pill has the same damaging influence on vaginal flora as antibiotics. Steroids in the pill have an ability to suppress the immune system and change the composition of bodily flora. Unfortunately, in our modern society women are put on the pill at a very early age, and by the time they are ready to have children they have been taking these drugs on a regular basis for years, which would have a profound effect on the composition of their bodily micro-flora.

Many other drugs have a damaging effect on vaginal flora, particularly steroids, sulphonamides, some non-steroid anti-inflammatory preparations and others.

Apart from drugs there are some other influences which can change the composition of vaginal flora, for example poor diet, infections, personal care products and prolonged stress. But here we have to talk about the most important question: where does the vaginal flora come from?

The medical science shows that the flora in the vagina comes from the gut. What lives in the woman's bowel will live in her vagina. For example, in women with recurrent thrush, no matter how many powerful anti-fungal topical preparations are used, the thrush always comes back. It comes back because the fungus which causes it, called *Candida albicans*, lives in this woman's bowel. Until she gets rid of it in the bowel, she is not going to be free from vaginal thrush. But why does this woman have an overgrowth of fungi in her bowel? Because she does not have a healthy gut flora to protect her from this fungus and many other microbial invaders. This woman has a condition, called Gut Dysbiosis. She will not only have an overgrowth of *Candida albicans* in her gut but lots of other pathogenic microbes, causing many other health problems.

Amongst all the parents of GAPS children I have met, the mother always invariably has signs of chronic Gut Dysbiosis. Most mothers have been taking the contraceptive pill for years before having children. Many mothers have had numerous courses of antibiotics. Many of them have not been breastfed as babies and their mothers show typical symptoms of Gut Dysbiosis. Almost every one of them has one or more health conditions which are typically associated with abnormal gut flora. The most common health problems which mothers of GAPS children suffer from are: digestive disorders, asthma, eczema, hay fever and other allergies, migraines, PMS, arthritis, skin problems, chronic cystitis and vaginal thrush. These conditions seem to be unrelated, but they are all children of one parent – Gut Dysbiosis.

What about fathers? In many cases fathers of GAPS children also suffer from digestive problems, asthma, eczema, migraines and skin problems, which indicates that they do not have a normal gut flora. Of course the father is a great contributor to a mother's vaginal flora through regular sexual contact. In fact, in those rare cases when the mother did not show any signs of Gut Dysbiosis the father was severely affected by it. Having abnormal gut flora the father would have abnormal flora in the groin, which he would regularly share with his wife. Then the wife would pass that flora to the baby at the time of birth.

So, what happens after the baby is born? The most important thing that should happen is breastfeeding. Breast milk, particularly colostrum in the first days after birth, is vital for appropriate population of the baby's digestive system with healthy microbial flora. It is known that bottle-fed babies develop completely different gut flora to the breast-fed babies. That flora later on predisposes bottle-fed babies to asthma, eczema, other allergies and other health problems. We all know that breast is the best! However, most things that are floating in a mother's blood will also be in her breast milk. A mother with abnormal gut flora will have a whole host of toxic substances, which are produced by pathogenic microbes in her gut and maldigested foods absorbed into her bloodstream. These toxins will be excreted in her breast milk and fed to her baby. In particularly severe cases, mothers of GAPS children could not breastfeed their babies because the baby would refuse the breast or just fall asleep after the first few mouthfuls of the breast milk. We know that some of the toxins, which are produced by abnormal gut flora, have the chemical structure of opiates, such as morphine and heroin. If the baby gets these opiates in the breast milk then it is quite understandable why the baby falls asleep after the first few mouthfuls. Another reason for the baby to refuse breast is milk allergy. In a woman with Gut Dysbiosis the gut lining is damaged and leaky. It allows through partially digested proteins and antigens. Milk antigens have been detected in breast milk. I have seen a few cases when the baby took to the breast after the mother removed dairy foods from her diet. A lot of cases of severe eczema in babies can also be relieved by this measure.

On the positive side, however, the mother would also develop antibodies to her pathogenic flora in the gut. These antibodies too will be excreted through her milk and fed to her baby. So, if the baby has inherited abnormal gut flora from the mother, this flora will be controlled by antibodies in the breast milk while the baby is breastfed. When the breastfeeding stops, however, this protection stops as well. A lot of parents of GAPS children can time the start of health problems in their child to stopping breastfeeding: ear infections, digestive problems, eczema, etc. It is possible that the baby has developed an abnormal gut flora, which was controlled by antibodies in breast milk, so its own immune system has not developed any protection against this abnormal gut flora. On the contrary, there is a lot of evidence to suggest that the baby's immune system accepts these pathogenic microbes in the gut as something normal because that is all it has known from the beginning and does not recognise these microbes as foreign and does not attack them. As a result, after the breastfeeding stops there is an explosion of growth of abnormal bacteria, viruses and fungi in the baby's digestive system. In different children it takes a different length of time, depending on the individual composition of the gut flora, severity of Gut Dysbiosis and the diet of the child.

Coming back to the health of the parents of GAPS children, when I ask questions about the health of their child's grandparents, particularly on the mother's side, it becomes obvious that we have generations of people with compromised gut flora. This damage becomes deeper in every generation. The era of antibiotics, contraceptive pill, breastfeeding going out of fashion and drastic changes in diet have all contributed to this phenomenon. Doctors have known for centuries that unhealthy parents produce unhealthy children. The mother's body is a home for the growing baby for nine months and a source of nourishment and care for months after the birth. So, the mother's health is particularly important for the health of the baby. In our modern society we have generations of women, whose health has been compromised by our modern life styles. Should it, therefore, come as a surprise to us that we have epidemics of autism, ADHD, dyspraxia, dyslexia, asthma, eczema, allergies, diabetes and many other health problems in our children?

There is another important factor which makes children vulnerable – the toxic load which the child is born with. What is it? For years we believed that the placenta in a pregnant woman protects the foetus from any toxins which the woman might have in her body. Recent studies show that we were wrong. The foetus accumulates most toxins which the mother is exposed to. Mercury from amalgam fillings, toxins coming from food and environment and toxins produced by abnormal gut flora in the mother have a good chance of accumulating in the foetus. Depending on how toxic the mother is during pregnancy different babies are born with a different toxic load. A baby with a high toxic load will start its life at a disadvantage, being more vulnerable to various environmental influences: vaccinations, infections, food, drugs, etc. That is why the old wisdom of treating pregnancy with respect is so important. A pregnant woman has to be extremely careful what she puts into her mouth and on her skin. A good quality diet, plenty of rest, plenty of clean, fresh air and gentle physical activity in the fresh air are all vitally important. Protecting pregnant woman from exposure to any man-made chemicals, tobacco smoke, radiation, drugs, etc., will help her produce a child with a low toxic load in its little body, which will give it a good start in life.

What about other children in the family? In my clinical experience the siblings of autistic, hyperactive and other GAPS children are almost invariably affected by abnormal bodily flora and conditions which are caused by it. The most common ones are eczema, asthma, digestive problems and anaemia. Less common are attention deficit with or without hyperactivity, dyspraxia, dyslexia and autism. Of course, these children have inherited the same flora as their GAPS sibling. But due to genetic differences, a different toxic load at birth and various other factors, their bodily dysbiosis, and the toxicity which it produces, manifests itself differently. Well-functioning gut flora is the major regulator and housekeeper of our immune system. Allergies like eczema and asthma are the result of a malfunctioning immune system, and the most common conditions I see in the siblings of autistic children, for example.

Digestive problems are usually not as severe in the siblings, as in their GAPS brother or sister. Nevertheless, they are quite common, which is not surprising considering that they got their gut flora from the same mother as their more severely affected sibling.

Anaemia is something that is not readily recognised in connection with autism, eczema, asthma, ADHD, schizophrenia and other GAPS disorders. And yet the majority of GAPS children I have seen look pale and pasty and their blood tests show typical for anaemia changes. However, when you look at the mothers and siblings of these children, they almost without exception look just as pale and pasty. The reason for that is that most people with abnormal gut flora have various stages of anaemia. We have already discussed why it happens in the previous chapters. Here I would just say that anaemia, even mild, is not something to be taken lightly as it comes with a constant feeling of tiredness, lack of energy and stamina and difficulties in concentration, completing daily tasks and learning.

On the whole, having met many families with GAPS children, I usually find that the whole family needs treatment. The most fundamental purpose of treatment has to be normalising the gut flora and addressing nutritional deficiencies. As the whole family gets healthier, the parents have more energy and stamina to deal with their child's problems and to bring up their other children. A family is a living organism and has to be seen and treated as a whole. In our struggle to help our GAPS children it is very easy for us, parents, to neglect ourselves. But, at the end of the day, a strong healthy family is what we are all about. Isn't it?!

8. Vaccinations:
Does MMR Cause Autism?

The human mind is like an umbrella –
it functions best when open.
Walter Gropius, 1965

When talking about autism it is impossible to avoid the issue of the MMR vaccine and vaccination in general. In my practice I see some parents of autistic children who link their child's disorder with the MMR (Measles, Mumps and Rubella) vaccine where a majority cannot make this connection. An equal number of families connect their child's regression with DPT (Diphtheria, Pertussis and Tetanus) vaccination. Following research by Dr Wakefield there has been a great deal of publicity on this subject. The British government has put a lot of effort and money into convincing the public that the MMR vaccine is safe. While the MMR vaccine was in the limelight, other vaccines got questioned as well, due to the fact that many of them contain a preservative called Thimerosal, a Mercury compound, and many other toxic and questionable substances. DPT vaccine containing Thimerosal has been banned in many countries. However, in other countries a fair amount of old formula, containing Thimerosal, may still be injected into babies. Many vaccines are new and have not been tested for long enough, yet apparently the number of complications from these vaccines is much higher than anybody would expect. On top of all this we have to remember that vaccines are commercial products made with profit in mind. Is it true that the £3 million which the UK government spent on MMR promotion was paid for by the companies who have a commercial interest in this vaccine?

So, does MMR cause autism?

I do not believe that things are that simple. Here we have to look at vaccination as a whole.

Let us have a look at what is happening to children in our modern society. If you look around, how many healthy children do you see?

Childhood asthma, eczema, diabetes, allergies, hay fever, digestive disorders, ADHD and autistic spectrum disorders have all gained epidemic proportions! The majority of siblings of autistic children have eczema, asthma or another one of those disorders. And though all these health problems appear to be different, they have one thing in common – a compromised immune system. A compromised immune system is not going to react to environmental insults in the normal way! Vaccination is a huge insult to the immune system. The manufacturers of vaccines produce them for children with normal immune systems which will react to these vaccines in a predictable way. However, in our modern society with our modern way of life, we are rapidly moving to a situation where a growing proportion of children do not have a normal immune system and will not produce an expected reaction to the vaccine. In some of these children vaccination, putting an enormous strain on an already compromised immune system, becomes that "last straw which breaks the camel's back" and brings on the beginning of autism, asthma, eczema, diabetes, etc. In other children, whose immune system is compromised to a lesser degree, vaccination will not start the disorder, but it will deepen the damage and move the child closer to it. However, if the child's immune system is severely compromised, then the child will get ill even if vaccinations are completely avoided. Today, following all the publicity on this issue, many parents do not vaccinate their children at all. In my clinic I see a growing number of GAPS children who have not been vaccinated. Yet they suffer from autism, ADHD, asthma, eczema and other GAPS problems. It is the state of the child's immune system that appears to be the decisive factor, not the vaccines.

So while MMR and other vaccines may not be the direct cause of autism, in immune-compromised children they can do a lot of harm and in some children may well provide the trigger which starts the disorder.

Following all the scandals around vaccinations it is no surprise that a lot of people around the world believe that we should abandon childhood vaccinations altogether. What these people forget is that before the vaccination era it was quite normal for every family to lose one, two, three and sometimes even more children to childhood infections, like measles, rubella, mumps and others. This is the natural selection law, which Mother Nature has imposed on all living creatures on

Earth. No animal would have all of its young survive. In fact in many species most babies in the litter die, with only the strongest surviving. This law of natural selection ensures that the planet is populated by the best and the fittest in each species. In our modern world we humans are not prepared to obey this law. No mother would allow her child to perish, when there are ways to let the child live, despite the fact that this child may not be the best and the fittest she can produce. Childhood infections are one of the tools of natural selection. Children who survive them come out healthier with stronger immune systems; weak children are not supposed to survive them. Vaccinations are one of those ways we humans have invented to allow our weaklings to survive. So, we cannot abandon vaccinations altogether unless we are prepared to obey the laws of Nature. We have to come up with a more rational approach to vaccinations.

Vaccinations, which saved the lives of millions of children worldwide in the last century, are becoming dangerous thanks to changes in our life styles. The number of immune-compromised children in developed countries is enormous and growing every day. It is time for the medical profession and governments to review their attitude to vaccinations. The rule to vaccinate everybody has to change!

In this book I propose the following procedure: a comprehensive immunological survey should be performed on every baby before a decision about vaccination is made. This survey should include:

1. A questionnaire to assess the health history of the parents and the infant.
2. A comprehensive stool and urine analysis to assess any risk of gut dysbiosis in the baby.
3. A test to assess the infant's immune status.

These questionnaires and tests have to be put into an appropriate pre-vaccination panel for all babies and the results of this survey have to play an essential part in the process of deciding which of the following steps to take:

•   No vaccinations at all. An infant born to a mother with ME, fibromialgia, digestive problems, asthma, eczema, severe allergies, autoimmune disorders or neurological problems should not be vaccinated. An infant presenting with eczema, asthma, digestive problems or any other disorder which would indicate compromised gut flora and immunity should be a red flag not to vaccinate! Younger siblings of autistic children, children with severe eczema, asthma, allergies, ADHD, epilepsy and insulin dependant diabetes should not be vaccinated. At a later age these children can be retested, and in those cases where the child does not have immune deficiencies, vaccination with single vaccines only may be considered. These single vaccines should be spaced at least six weeks apart.

- Delayed vaccination until the results of the tests are better. This would apply to infants who have generally healthy mothers and do not present with any particular health problems, but on testing show abnormalities in their immune systems. These children should be retested every six to eight months and vaccinated with single vaccines only when they are ready.
- Standard vaccination protocol with single vaccines only. This would apply to healthy infants who have healthy parents and whose tests show normal immune development.

These are just initial guidelines, which need to be worked on in order to set an appropriate vaccination protocol. Those £3 million which the British government spent on promoting MMR might have been just enough to develop such a protocol, and, in my opinion, be a much more worthwhile investment in the future health of our nation.

Concerning our current standard vaccination protocol there is a strong argument to administer single vaccines only rather than combined vaccines, like MMR and DPT. In a natural situation a child would never be exposed to measles, mumps and rubella at the same time. Indeed, in those extremely rare occasions in the past when two of these infections happened at the same time, the medical literature describes impaired physical and mental development in the child. Of course the proponents of the combined vaccines would say that millions of children around the world were vaccinated this way without any ill effects. However, in view of GAPS conditions reaching epidemic proportions we have to review our old policies. It is very likely that combined vaccines will have to be abandoned altogether.

9. Schizophrenia

Schizophrenia is that big bag, where psychiatrists put all the patients who are difficult to understand. There is a considerable overlap between depression, bipolar disorder, obsessive-compulsive disorder, dyslexia and schizophrenia. Quite often a patient would be diagnosed as bipolar only to be later re-diagnosed as schizophrenic. Depression is often the only symptom present in a patient for years before other symptoms of schizophrenia develop. Members of the family of a schizophrenic patient often suffer from dyslexia, dyspraxia, depression, bipolar disorder, autism, ADHD and obsessive-compulsive disorder. Just as with childhood learning disabilities we see that psychiatric patients do not fit neatly into our diagnostic boxes. Is it because we are missing some underlying problem, which may be causing all these different conditions in different people?

The only treatment modern psychiatry can offer schizophrenic patients is antipsychotic drugs. The use of these drugs is often based on trial and error, and though in many cases they do control psychotic symptoms, they have serious side effects and do not cure the patient. Like most drugs used in modern medicine, they are symptomatic, which means that they only reduce the symptoms without treating the disease. On average anti-psychotic drugs reduce symptoms only by 15–25 %, which means that 75–85 % of symptoms are left unresolved.

Before the era of pharmaceuticals ruling medicine, psychiatrists routinely recorded that psychiatric patients not only had psychiatric problems, but were also very ill physically. The most common physical problems were digestive, cardio-vascular, diabetes, lung and urogenital infections, autoimmunity and other signs of immune abnormalities. In an old *Textbook of Psychiatry* by Henderson and Gillespie, published in 1937, it is clearly stated: "A thorough physical examination is absolutely essential in every case – schizophrenics are commonly poorly nourished". Recent research proves it to be correct. Deficiencies in vitamins (such as niacin or B3, B6, B12, B1, folic acid, vitamin C) and many minerals (such as magnesium, zinc, manganese, etc) are routinely recorded in schizophrenic patients. A Canadian doctor, the late Abram Hoffer, has successfully treated thousands of schizophrenic patients with supplementation of B3, B12, folic acid and vitamin C. An American doctor, Carl Pfeiffer, has studied more than 20,000 patients and showed that treating them with nutritional supplementation and diet can be far more effective than using prescription drugs.

Why do schizophrenic patients have nutritional deficiencies? We already know that the answer will be found only in their digestive systems. A French psychiatrist, Phillipe Pinel, almost 200 years ago wrote, "the primary seat of insanity generally is in the region of the stomach and intestines". US professor Curtis Dohan, MD, devoted many years to researching what connection digestive abnormalities in schizophrenic patients may have with their psychological state. It had been noticed previously that there is a considerable overlap between coeliac disease and schizophrenia and Dr Dohan found that symptoms of schizophrenia could be dramatically relieved by cutting all grains out of the diet. He also found that some cultures in the South Pacific, which never consumed grains, had no schizophrenia. Only when they adopted a Western diet full of grains did they start getting cases of schizophrenia. Another good example is Ireland, where people did not consume wheat until the potato famine in 1845. Before then there were no cases of schizophrenia or coeliac disease recorded in Ireland. Since adopting wheat as a staple food the Irish have one of the highest incidences of coeliac disease and schizophrenia in the world. In the late 1970s it was discovered that gluten from grains and casein from milk can be turned into opiates in the digestive system, which absorb into the blood, cross the blood–brain barrier and affect the brain. These opiates were found in the urine of schizophrenic patients and those with depression and autoimmune conditions. Later on Dr Reichelt in Norway and Dr Shattock in the UK found the same compounds in the urine of autistic children. That is how schizophrenia and autism found themselves in the same company. It became clear that both groups of patients could not digest gluten from grains and casein from milk.

Schizophrenic patients usually develop psychotic symptoms in their teens or early twenties. However, when I talk extensively with the parents of these patients, a picture of GAPS emerges. Mothers of these patients almost invariably have abnormal gut flora and associated disorders. This means that she would pass her abnormal flora to her baby. A large percentage of schizophrenic patients were not breastfed as babies, which would further compromise their digestive flora and immune system. From their childhood health history it becomes clear that the patients were physically ill long before developing psychotic symptoms. Digestive problems, allergies and reactions to food, eczema, asthmatic episodes, malnourishment, lack of stamina, hyperactivity, attention deficit, dyspraxia, dyslexia, fatigue, irritability, poor sleep, night terrors were all common. All these symptoms indicate that the child had abnormalities in gut flora with all the usual consequences: malnourishment with multiple nutritional deficiencies, compromised immunity and toxicity, coming from the gut. The mixture of these toxins obviously was not right for making the child autistic for example, but was enough to cause other problems. In these cases schizophrenia does not come from nowhere, it comes out of GAPS.

Seeing that schizophrenic symptoms usually appear around puberty, it is reasonable to suspect that puberty plays some role in the onset of schizophrenia. It is possible that the hormonal turmoil of puberty in some way interacts with the toxins in the child's body and tips the child into a psychotic state. It is also possible that the hormones open the blood–brain barrier for some of the toxins, which were in the child's body all his/her life, but could not get into the brain before. Another interesting possibility is something wrong happening in the maturation processes of the brain. Apparently through different stages of growth the brain prunes its receptors. The most active pruning goes on around two years of age and at puberty. It is possible that at puberty opioid peptides and other toxins escaping the gut of the youngster interfere with this natural pruning process and tip the brain into psychoses. Hopefully, future research will explain these issues. What is obvious is that psychotic manifestation is only a progression of the physical problems in the child's body, and not a new disease appearing out of nowhere!

The toxicity produced by abnormal microbial mass in the patient's digestive system affects the brain and causes the symptoms of schizophrenia. So, in order to help the patient we need to get rid of this toxicity. In order to do that we need to treat the patient's digestive system.

In my clinical experience the same nutritional management that I prescribe for GAPS children works very well for schizophrenic patients.

I believe this happens because this nutritional management heals the gut lining and re-establishes normal gut flora. As a result, the patient starts digesting and absorbing food properly. The gut stops being the major source of toxins in the body and becomes the major source of nourishment, as it is supposed to be. As the nutritional deficiencies and toxicity go away the psychotic symptoms go away with them.

What about the medication?

This is a very important point that has to be taken into account. It is very rare to see a psychiatric patient who is not taking anti-psychotic medication. Anti-psychotic drugs change the biochemistry of the brain and, according to the latest research, even the structure of the brain. Recent publications in the *Lancet* and the *American Journal of Psychiatry* suggest that long-term use of neuroleptic drugs cause brain atrophy (shrinkage). It is not known yet whether these changes are reversible. On top of that, anti-psychotic drugs have a long list of unpleasant side effects and, in essence, are toxic. So, it is a logical desire of any patient to come off the drugs as soon as possible. However, as we detoxify the patient through nutritional management it is important not to change his/her medication until the patient is ready for it. I will explain why. When we are sure that through diet and supplementation the patient's physical and mental state has dramatically improved and is stable, we can consider removing the medication. Despite the fact that the pharmacological companies which produce neuroleptics allow patients to stop these drugs abruptly, there is a considerable amount of published clinical evidence to show that *anti-psychotic drugs must be removed very slowly and very carefully.* Sudden removal of these drugs can cause a severe withdrawal reaction because the brain's biochemistry and structure need time to re-adjust to life without the drug. When the drug is stopped abruptly, unfortunately the withdrawal reaction is very often seen as a relapse of the disease itself, and the patient is promptly put back on the drugs. It is vitally important to work closely with the patient's psychiatrist in order to reduce the dose of the drug very slowly and very gradually in order to avoid the withdrawal reaction. Depending on the dose of the drug and how long the patient has been taking it, this period can take months, sometimes years (if the patient was on a cocktail of drugs). Typical symptoms of withdrawal are to be expected in this period: nausea, vomiting, absence of appetite, headaches, lethargy, lack of energy, sleep disturbances and mood swings. One of the side effects of a lot of neuroleptic drugs is weight gain and water retention. So, weight loss is also to be expected on withdrawing these drugs. Though the weight loss can be quite rapid, it usually comes down to the normal range for the person and should not cause any particular worry.

I would like to emphasise again that it is important to build up the patient nutritionally first and remove the cause of the problem – the GAPS – before starting the process of drug withdrawal. It is very important for the patient and his/her carers to understand that in this period of drug withdrawal it is vital to stick to the GAPS Nutritional Programme rigidly! This is not a good time to be relaxed with diet and supplementation! After the drugs have been safely removed and the patient has been stable for at least a year on an occasional basis different foods (not allowed on the GAPS diet) can be tried, but not earlier.

Pellagra

There is a certain group of schizophrenics who may be not schizophrenic at all but pellagrines. Pellagra is a deficiency of vitamin B3 (niacin or niacinamide). The typical symptoms of pellagra can look very much like schizophrenia: delusions, hallucinations, confusion, headaches, anxiety, depression, irritability with a lot of physical symptoms: dermatitis, chronic diarrhoea and inflammation of mucous membranes. It used to affect poor populations whose diet was mainly corn-based. Until the real cause of this disorder was discovered pellagrines were treated almost like lepers. People believed that pellagra was infectious and contagious until it was discovered that a diet rich in vitamin B3 completely cures it. A Canadian psychiatrist, Dr Abram Hoffer, has helped thousands of patients with schizophrenia by simply supplementing their diet with large doses (2–4 g a day) of vitamin B3. Later on he added vitamin C and some other nutrients to his treatment protocol.

The GAPS Nutritional Protocol will supply the patient with a lot of vitamin B3. However, based on Dr Hoffer's research, I believe that schizophrenics, in addition to following the GAPS Nutritional Protocol, for the first few weeks should supplement vitamin B3: niacin or niacinamide, 1–2 grams twice a day. Niacin causes flushing of the skin for 15–25 minutes. This is a benign reaction and should not alarm the patient. If it is a problem then "non-flush" niacin is available. It is always best to administer treatment under professional supervision.

On the whole there is a general opinion that schizophrenia is incurable. That is what the patients and their relatives are usually told at the time of diagnosis. However, according to the experience of doctors, like Abram Hoffer, Curtis Dohan, Carl Pfeiffer and many other medical practitioners, who treated their patients with nutrition, schizophrenia is not incurable at all. There are thousands of patients around the world who have recovered completely through using appropriate diet and nutritional supplementation. Nutritional treatment is the way forward for these patients and more and more psychiatrists are becoming aware of it. However, the way official psychiatry is presently organised, it is the patients and their families who have to administer nutritional treatment. It is not an easy undertaking, but extremely rewarding. As one of my patients said recently: "You were right about the diet! I feel absolutely normal now. I am going to stick to my diet and supplements religiously!"

10. Epilepsy

In my experience about 30% of children with learning disabilities suffer from various fits, most commonly autistic children. Some have absences, some have full grand mal seizures, some have various involuntary movements, tics and spasms, some suffer from Tourette-like symptoms, some have head bobbing and periodic shaking of the whole body or jittery movements. Some children have fits of crying and tantrumming, where nothing the parents do can stop the fit. As one mother put it "I know it is some sort of fit, like a seizure. We can't get through to him, I don't think he can even hear us, he just has to complete the fit; nothing can stop it. We just have to leave him to it, and when the fit is finished he stops himself". After the fit the children are usually sleepy or "floppy", or very tired or distressed.

There are many forms of epilepsy; the classification is very long and complex. On top of that there are many other conditions which may look like seizures but are not considered "true" epilepsy (jitteriness, benign myoclonus of early infancy, benign paroxysmal torticollis, gastro-oesophageal reflux in infancy, shuddering attacks, startle disease, paroxysmal vertigo, tics and ritualistic movements, paroxysmal choreoathetosis, pseudoseizures, anxiety states, drug-induced dystonia, blue breath-holding attacks, pallid syncopal attacks, vasovagal syncope, simple faints, migraine, narcolepsy, head bobbing or banging, night terrors, etc.). There are many factors that can cause an epileptic seizure: fever, kidney or liver failure, electrolyte imbalances, low blood sugar, lack of oxygen, low level of calcium in the blood, hormonal abnormalities, various errors in metabolism, drug introduction, drug withdrawal, trauma, brain tumour, vascular malformations in the brain, strokes and toxins. The majority of epilepsy, particularly in children, is classified as idiopathic, which is a medical term meaning "we have no idea what causes it". With all our modern medical science we still do not know what exactly makes the brain create an electrical storm, which shows itself as an epileptic seizure. Epilepsy is common amongst children and adults with learning disabilities. The statistics vary, but the majority of doctors agree that in mild disabilities around 10% of patients have epilepsy, in severe cases around 50%, though some practitioners state numbers as high as 80% in severe autism.

Unfortunately, since the invention of anti-epileptic drugs, mainstream medicine does not seem to be interested in finding out what causes epilepsy in every individual case: the patient is given a prescription and told to take the drugs more or less permanently. It is a fact that at least 70% of children who had a single seizure will never have another one. Yet, many of these children are put on drugs. Anti-epileptic drugs work by suppressing brain activity: they neither cure the condition no do they prevent susceptibility to seizures. They do not work in everyone, generally drugs are able to control seizures to various degrees in about 70% of cases and they have side effects. When a young child is put on long-term anti-epileptic medication the child is condemned to a plethora of side effects that influence the child's mental and physical development. On top of that, due to suppression of the brain activity, these children are not able to learn well, they do not do well academically or socially and their personality changes. These children sleep a lot and when they are awake they are usually dull company: I have lost count of the loving parents who described their child as a "zombie" due to anti-epileptic medication. The way the health system is structured the parents are locked into repeat appointments, where the child has to visit their epilepsy treatment team every few months to review the drug prescription. If the parents do not turn up for appointments or do not administer the drug to the child, they feel that they will get into trouble with the authorities. In many patients the seizure control is only partial; there are many cases where the seizures do not disappear with drug treatment but change their character and can become more severe and distressing. When drugs fail, the patient may be offered brain surgery or vagus nerve stimulation.

It is still a mystery how many anticonvulsant drugs work, so the drugs are often used on a trial and error basis: if one drug does not work a second one is added, if that does not work a third drug may be added, despite the fact that most experienced doctors know that if two drugs do not work, adding more drugs is not likely to improve the situation. The first-line treatment for children is usually sodium valproate (Epilim) for generalised epilepsies and syndromes, and carbamazepine

(Tegretol) for partial seizures and syndromes. Sodium valproate has a long list of side effects: digestive problems, nausea, ataxia, tremors, hair loss, increased appetite and weight gain, problems with blood coagulation, impaired liver and kidney functions, oedema, amenorrhoea, skin rashes, pancreatitis and blood cell abnormalities. Carbamazepine has similar side effects plus dizziness, drowsiness, headaches, confusion and agitation, double vision, anorexia, fever, heart problems, lymph node enlargement, hepatitis and acute kidney failure. Other drugs frequently used in adults and children are phenytoin, lamotrigine, ethosuximide, phenobarbitone, clobazam, vigabatrin, nitrazepam, steroids, acetazolamide and gabapentin. They all have a long list of side effects and almost every one has a caution: "avoid sudden withdrawal!", which means that these drugs are addictive. Many anti-epileptic drugs cause bone structure abnormalities and bone fractures as they interfere with normal bone metabolism. Some drugs (phenytoin, primidine and phenobarbital) deplete folic acid in the body, so many side effects of these drugs are similar to symptoms of severe folic acid deficiency. Considering that seizures are also known to deplete the body of folic acid, adding these drugs can have very serious consequences unless the person is supplemented with this vitamin. Long-term phenytoin is known to cause B1 (thiamine) deficiency, which in itself can cause seizures. Seizures are also known to deplete vitamin B6 in the body. Many older textbooks point out that patients with epilepsy are deficient in vitamin B6, so before any drugs are considered it is recommended to give the person B6 injections first. Indeed there are published cases where epilepsy was resolved by vitamin B6 injections alone. Unfortunately, modern treatments do not include this vitamin. In order for the body to activate B6 it needs zinc, so supplementing zinc will improve the efficacy of B6 treatment, as people with epilepsy are known to be deficient in zinc. Every seizure places enormous demands on the nutritional status of the body, leaving the person depleted of many nutrients. People with epilepsy are known to have nutritional deficiencies, most commonly in folic acid, vitamin B6, thiamine, other B vitamins, essential fatty acids, amino acids, magnesium, zinc, manganese, selenium, fat-soluble vitamins and other nutrients. The deficiencies are particularly severe straight after the seizure. There are cases of epilepsy published that show it can be treated successfully with nutritional supplements and diet alone. Indeed, dietary treatments were the first and the only successful treatments used for epilepsy before anticonvulsant drugs were invented.

Treating epilepsy with diet

From antiquity starting with Hippocratis and Galen epilepsy has been treated with fasting. Various physicians at the beginning of the 20th century also tried treating epilepsy with fasting. Bernard Macfadden, Hugh Conklin, Dr McMurray and others reported that many of their patients were never afflicted by fits again after completing a 21-day fast, particularly if followed by a low carbohydrate diet. They acknowledged that children generally recovered better than adults. The problem is that one cannot fast forever and in many cases the seizures returned when the fast ended, so the search for a suitable diet to replace fasting was on the way. In 1921 it was discovered that fasting changes body metabolism: the liver uses body fat to produce substances called ketone bodies (hydroxybutyrate, acetoacetate and acetone), which can cross the blood-brain barrier and provide the brain with energy. Normally the brain uses glucose as an energy source, but in fasting glucose is not available, so the brain switches to using ketone bodies instead. It was assumed that it is the ketone bodies that stop the seizures, and so a search for a diet that can produce ketone bodies began. Such a diet was developed in the 1920s at the Mayo Clinic in the USA called "the ketogenic diet", it severely restricted carbohydrates and proteins and replaced them with fat. Again the best results were obtained with children: the Mayo Clinic reported that initial use of the diet produced seizure control in 95% of patients with 60% becoming seizure-free. The diet won immediate interest and acceptance in the medical community. However, from 1938 onwards anticonvulsant drugs were discovered and the diet gradually got forgotten. The anticonvulsant drugs work in about 70% of cases, which leaves out quite a large group of patients, so interest in the ketogenic diet revived again in the 1990s. Thankfully, since the 1930s work on the ketogenic diet continued at Johns Hopkins Hospital in the USA and the model this hospital developed has become the classic ketogenic diet.

The classic ketogenic diet provides a 4:1 ratio of fat to the combined weight of carbohydrate and protein, which is called a ketogenic ratio. The meals largely consist of heavy cream, butter, eggs, meats and very small amounts of non-starch vegetables and fruit. Every meal has to be carefully calculated under the supervision of a trained dietician and the diet has to be initiated in the hospital. As the diet does not provide all the nutrients for the body, supplements have to be taken. The diet has side effects: most common are constipation, low-grade acidosis, hypoglycaemia, retarded growth in children, bone fractures and kidney stones. In adults common side effects include weight loss, constipation and menstrual problems. The latest meta-analysis of 19 studies into the effectiveness of ketogenic diet has concluded that half of the patients achieve a 50% reduction in seizures and a third achieve a 90% reduction. If successful, the diet has to be followed for two years at least, in many cases much longer. About 10% of children on the ketogenic diet become seizure free and once they have had no fits for 6 months, the diet can be discontinued. Unfortunately, in about 20% of patients seizures return when they stop the diet. Some children are able to reduce or remove anticonvulsant medication, but many have to continue taking it. These numbers have to be seen in the light of modern times, when the first-line treatment for any newly diagnosed child is drugs. Only drug-resistant children are offered the ketogenic diet, usually as a last resort. If the diet was the first-line treatment instead of drugs, the numbers could be very different: possibly the same as the numbers reported by the Mayo Clinic in the 1920s.

Another variation of the ketogenic diet was developed in the 1970s – the **MCT diet**, based on oil made of medium-chain triglycerides (MCTs). The MCT oil induces ketosis better than traditionally used cream and butter (which contain largely long-chain triglycerides). MCT diet provides 60% of calories as MCT oil, which is a highly refined product and not very palatable. On top of that it can cause a lot of digestive problems, including diarrhoea, cramps and vomiting. However as MCT oil is better at producing ketone bodies, more protein and carbohydrates can be added to the menu. Both the classic ketogenic diet and the MCT diet are considered to be equally effective at controlling seizures. As it is easier for dieticians to do the dietary calculations with MCT oil, this version of the diet has become popular in many clinics.

As the search for an effective diet continued, another variation on the theme has shown that ketone bodies may not be the most important part of the seizure control. Around 2003 many patients found that following the induction phase of the Atkins diet controls seizures. Based on this information the team at the Johns Hopkins Hospital modified the Atkins diet to suite the purpose. The ketogenic ratio in the **Modified Atkins Diet** in only 1:1 and does not have to be constantly maintained. Compared to the classic ketogenic and MCT diets the Modified Atkins Diet places no limits on protein and calories and it can be implemented at home without involving dieticians or hospital stays. There are few side effects and preliminary studies show that Modified Atkins Diet can give the same or even better seizure control than the classic ketogenic or MCT diets.

Going even further away from ketosis, a **Low Glycemic Index Treatment (LGIT)** has been developed to control seizures. Although it is also a high-fat diet, the LGIT allows more carbohydrate than the ketogenic diet or Modified Atkins Diet, as long as the carbohydrates are of low-glycemic index. This diet does not require hospital stay or intensive dietician support, it has few side effects and produces similar results to the Modified Atkins Diet.

How do the diets work?

It is still considered to be a mystery how the ketogenic diet works. The initial assumption that it is the ketone bodies that reduce the seizure activity proved to be wrong, as the level of ketones does not correlate with an anticonvulsant effect. It appears that ketone bodies are just used by the brain as an energy source while the body is dealing with the real cause of the seizures. In my opinion, what unites all these diets is the low carbohydrate content, in particular the exclusion of heavy starchy complex carbohydrates. The GAPS diet does the same: all starch and complex carbohydrates are removed. As we have discussed in this book, carbohydrates, particularly starch and refined sugars, feed pathogens in the body: in the gut and everywhere else. By severely restricting carbohydrates in the diet the activity of pathogens in the body is also severely restricted.

From the beginning of its existence the "side effect" of GAPS

Nutritional Protocol in many of my patients was the disappearance of fits, seizures, tics, spasms and involuntary movements, whether truly epileptic or not. In many children the fits just stop and never come back, in others the severity and frequency of seizures reduce gradually to stop altogether or stabilise at some manageable level. My clinical experience has led me to a simple conclusion: the majority of epileptic seizures are the result of two factors, which work in combination:

1. Damaged gut wall. A damaged "leaky" gut wall lets in a plethora of very toxic substances that reach the brain and trigger the seizures, fits, tics, spasms, involuntary movements, etc. The toxins are produced by the abnormal gut flora, and the mixture of toxins can be quite individual, depending on what kind of pathogens the person has in the gut. The damaged gut wall also lets through partially digested foods, activating immunity and creating food allergies and intolerances, which in themselves can manifest as seizures, fits, tics, spasms and involuntary movements. I have children in my clinic who only have fits after eating particular foods.

2. Nutritional deficiencies (which we have discussed earlier). In a person with abnormal gut flora the gut is in no fit state to digest food properly and to nourish the body. Deficiencies in folic acid, B6, manganese and B1 have been recorded as causing seizures. Other nutritional deficiencies, such as in magnesium, zinc, amino acids, fatty acids and fat-soluble vitamins, have not been studied as well yet in relation to epilepsy, but they may be just as important. A person with abnormal gut flora always has nutritional deficiencies: they are an integral part of GAPS.

A very small percentage of seizures is triggered by a physical focus in the brain, such as a tumour, a vascular malformation or a scar left after trauma, infection, or a stroke. But even in these cases, when the diet is changed to remove nutritional deficiencies and reduce the level of toxicity getting into the brain of the person, the seizures reduce in frequency or disappear altogether. Some seizures can be triggered by environmental toxins, which the person has become particularly sensitive to, getting in from the outside. I have a mildly autistic child in my clinic who has grand mal seizures only when he is exposed to the smell of paint, when the woodwork in the house has been freshly painted. These cases are rare; the majority of cases, in my experience, are due to the GAP Syndrome, particularly in children. These are the cases which our mainstream medicine classifies as idiopathic.

GAPS Nutritional Programme has been designed to take control of pathogens in the gut and to heal the gut. As the gut wall heals, the level of toxins and partially digested foods getting through drops dramatically, so the brain has a chance to start functioning normally. At the same time GAPS diet provides highly nutritious foods, while making the digestive system fit enough to digest them; these factors quickly remove nutritional deficiencies which could have been contributing to seizure activity.

Let us have a look at a typical case study, which demonstrates this situation very well.

A seven year-old boy M. had a typical GAPS health history. Both the parents were affected by abnormal gut flora. In the first year of life M. was breastfed and showed normal development. However, he suffered with colic and when solids were introduced he reacted to many foods with diarrhoea, while some foods made him constipated. M. was also susceptible to colds and chest infections, which were treated with homeopathy; antibiotics were generally avoided. The parents were aware of the dangers of vaccinations and did not vaccinate M., apart from polio and tetanus. In the second year of life M. developed normally and was mentally and physically advanced for his age, he was very bright and well co-ordinated. However, his digestion still remained vulnerable: his stools were irregular and he would get bloated. After his second birthday he slowly started limiting his diet in a typical GAPS fashion to starchy and sweet foods, refusing everything else. By the age of three M. has limited his diet to bread, humus, sweets, snack bars, sweet baked goods, cheese, sweet yoghurt, apples, pears, crisps, raisins and bananas. His digestion worsened: he started getting abdominal pains and his stool looked green and smelled of rotten fish. M. became quite thin and very pale with dark circles under his eyes. Around age three M. started lining up toys, getting obsessed with things and becoming more distant. The parents worried that he was developing autism and tried GFCF diet with M. for six months with no effect. At the age of three and a half, after a cold with high temperature, M. became clumsy and hyperactive, and even fussier with food. Then he started having absences, which initially were not recognised as seizures: he would roll his eyes up for a few seconds, freeze and become unresponsive. Shortly after that he had his first grand mal seizure. A diagnosis of Idiopathic Generalised Epilepsy followed and Sodium valproate (Epilim) was prescribed, which changed the nature of the fits: M. started having 10–15 petit mal seizures per day. The seizure would start from an aura of M. walking fast in circles, fully conscious, then he would go into slow-motion involuntary movements. The dose of Epilim was increased, which did not have an effect, so the dose was increased again. The seizures changed to absences and their number reduced to 2–4 a day, but periodically M. would have up to 15 absences per day. Since starting the medication at the age of three and a half M. has regressed in his learning ability and development: at the age of seven he could not read, was listless or fidgety, unsettled, at times hyperactive and aggressive towards children at school. His attention span was low and he was not coping with the school curriculum. His social skills were poor and he could not make friends, he only played with his four year-old sister on her age level and on his terms. At the age of five M. was diagnosed with Asperger's syndrome. When I first met M. he was tall and thin and looked pale with dark circles around his eyes. He was hyperactive with low attention span, could not stay still and his language was delayed. His digestion was poor, stools abnormal and he was slightly bloated.

The GAPS diet was implemented, starting from the Introduction diet. By the time M. was on the Full GAPS diet he had become much calmer with better focus and better ability to learn. His digestion improved, he was having normal stools and no more abdominal pain. However, the frequency of absences did not change, and the parents felt that medication was actually causing the seizures. M. was taking 800mg of Sodium valproate (Epilim) per day, and we started slow dose reduction of this drug. It took a month to reduce the dose down to 600mg per day: M. became much calmer and "more himself", his concentration span improved and the school teachers commented that his behaviour had improved. But most importantly, his seizures reduced in numbers. As we continued reducing the dose of Epilim, so the seizure frequency continued reducing. It took about 18 months to stop the medication completely. The process was slowed down by a couple of "tummy bugs" with diarrhoea, and a few occasions when M. cheated on the diet, which increased the seizure activity temporarily. By the time the drug had been completely removed M. had one or two very mild absences per week, so mild that only the parents could spot them. M became calm, and his concentration span and his behaviour became normal. He was still behind his peers in his learning, but was working hard to catch up. He looked well, was full of energy and had no digestive problems anymore.

Let us discuss this case. This little boy had inherited compromised gut flora from his parents from the start of his life, and despite the fact that M. was breasfed and antibiotics and vaccinations were avoided, the abnormal gut flora was there causing mild digestive problems. It is typical for a child with abnormal gut flora to start limiting their diet to starchy and sweet foods, refusing all savoury meals (for an explanation please look in the chapter *It's feeding time*). Sweet and starchy foods feed the pathogenic microbes in the gut, allowing them to grow in number and damage the gut wall. At the same time these proliferating pathogens in the gut start producing large amounts of toxins, which absorb through the damaged gut wall into the bloodstream and get carried to the brain. As the gut function deteriorates, the foods do not get the chance to be digested properly before they absorb through the damaged gut wall. Once absorbed into the blood, these partially digested foods trigger very complex immune reactions (called food allergy or intolerance) which are capable of initiating seizures. The combination of toxins and partially digested foods (being dealt with by the immune system) flowing form the gut to the brain, cause the epileptic activity. This is what happened to M. in his third year of life: he entered the slippery slide of GAP Syndrome. Following the GAPS diet, starting from the Introduction part of it, allowed M. to heal his gut wall and alter his gut flora to the degree that he became practically seizure free. His anti-epileptic medication had to be stopped very slowly for two reasons: first, anticonvulsant drugs are addictive, and second, because M. cheated on the diet regularly. Despite slow progress the parents and M. were delighted with the outcome. They could now forget regular visits to the epilepsy clinics and lead a normal family life.

The majority of epilepsy cases in my clinic are children. However, I often receive emails from people all over the world, who have implemented the GAPS Nutritional Protocol on their own without any supervision. Here is one of these emails from Ms H., 40 years old:

"I have suffered from IBS for many years and have been diagnosed with celiac disease... I have also had temporal lobe epilepsy my whole life with spacing out, weird feelings, black-outs, distorted sights and sounds, and recently with muscle jerks, head turning, weird facial expressions, etc. I started your diet and most of what is wrong with me went away... I went off your diet a bit after having done it for one year: I stared eating rice and some refined sugar, and the jerks started again. I went back on the GAPS diet and the symptoms stopped."

In conclusion: it is a matter of personal choice for the patient or the parents of the patient how to approach epilepsy. Some people would never consider changing their diet and would rather choose drugs or surgery. Others want to get to the cause of the problem and try natural approaches. I think it is important to make an informed choice, rather than just accepting what your doctor tells you. As far as dietary treatment is concerned, it is generally easier to treat epilepsy, in children in particular, when there is no medication involved. I do believe that, wherever possible, diet should be the number one choice in childhood epilepsy, before drugs are considered. Children are developing every minute and every day: their bodies and their brains evolve and progress all the time, following an immensely complex programme, set in motion from birth. Modern medicine has little understanding of this divine programme, let alone any ability to alter it sensibly. Drugs interfere with your child's mental and physical development in a brutal and unpredictable way, which would affect your child for the rest of his or her life. I would like to quote Dr. John M. Freeman, MD, a world-renowned expert in treating epilepsy from prestigious Johns Hopkins Medical Institution in America: "We do not understand much about epilepsy. Little is known about the mechanisms by which seizures spread throughout the brain. We do not understand why seizures occur at one moment but not at another, or why one child's seizure threshold is lower than another's. To be truthful, little is known about how the various anticonvulsants work either." So, choosing a drug as a first-line treatment is not always the right way to go, though of course there are emergency cases where drugs are the most appropriate course of action. Choosing a diet may also not be easy. I have children in my clinic who started with the classic ketogenic diet and then switched to GAPS programme with good results. And I have children who start from the GAPS Nutritional Protocol with very good results. It all depends on the severity of the condition and individual circumstances of the patient.

Thankfully we live in a wonderful world where information is freely available! It has ever been easier to make an informed choice and to decide for yourself, what is right for you and your child.

Part Two: TREATMENT

The art of medicine consists in amusing the patient
while nature cures the disease.
Voltaire

A human body has an incredible ability to heal itself, given the right help. This is particularly true for children. I do not believe that any child, no matter how ill or disabled, is beyond improvement. When working in neurosurgery it never ceased to amaze me how remarkably well children's brains recover after some serious operations, when large parts of the brain were removed. The child would leave the hospital in a wheelchair and then come back for a yearly check-up with hardly any neurological deficit detectable.

However, Nature does not work fast. Getting ill can happen very fast, but recovery always takes much longer. I tell the parents of GAPS children and the carers of GAPS adults to brace themselves for at least two years of hard work. In some GAPS patients it takes longer. The purpose of the treatment is to detoxify the person, to lift the toxic fog off the brain to allow it to develop and function properly. In order to achieve that we need:

First: To clean up and heal the digestive tract, so it stops being the major source of toxicity in the body and becomes the source of nourishment, as it is supposed to be. *Second*: To remove toxicity, already stored in various tissues of the patient's body.

These two targets are achieved by means of GAPS Nutritional Programme. This programme has evolved through personal experience with my own child and clinical experience with hundreds of GAPS children and adults all over the world.

So, what does this programme involve?

The Nutritional Programme for Gut and Psychology Syndrome

1. Diet.
2. Supplementation.
3. Detoxification and life style changes.

In the next chapters we are going to look in detail at these three points. However, in addition to the nutritional programme there is another intervention which is extremely important to implement, particularly with children. This intervention is an appropriate education. It is beyond the scope of this book to discuss education. However, this is an important point to make: as the child starts to detoxify with the use of the nutritional programme he or she will be more capable of learning. Teachers and parents frequently comment on how much faster the child starts to progress through his or her educational programme when the GAPS Nutritional Protocol is implemented.

Diet
1. The Diet – a Discussion

Nowhere is there so much misunderstanding and confusion, as on the subject of diet. At one end of the spectrum there are plenty of medical professionals and other people, involved in caring for people with autism, schizophrenia, ADHD and other GAPS conditions, who will tell you that diet has nothing to do with these problems. At the other end of the spectrum there are a few books, mainly written by parents, about the miraculous effects of dietary changes on their children's condition. In between there are many families who have tried various dietary interventions with different results: from no effect to some improvement.

The amount of different information available on the diet for autism alone must be bewildering for the parents. The most heavily promoted is the gluten-free and casein-free diet. Then there are diets without salicilates and phenols. The anti-candida diet has to be taken into account, as GAPS people are without doubt affected by this yeast. Food allergies and intolerances are a big issue for many GAPS children and adults. And, as if all that is not enough, many parents of GAPS children have to battle with the fact that their child will eat hardly anything, as the majority of GAPS children are so finicky with food. Consequently, it is no surprise that many families try different dietary interventions for a while, see no results and drop the whole idea, joining the camp of cynics.

There is no doubt that appropriate diet is of paramount importance in treating any chronic degenerative disorder, including GAPS. But what diet?

Before we start talking about what is the appropriate diet for GAP Syndrome, we need to clear up some misunderstandings.

The Gluten Free and Casein Free Diet

In the previous chapter we talked in detail about research, done by Dohan, Reichelt, Shattock, Cade and others, where gluten and casein peptides, called **gluteomorphins** and **casomorphins**, were detected in the urine of autistic children, patients with schizophrenia, psychosis, depression, ADHD and some autoimmune disorders. These peptides have a similar chemical structure to opiate drugs and are thought to affect the brain in a similar fashion. The Gluten Free and Casein Free diet (**GFCF diet**) is based on this research. This diet has been very heavily promoted and has almost become the official diet for autism. Let us have a look at it in detail.

Gluten is a protein found in grains, mainly wheat, rye, barley and oats. Casein is a protein found in milk and milk products. The GFCF diet aims to remove all sources of these two proteins. The theory behind this diet is sound, the problem is the application. Autistic children, due to abnormalities in their gut flora, crave processed carbohydrates – the very foods that feed pathogens in their gut. The typical pattern of autistic development includes the fact that sometime in the first two years of life the child limits his/her diet to processed carbohydrates, dairy and sugar: breads, biscuits, cakes, sweets, crisps, breakfast cereals, pasta, milk and sweet yoghurts. In the majority of cases it is extremely hard to change the child's food preferences: he/she just will not accept any other foods. So, to transfer this child to the GFCF diet, processed carbohydrates containing gluten are replaced with gluten free processed carbohydrates, made with rice, sugar, potato starch, tapioca flour, soy, buckwheat flour, etc. This sort of food will feed the abnormal flora in the child's gut just as much as the previous diet did, perpetuating the vicious cycle of a damaged leaky gut and toxicity escaping from this leaky gut into the blood and brain. Of course, the fact that out of dozens of various toxins, flowing from the gut into the body, two toxins have been removed – gluteomorphin and casomorphins – does some good. In some children it has quite a noticeable effect. But unfortunately in the majority of cases it has very little or no effect at all, because the rest of the toxicity is still there, being produced by abnormal gut flora. As long as *Candida, Clostridia* and many other pathogens populate the gut, the inflammation will persist and the gut will stay leaky, allowing hundreds of different undigested and toxic substances into the body.

The fact that this kind of GFCF diet gained such a world-wide acceptance as *the diet for autism* is very unfortunate, because it addresses only a small part of the whole picture of autism: the gluteomorphins and casomorphins. As always, a lot of commercial companies jumped on the bandwagon, ready to supply GFCF pre-prepared foods, full of sugar, processed carbohydrates, denatured and altered fats and proteins and many other substances which autistic children must not have. Every publication on autism is full of advertisements for these foods, lulling the parents into a sense of false security: if it is GFCF it must be fine for my autistic child. Books are written full of recipes, based on these processed carbohydrates, sugar, altered fats and proteins. Websites and internet chat groups have been set up exchanging the same kind of recipes.....

This is just one of many examples in our human history of scientific data being used in the wrong way. There is no doubt that gluten and casein are better out of the diet of an autistic child. But these two substances are by no means the only decisive key to autism, schizophrenia and other GAPS conditions. The core issue, which we have to deal with, is the unhealthy gut ruled by abnormal microbes. An appropriate diet is an absolutely essential part of the treatment. But it is definitely not the GFCF diet, as we know it.

Phenols and salicylates

There is a theory that GAPS children and adults react to phenols and salicylates (a subgroup of phenols), so foods containing them should be out of their diet. Proponents of this theory advise cutting out pretty much all fruit, vegetables, nuts, seeds and oils. I don't know why they stop there because there is no food on this planet which does not contain phenolic compounds. All grains, meats, fish, eggs, milk, fruit, vegetables and plant matter are full of phenols.

Phenols are aromatic substances of small molecular weight. They give our foods their colour and flavour. They preserve foods in their natural state by protecting them from pathogens. They take an active part in the germination and growth of seeds and attract flower pollinators. They act as powerful antioxidants and detoxifiers, when introduced into our bodies. Many nutrients and active substances which are essential for us to have every day are phenols. Let's look at some of them.

- Vitamin C. Nobody can live without it.
- Vitamin K. Essential in blood clotting and many other bodily functions.
- Vitamin E. Essential for brain development and hundreds of other jobs in the body.
- Vitamins B1 (thiamin), B2 (riboflavin), B3 (niacin), B6 (pyridoxine) and folic acid are phenols. All these vitamins are essential for us to have every day if we are to remain alive at all.
- Amino acids – cholin, phenylalanine, tryptophan and others. Without them we would not be able to produce neurotransmitters for our brain and the rest of the nervous system.
- Some neurotransmitters themselves: dopamine, norepinephrine and histamine are also phenols.
- Gallic acid. Cutting out this phenol is the basis of the Feingold Diet or low salicylate diet. Gallic acid is found in about 70% of all foods including food colourings. Though food colourings, E-numbers and other food additives should be out of your GAPS patient's diet, cutting out 70% of all foods is rather punishing.

This list can go on. All natural proteins, fats and carbohydrates contain phenolic compounds. If we cut them all out we will have to starve.

However, there is no doubt that autistic children, as well as hyperactive, dyslexic, asthmatic, diabetic, schizophrenic patients and many other GAPS people do react to phenols and many other substances in food. Some people react to vegetables from the nightshade family (tomato, potato, aubergines/eggplant and all varieties of peppers). These reactions are very different from the classical allergy and cannot be described as allergic because they do not show the changes in the immune system typical of allergy. No clear scientific explanation for these reactions has yet been found. Here I would like to propose what I personally believe happens. Many food phenols have strong antioxidant and detoxifying abilities. Any naturopath, homeopath or doctor versed in natural medicine will tell you that before making you feel better any detoxifier initially makes you feel worse. This happens because we all have various toxins stored in the tissues of our bodies. When a detoxifying substance is introduced it washes toxins out of storage sites into the blood stream to be conjugated, taken to elimination organs and excreted in urine, sweat or bile. For those couple of hours, while these toxins are floating in your blood, being dealt with by the body, they cause symptoms. Depending on the nature of the toxin and individual susceptibilities these symptoms can be very different. They can vary from headaches and behaviour abnormalities to skin rashes and sneezing. So, in effect, what is happening is that the phenols from the food are trying to "clean you up". This phenomenon is called "detox reaction" or "Herxheimer reaction" and is typically observed in patients doing any detox programme. Stored toxicity does not just sit silently in the tissues of our bodies. It causes symptoms of chronic disease and lays down the ground for cancer formation. So detoxifying is an important thing to do. It has to be an ongoing process throughout our lives. Nature provided us with plenty of opportunity to do that by placing phenols and other powerful detox substances into all our foods.

GAPS children and adults are very toxic. Tests show that they store heavy metals, petrochemicals and other toxic substances in the tissues of their bodies, sometimes in frightening amounts. Many of these toxins are probably responsible for various physical and mental symptoms in GAPS patients. For example, there are great similarities in the clinical picture of acute poisoning with mercury, lead and other toxins, found in these patients, and the clinical picture of autism and psychosis. Based on these findings, there has been a lot of attention to heavy metal chelation in autism, the purpose of which is to take heavy metals out of the body. Anybody familiar with chelation knows that this process always involves the child going through a detox period, when autistic symptoms get worse and a lot of unpleasant new physical symptoms occur. Why? Because chelation drugs wash out stored heavy metals from the tissues into the blood to be taken out of the body. This "cleaning up" process causes symptoms, often quite severe.

There is no doubt that detoxification or elimination of toxic substances has to be an integral part of the treatment for GAPS patients. Natural phenols found in foods are Nature's way of eliminating toxins from the body on a daily basis. So, the last thing we should do is to cut them out of the diet. Of course, in the process of "cleaning up" they will cause the "detox reaction". Most phenols in the foods will not cause a severe reaction (unless the patient has a true allergy to a particular food). The child or adult may experience worsening of behaviour and sleep, more self-stimulation, more hyperactivity and mood swings. This period is temporary and most patients survive it very well. As the body starts to detoxify, the negative reaction usually goes away. If your GAPS child or adult is particularly sensitive to some food, cut it out of the diet for 4–6 weeks and then introduce it slowly, starting with tiny amounts and gradually increasing them. This way you can keep the detox reaction under control. The important thing is to make sure that the person has not got a true allergy to that particular food, which can be tested for in most medical facilities.

Clinical experience shows that when the patient has been put on the appropriate diet for GAPS, his/her sensitivity to phenols changes: foods which the patient used to react to do not cause reaction any more. The diet, which we will be talking about later, has an ability to heal the gut lining, so the toxins and maldigested foods, which used to leak through, do not leak any more. So, the mixture of toxins, which the body has to deal with, gets greatly reduced. And with it the reactions to detoxifying phenols also change. Generally, as the gut heals, the reactions to many phenolic compounds, as well as many food intolerances, go away. As you "fix the leak" there will be less "cleaning up" going on in the body and hence fewer symptoms associated with it.

In the meantime there is an amazingly effective way to deal with sensitivity to phenols and other food compounds. It will also deal with true allergies to foods. This way is Neutralisation. The method of neutralisation was first discovered in 1979 by Dr Robert Gardner from Brigham Young University. He found that just a few drops of small water dilutions of pure phenolic compounds would completely neutralise allergic reactions to foods. No explanation has yet been found for how this method works, but there is data to show that it can work remarkably well. In every individual case a particular neutralising dose has to be found, which then will be given to the patient as drops under the tongue. Today neutralisation has become a well-established method of treating allergies and food sensitivities, and in most developed countries there are allergy specialists who can do it. There are number of neutralisation or desensitisation techniques already used, such as bio-resonance therapy, EPD (Enzyme Potentiated Desensitisation), incremental immunotherapy, NAET (Nambudripad's

Allergy Elimination Technique), chirokinetic therapy and homeopathy. None of the methods work for everybody, but all of them have some success record. Neutralisation may allow your GAPS child or adult to have the foods he or she used to react badly to, without any limitations.

In conclusion, there is no need to deprive children and adults with autism, ADHD, schizophrenia, dyslexia, dyspraxia, etc. of fruit, vegetables, nuts and many other phenol-containing foods. They are full of nourishment and will help your GAPS patient to detoxify quicker in order to achieve his or her full potential.

"We had bad experiences with phenols. Tom used to get red ears, would become irritable, basically "off the wall". When we started the diet (she means the correct diet for GAPS) we tried the phenol foods again. Now we have no phenol problems. Hooray!"
Tom's mother,
(Correspondence via e-mail)

The anti-candida diet

As we discussed earlier the era of antibiotics and steroids gave yeasts and moulds a special opportunity. These ubiquitous micro-organisms always lived in our bodies. However, in a healthy body they are controlled by the beneficial bacteria and do us no harm. As these good bacteria get destroyed by antibiotics and other modern influences, yeasts get out of control and turn from a harmless neighbour into a terrible menace. One particular family of yeasts, called *Candida*, has received the most attention. It is a large family of fungi which cause a commonly known problem, called "thrush". When that happens *Candida* transforms from its harmless one-cell state into an invasive active state, when it grows long stringy hyphae and puts "roots" through the tissues of the body. This sort of growth can happen in the digestive system and many other internal organs, producing a whole host of toxic substances, alcohol and acetaldehyde being some of them. Pretty much every chronic degenerative disorder has been connected to *Candida* overgrowth from arthritis and digestive problems to ME, MS, Chronic Fatigue Syndrome, fibromyalgia, neurological disorders and cancer (T. Simoncini, 2000). GAPS children and adults, almost without exception, are seriously affected by *Candida* species and possibly by other fungi.

As *Candida* and other yeasts thrive on sugars, the anti-candida diet aims to remove all food sources for these pathogens: sugar and everything that contains it, fructose, maltose, lactose and other sugars, including maple syrup and honey. Fruit is excluded, as it is viewed as a source of simple sugars. As *Candida* overgrowth can cause an allergy to other fungi and moulds, all fungi and fermented foods are also eliminated: yeast and baked foods made with yeast (breads, pastries, etc.), soured milk products, all cheeses, all fermented beverages, vinegar, malt, mushrooms, tea and coffee, dried fruit and fruit juices. However, grains are not excluded from the diet: corn, barley, wheat, rye, millet, oats, rice, etc. and foods made out of them, as long as they do not contain yeast. Starchy vegetables are not excluded either: potato, yams, sweet potato and Jerusalem artichoke.... And this is where the problem is. Let us see why?

Candida is never alone in the digestive system. It lives in company with some 500 or more different microbes which can cause disease. And indeed, when the gut flora of a GAPS patient is tested, apart from *Candida* there are many other pathogens detected, *Clostridia* family being the most common one. These pathogens and their toxins damage the gut lining, making the enterocytes (major digesting and absorbing cells of the gut) unable to perform their duties of splitting up carbohydrates into small enough molecules to be absorbed. The result is that complex carbohydrates, those found in grains and starchy vegetables, do not get digested and become food for the pathogenic flora. They undergo fermentation and putrefaction in the gut, instead of proper digestion, and become a source of toxins, which further damage the gut wall and undermine the immune system. The majority of pathogens, including different bacteria, fungi, protozoa and worms, feed on undigested carbohydrates.

The anti-candida diet, in combination with the GFCF diet and often with the phenol-free diet, is promoted for autistic children. In practise what it boils down to is lots of rice and things made out of it, potato, potato crisps, gluten free breads, biscuits and other baked goods, as autistic children crave processed carbohydrates. Unfortunately, these carbohydrates will allow their inflamed and damaged gut to stay inflamed and damaged, keeping up the toxicity in the body. That is the very toxicity which makes these children autistic.

So, what exactly should GAPS people avoid in their diet?

To understand that we need to look at how foods are absorbed in our human digestive tract. The absorption of digested foods happens in the small intestine, mainly in its first two parts: the duodenum and jejunum. The walls of these parts of the digestive system form tiny finger-like protrusions, called villi, to increase the absorptive surface. These villi are lined by the cells, called **enterocytes**. These are the cells which absorb our food and pass it into the bloodstream to nourish our bodies. (Fig 3)

The importance of these cells to our health simply cannot be over-estimated. These cells are born at the base of the villi and through the course of their short life travel to the top of the villi, slowly getting more mature on the way. When they reach the top of the villi they are shed off, because by then they have performed so much work that they have become old and worn out. This process of constant renewal of enterocytes is ruled by the beneficial bacteria, which live on them. As already mentioned in the chapter on gut flora, the beneficial bacteria ensure that enterocytes are healthy and capable of performing their jobs. When the beneficial bacteria are not there and the absorptive surface of the intestine is populated by pathogenic microbes instead, the enterocytes cannot be healthy and cannot perform their duties. Animal research shows that in the absence of good bacteria enterocytes change their shape, their travel time to the top of the villi becomes too long which can turn them cancerous. But most importantly, they become unable to perform their jobs of digestion and absorption of food. Let us have a look at how enterocytes absorb different groups of nutrients: carbohydrates, proteins and fats.

Carbohydrates

All carbohydrates are made of tiny molecules, called *monosaccharides*. There are many of them. The most common ones are **glucose, fructose**

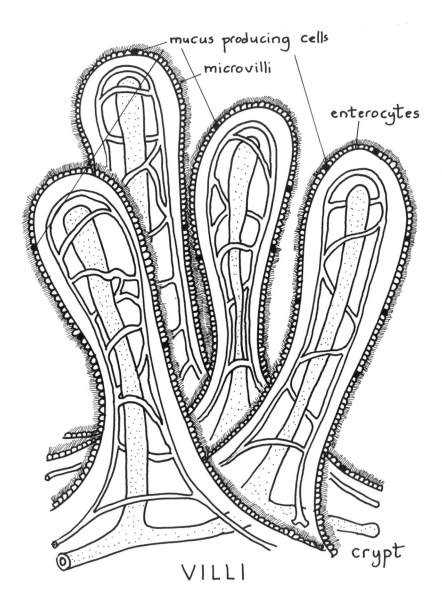

mucus producing cells

microvilli

enterocytes

crypt

VILLI

Fig 3   The absorptive surface of intestines

and **galactose**. These *monosaccharides* or *monosugars* can easily penetrate the gut lining; they do not need digestion. Glucose and fructose are found in abundance in fruit and vegetables. Honey is made of fructose and glucose and does not require much digestion. Galactose is found in soured milk products, like yoghurt. *Monosugars* from fruit and some vegetables are the easiest carbohydrates for us to digest and should be the main form of carbohydrate in the diet of any person with a digestive disorder.

The next size carbohydrates are *disaccharides* or *double sugars*, made out of two molecules of monosaccharides. The most common ones are **sucrose** (the common table sugar), **lactose** (the milk sugar) and **maltose** from digestion of starch. These *double sugars* cannot be absorbed without quite a bit of work on the part of enterocytes. The tiny hairs (microvilli) on the surface of enterocytes, called the brush border, produce enzymes called *disaccharidases,* which break down the double sugars into monosaccharides to be absorbed. This is where the biggest problem lies for people with digestive disorders. The sick enterocytes lose their ability to produce brush border enzymes. As a result, double sugars, like sucrose, milk sugar lactose and products of starch digestion cannot be split into monosugars, and hence cannot be absorbed. They stay in the gut becoming major food for pathogenic bacteria, viruses, *Candida* and other fungi, getting converted into a river of toxic substances which damage the gut wall even further and poison the whole body. Deficiencies in disaccharidases almost always accompany all sorts of digestive disorders. Recent studies performed by Dr K. Horvath in Maryland University and Dr T. Buie in Harvard confirmed these deficiencies in autistic children. So, double sugars or disaccharides have to be out of the diet for GAPS children and adults in order not to feed abnormal flora and to allow the villi time to recover by shedding off sick enterocytes and building a layer of healthy ones.

We have mentioned maltose – the result of **starch** digestion. Apart from sugar (sucrose) starch is the main form of carbohydrates we consume. All grains and some root vegetables (potato, yams, sweet potato, Jerusalem artichoke, cassava) are very rich in starch. Starch is made of huge molecules with hundreds of monosugars connected into long strands with many branches. Digestion of starch requires quite a bit of work on the part of the digestive system and apparently even in healthy people, due to its complex structure, a lot of starch goes undigested. Undigested starch provides a perfect food for pathogenic flora in the gut, allowing it to thrive and produce its toxins.

Whatever starch does get digested, the result of this digestion is molecules of *maltose*. Maltose is a double sugar which cannot be absorbed without being split up into monosugars by the enterocytes. In a person with abnormal gut flora enterocytes are not able to split double sugars, so maltose goes undigested, unabsorbed and falls prey to the abnormal microbes. To allow the enterocytes to recover and to stop feeding abnormal gut flora, starch has to be out of the diet for GAPS children and adults. It means no grains or anything made out of them and no starchy vegetables. Clinical practice shows that when the gut has been given a long enough period without double sugars and starch, it has a good chance of recovery. Once this recovery takes place, the person can start having grains and starchy vegetables again without any ill effects.

Of course, nothing in Nature is black and white. Most fruit, particularly when unripe, contain some sucrose, which is a double sugar. That is why it is very important to eat *ripe* fruit. Most vegetables and some fruit contain a little bit of starch. However, the amounts of sucrose and starch in fruit and non-starch vegetables are tiny compared to grains, starchy vegetables and table sugar. In the majority of people with digestive disorders their gut lining can cope with these tiny amounts of sugar and starch from fruit and non-starch vegetables.

Proteins

As a result of digestion in the stomach by an enzyme called Pepsin and in the duodenum by pancreatic protein-digesting enzymes, proteins reach enterocytes in the form of peptides. Peptides are small chains of protein, made of amino acids, and normally should not be absorbed until they are broken down into single amino acids. This process is accomplished by enterocytes. On their hairy surface (the brush border) healthy enterocytes have peptide digesting enzymes, called Peptidases. Each peptidase is specific to a certain peptide chain and even to a certain chemical bond in this chain. These enzymes break the peptides down into single amino acids, which then get absorbed. In a child or adult with abnormal gut flora enterocytes are sick. They are unable to produce many different peptidases and to accomplish this last step in protein break down and absorption of amino acids. At the same time the pathogenic bacteria, fungi and viruses damage the gut wall, allowing undigested peptides to leak through. We already know two proteins which do not get broken down properly and get absorbed as peptides: gluten from grains and casein from milk. There may be more proteins, which we have not studied yet and which may not be digested properly and absorbed as peptides. Hopefully, future science will show.

In the meantime, proteins are essential for us to have, particularly for a growing child. The best sources of easy-to-digest and very nourishing proteins are eggs, meats and fish. For GAPS children and adults it is important to eat easily digestible proteins to make the work as easy as possible for their digestive systems. The way we cook meats and fish has an effect on their digestibility: boiled, stewed and poached meats and fish are much easier to digest, than fried, roasted or grilled. Eggs are one of nature's treasure chests of excellent quality protein, most B vitamins, zinc and many other useful nutrients. Unless the patient shows a clear allergy to egg, eggs should be an important part of the diet.

Fats

To be absorbed fats require bile. The enterocytes do not have to do much work in absorbing fats, as far as we know. That is why the clinical practice shows that people with digestive disorders tolerate fats quite well. However, there is a problem in a person with abnormal gut flora. The gut lining is a mucous membrane. Any mucous membrane, when under attack from pathogens produces a lot of mucous to protect itself. In people with digestive disorders mucus production is excessive. These large amounts of mucus interfere with digestion of food including fats. Mucus coats food particles and does not allow bile and digestive enzymes to get to them. As a result a lot of fat goes undigested and often comes out as pale greasy stools. This impaired absorption of fats also causes deficiencies in fat soluble vitamins: A, D, E and K. Clinical experience shows that when starch and double sugars are out of the diet for a long enough period, the production of mucus normalises and, as a result, the absorption of fats improves.

To summarise:

A GAPS patient has to avoid:

- All grains and anything made out of them: wheat, rye, rice, oats, corn, maize, sorghum, barley, buckwheat, millet, spelt, triticale, bulgur, tapioca, quinoa, cous-cous (some of them are not strictly grains, but are commonly perceived as such, so we have listed them here). This will remove a lot of starch and all gluten from the diet. In fact removal of all grains makes the diet truly gluten free.
- All starchy vegetables and anything made out of them: potato, yams, sweet potato, parsnip, Jerusalem artichoke, cassava, arrowroot and taro.
- Sugar and anything that contains it.
- Starchy beans and peas: soybeans, mungbeans, garbanzo beans, bean sprouts, chick peas, faba beans.
- Lactose and anything that contains it: fluid or dried milk of any type, commercially produced yoghurt, buttermilk and sour cream, processed foods with added lactose.

For a full list of foods to avoid see the next chapter.

No processed foods, please!

"Do you know what breakfast cereal is made of?
It's made of all those little curly wooden shavings
you find in pencil sharpeners!"
Roald Dahl, 1964,
(Charlie and the Chocolate Factory)

We live in an era of convenience foods, which are very processed foods. When Mother Nature made us humans, she at the same time provided us with every food we need to stay healthy, active and full of energy. However, we have to eat these foods in the form Nature made them. It is when we start tampering with natural foods that we start getting into trouble. Any processing that we subject the food to, changes its chemical and biological structure. Our bodies were not designed to have these changed foods! The more food is processed, the more nutrient depleted and chemically altered it becomes. Apart from losing its nutritional value, processed food loses most of its other properties: taste, flavour and colour. So, to compensate for that various chemicals are added: flavour enhancers, colours, various E numbers, additives and preservatives. Many of these chemicals have been conclusively shown to contribute to hyperactivity, learning disabilities, psychiatric disorders and other health problems. Natural foods do not keep very well, so the industry has to change them to prolong their shelf life. So, natural foods get subjected to extreme heat, pressure, enzymes, solvents and countless number of various other chemicals, fats get hydrogenated and proteins get denatured. Natural foods get changed into various chemical concoctions, which are then packaged nicely and presented to us as "food". "Food" made to suit commercial purposes where health considerations never enter the calculation. The manufacturers are obliged to list all the ingredients on the label. However, if the manufacturer uses an ingredient which has already been processed or made from processed substances, this manufacturer is not obliged to list what that ingredient was made from. So, if you are trying to avoid something in particular, like sugar or gluten for example, reading an ingredient list may not always help you.

If we look at the supermarket shelves, we will see that the bulk of processed foods are carbohydrates. All those breakfast cereals, crisps, biscuits, crackers, breads, pastries, pastas, chocolates, sweets, jams, condiments, sugar, preserved fruit and vegetables, frozen pre-cooked meals with starches and batter are highly processed carbohydrates. We will examine some of them in detail. But first, let's look at them as a group.

Generally all carbohydrates in foods get digested and absorbed as glucose. Nature provides us with plenty of carbohydrates in the form of fruit, vegetables and grains. When we eat them in their natural untampered form, the carbohydrates in them get absorbed slowly, producing a gradual increase in blood glucose, which our bodies are designed to handle. Processed carbohydrates get absorbed very quickly, producing an unnaturally rapid increase in blood glucose. Blood glucose is one of those factors which our bodies go to great lengths to keep within certain limits, because both high and low values are harmful. A rapid increase in blood glucose, called **hyperglycaemia**, puts the body into a state of shock, prompting it to pump out lots of insulin very quickly to deal with the excessive glucose. As a result of this over-production of insulin, about an hour later the person has a very low level of blood glucose, called **hypoglycaemia**. Did any of you notice that after eating a sugary breakfast cereal in the morning you feel hungry again in an hour. That is hypoglycaemia. What do people usually have at that time in the morning to satisfy their hunger? A biscuit, a chocolate bar, a coffee or something like that, and the whole cycle of hyper–hypoglycaemia begins again. This up and down blood glucose roller coaster is extremely harmful for anyone, let alone GAPS children and adults. It has been proven that a lot of hyperactivity, inability to concentrate and learn, aggression and other behavioural abnormalities in school children are a direct result of this glucose roller coaster. The hyperglycaemic phase produces a feeling of a "high" with hyperactive and manic tendencies and self-stimulation in autistic children, whilst the hypoglycaemic phase makes them feel unwell, often with a headache, bad mood, tantrums, aggression and general fatigue with excessive sweating. (Fig 4)

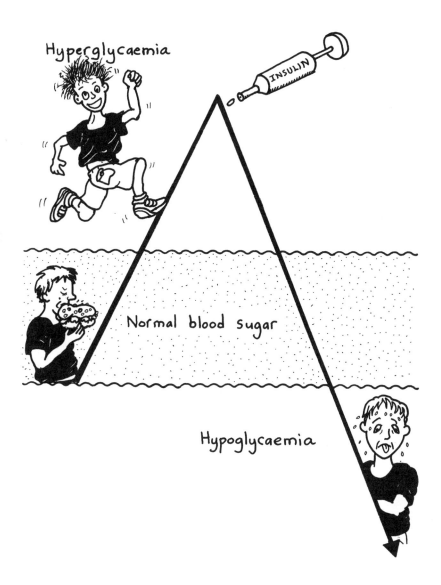

Fig 4   Blood-glucose roller coaster

Another important point about processed carbohydrates is their detrimental effect on the gut flora. We have talked in detail about the crucial role played by the normal gut flora in our health. Processed carbohydrates feed pathogenic bacteria and fungi in the gut, promoting their growth and proliferation. Apart from that they make a wonderful glue-like environment in the gut for various worms and parasites to take hold and develop. All these micro-creatures produce toxic substances that pass into the bloodstream and literally "poison" the person. The more processed carbohydrates – with or without gluten – you give your GAPS child or adult, the more "toxic" he or she will become and the more autistic, schizophrenic, hyperactive or other symptoms you will see.

In the previous chapters we have looked in detail at the state of the immune system in GAPS patients. Compromised immunity plays an important role in GAPS development. By negatively altering the gut flora processed carbohydrates play an important part in damaging the person's immune system. However, on top of that, there is ample evidence showing that processed foods, particularly processed carbohydrates and sugar, directly weaken the functioning of macrophages, natural killer cells and other white blood cells and undermine systemic resistance to all infections. An immune-compromised person who has sugary drinks and crisps daily, will worsen their immune system's condition by these food choices.

Let us have a look at some of the most common forms of those processed carbohydrates.

Breakfast cereals

They are supposed to be healthy, aren't they? That is what numerous TV advertisements tell us. Unfortunately, the truth is just the opposite.

- Breakfast cereals are highly processed carbohydrates, full of sugar, salt and other unhealthy substances. A bowl of breakfast cereal will start your child's day with the first round of the blood sugar roller coaster with the all too familiar behaviours for you to deal with.
- Being a great source of processed carbohydrates, breakfast cereals feed abnormal bacteria and fungi in the gut, allowing them to

produce a new portion of their toxins perpetuating the vicious cycle of GAPS.

- What about fibre? The manufacturers claim that with a bowl of their product you will get all the fibre you need. Unfortunately it is the wrong kind of fibre for GAPS patients. The fibre in breakfast cereals is full of phytates – substances that bind essential minerals and take them out of the system, contributing to a patient's mineral deficiencies.

- There has been an interesting experiment performed in one of the food laboratories. They analysed the nutritional value of some brands of breakfast cereals and the paper boxes in which these cereals were packaged. The analysis showed that the box, made of wood pulp, had more useful nutrients in it than the cereal inside. Indeed, breakfast cereals have got very low nutritional value. To compensate for that the manufacturers fortify them with synthetic forms of vitamins, claiming that by eating your morning bowl of this cereal you will get all your daily requirements of those vitamins. Well, the human body is not that simple; it has been designed to recognise and use natural vitamins, coming in natural food form. That is why synthetic vitamins have a very low absorption rate, which means that most of them go through and out of your digestive tract without doing you any good. Then, whatever amount of those vitamins does get absorbed is often not recognised by the body as food and gets taken straight to the kidneys and excreted in urine. We have a new syndrome in our modern pill-popping society – a syndrome of expensive urine.

So, no matter what the advertisements say, there is nothing healthy in breakfast cereals for the GAPS child or adult.

Crisps and chips and other starchy snacks

Crisps, chips and popcorn, a backbone of children's diet nowadays, are highly processed carbohydrates with a detrimental effect on the gut flora. But that is not all: they are saturated with vegetable oil, which has been heated to a very high temperature. Any vegetable oil that has been heated has got substances called trans-fatty acids, which are unsaturated fatty acids with an altered chemical structure. What they do in the body is to replace the vital omega-3 and omega-6 fatty acids in cellular structure, making the cells dysfunctional. Consuming trans-fatty acids has a direct damaging effect on the immune system. They are known to increase the activity of Th2 and weaken Th1 immunity. As you remember, the Th1 immunity is already suppressed in many GAPS patients and Th2 is overactive. Cancer, heart disease, eczema, asthma and many neurological and psychiatric conditions have been linked to trans-fatty acids in the diet. For a full story about fat processing please look in the chapter: *Fats: the Good and the Bad.*

Recently another strong argument appeared against consuming crisps and chips:

The acrylamides story

In the spring of 2002 the Swedish National Food Administration and Stockholm University reported that they had found highly neurotoxic and carcinogenic substances in potato crisps, French fries, bread and other baked and fried starchy foods. These substances are acrylamides. Scientists in Norway, UK and Switzerland have confirmed this finding. They found particularly high levels of acrylamides in starchy foods, fried or baked at high temperatures. Recently, instant coffee has been added to the list of foods containing these highly dangerous substances. The World Health Organisation, United Nations Food and Agriculture Organisation and the US Food and Drug Administration have set a plan to identify how acrylamides are formed in foods and what can be done to eliminate them, since they can cause cancer, neurological damage and infertility. Acrylamides are so harmful to health that there are certain maximum limits set for these substances in food packaging materials. For years government agencies paid a lot of attention to controlling the amount of acrylamides in the plastic food packaging, but nobody looked at the food inside that packaging. Now it has been discovered that some foods inside these plastic packets have incredibly high amounts of acrylamides, way above all allowed limits. The acrylamides story provides another reason for the GAPS child or adult to avoid crisps, chips and other starchy snack foods.

Wheat

Cutting out gluten is recommended for autism, schizophrenia and coeliac disease, so gluten-free wheat products become a major part of their diet. But let us have a look at wheat as a whole – with gluten or without it. Virtually nobody buys wheat as a grain and cooks it at home, we buy foods made of wheat flour. The flour arrives at bakeries in pre-packaged mixes for different kinds of breads, biscuits and pastries. These mixtures are already processed with the best nutrients lost. Then they are "enriched" with preservatives, pesticides to keep insects away, chemical substances to prevent the flour absorbing moisture, colour and flavour improvers and softeners – just to mention a few. Then the bakery makes breads, pastries, cakes, biscuits, etc., out of these chemical cocktails for us to eat. The producer is quite happy to take the gluten out of these mixtures and make gluten-free products. So, you will get all the processed carbohydrate with all the chemical additives in it, but this time without gluten. Once swallowed, a piece of white bread turns into a glue-like mass, which feeds parasites and pathogenic bacteria and fungi in the gut, contributing to the general toxic overload a GAPS patient already has. Being a staple in the Western world, wheat is also a number one cause of food allergies and intolerances.

Sugar and anything made with it

Sugar was once called a "white death". It deserves 100% of this title. The consumption of sugar in the world has grown to enormous proportions in the last century. It is estimated that an average Western person consumes about 160–200 lb. of this highly processed substance per year. Sugar is everywhere and it is hard to find any processed food without it. Apart from causing the blood glucose roller coaster and having a detrimental effect on the gut flora, it has been shown to have a direct damaging effect on the immune system, which is already compromised in GAPS patients. On top of that, to deal with the sugar onslaught, the body has to use available minerals, vitamins and enzymes at an alarming rate, finishing up being depleted of these vital substances. For example, to metabolise only one molecule of sugar the body requires around 56 molecules of magnesium. Consumption of sugar is a major reason for widespread magnesium deficiency in our modern society, leading to high blood pressure, neurological, immune and many other problems. A GAPS patient is already deficient in magnesium and many other vital nutrients and should not have sugar in any form. Cakes, sweets and other confectioneries are made with sugar and wheat as the main ingredients, plus lots of chemicals like colours, preservatives, flavourings, etc. It goes without saying that they should be out of the diet (with or without gluten).

Soft drinks are a major source of sugar in our modern diets, not to mention all the chemical additives. A can of soda can contain from 5 to 10 teaspoons of sugar. Fruit juices are full of processed fruit sugars and moulds. Unless freshly pressed, they should not be in your diet either. Aspartame, a sugar replacement in so-called "diet" drinks, has been found to be carcinogenic and neurotoxic and most definitely should be avoided by GAPS children and adults. The industry keeps coming up with new processed and artificial sweeteners (xylitol, corn syrup, agave syrup, other syrups, etc.). None of them can be trusted and it is essential for GAPS patients to avoid them all.

Sugar and wheat are so insidious that it can be very hard to find any processed food on the supermarket shelves without them.

To summarise, any GAPS patient, whether autistic, schizophrenic, hyperactive, dyslexic, asthmatic, etc., should have no processed foods at all in his/her diet. All foods should be bought fresh, as close to the way Nature made them as possible, and prepared at home. A digestive tract is a long tube. What you fill that tube with has a direct effect on its well being. A GAPS digestive system is damaged and very sensitive. You cannot trust any food manufacturer to fill it. You have to fill your GAPS child's (or GAPS adult's in your care) digestive system yourself by freshly cooked nourishing food, where you are in control and in charge of what the exact ingredients are and how they are processed.

No soya, please!

Soya is a very big business, particularly in the USA. A large percentage of the industry uses genetically modified soya. Soya is cheap to produce and, following some research suggesting that it may be beneficial for menopausal women, the whole market has exploded with soya products. It can be found in many processed foods, margarines, salad dressings and sauces, breads, biscuits, pizza, baby food, children's snacks, sweets, cakes, vegetarian products, dairy replacements, infant milk formulas, etc. Is there a problem with that? Let us have a look at some facts.

1. The perceived benefits to menopausal women, seen in Japan and other Eastern cultures are due to the form in which soy is traditionally used: as a whole bean or fermented as a soy sauce, natto, miso and tempeh. The form in which soya is used in the West is called *soy protein isolate*. How is it made? After removing the fibre with an alkaline solution the soybeans are put into large aluminium tanks with an acid wash. Acid makes the soybeans absorb aluminium, which will remain in the end product. Aluminium has been linked to dementia and Alzheimer's disease and indeed there has been a lot of publicity recently linking soy consumption with these mental disorders. After the aluminium-acid wash the beans are treated with many other chemicals including nitrates, which have been implicated in cancer development. The end product is an almost tasteless powder, easy to use and add to any food. Up to 60% of processed foods, including soya milk and soya infant formulas, contain this powder.

2. Soya is a natural goitrogen. What does this mean? It means that soya has an ability to impair iodine absorption and reduce thyroid function. Due to various toxins found in GAPS patients they are, almost without exception, hypothyroid, which means that their thyroid function is already impaired. Low thyroid function has very serious implications for a growing child, including abnormalities in brain development and maturation. Having soya in the diet will reduce the child's thyroid function even further.

3. Soya beans have a very high concentration of phytates. These substances are found in all grains as well, particularly in their bran. Phytates have a great ability to bind to minerals and prevent them from being absorbed, particularly calcium, magnesium, iron and

zinc. We already know that GAPS children and adults are deficient in these vital minerals. Adding soy to their diet would make these deficiencies even worse.

4. Great Plains Laboratory, which has performed allergy testing on a large number of autistic children, found that almost every child had extremely high allergies to soy. Based on their experience the head of the laboratory Dr W. Shaw directly advises against the use of soy in autistic children.

5. Soy has gained its popularity as a treatment for menopause because it contains natural oestrogens or phytoestogens. These substances may be useful for menopausal women, but not for small children. There is a growing concern among health professionals about the amount of phytoestogens infants and small children might be getting from soya milk and infant formulas. Again, due to toxicity in their bodies, the whole hormonal balance is already upset in GAPS children. Adding another interference in the form of phytoestogens does not seem like a good idea.

More than 90% of world soy production is genetically modified, which is rarely labelled as such. So, whichever way you look at soya it is best to be avoided by GAPS patients. When the GAPS Programme has been completed traditional fermented soy products can be used: natto, miso and soy sauce. Just make sure that the soya beans they were made from are organically grown and not genetically modified.

A letter from a parent (23 November 2003)

Walker was three and a half years old [when he] was diagnosed with moderate to severe autism and dyspraxia. He was non-verbal and the specialists were telling us that he may never speak.

We followed the advice of researchers and put him on a strict gluten/casein (gf/cf) free diet. We did have success with this, but felt there was more that could be done. It wasn't until I consulted with you about a nutritional plan for Walker that I realised we had a long way to go in terms of eating healthy and healing Walker's gut! The ironic thing was that we always considered our family as being relatively health-conscious. Upon analysing our diet, I quickly realised that we had fallen into the trap of eating nothing but processed, chemically treated, convenience food. We began to follow your advice by eating foods in their natural, raw state and saw almost immediate changes in Walker. Within a few weeks, Walker spoke his first sentence and the rest is history!

The nutritional advice you gave us was invaluable to Walker's recovery.

I use the word "recovery" here because, as of today, my son (who is now five years old) is attending mainstream school and has many friends. In fact, he's a social butterfly! He is learning at a normal rate and his autism and dyspraxia are almost undetectable!! Anyone who knew Walker two years ago cannot believe the "transformation" which has taken place. How could a boy who was completely emotionless and cut off from the world be the same boy he is today? It's just amazing. When I talk to people about "diet and nutrition" today, they don't quite understand how food can affect a person in that way. After all, it is quite difficult for someone who hasn't seen what we've seen to fully comprehend his miracle in its entirety!

Although there are many books written on special diets for children with autism, ADD, ADHD, etc., (and I've read them all) I haven't come across one that is similar to the nutritional advice you suggested for Walker. In fact, I've found many of these books suggesting foods that I know would actually cause Walker great harm. The older research that specifically talks about a strict gf/cf diet is just the tip of the iceberg... there is much more to this story! I get very frustrated when I see many families following this advice and buying "processed" gf/cf products that contain many other harmful ingredients. These are often the same parents who are elated to discover that Diet Coke and potato crisps are gf/cf and go out and buy them in bulk!! Ugh!

Holly Branch, mother of Walker
Surrey, UK

2. The Appropriate Diet for GAP Syndrome

We have concentrated on some diet aspects in the previous chapter. Now, let us discuss what is the right diet for GAPS people.

GAP Syndrome essentially is a digestive disorder and should be treated as such. There is no need to re-invent the wheel when it comes to designing a diet for digestive disorders. There is a diet already invented, a very effective diet with a more than 60-year excellent record of helping people with all sorts of digestive disorders, including such devastating ones as Crohn's disease and ulcerative colitis. This diet is called **Specific Carbohydrate Diet** or **SCD** for short.

SCD was invented by a renowned American paediatrician Dr Sidney Valentine Haas in the first half of the 20th century. Those were the good old days, when doctors used to treat their patients with diet and natural methods. Carrying on with the work of his colleagues Drs L. Emmett Holt, Cristian Herter and John Howland, Dr Haas has spent many years researching the effects of diet on celiac disease and other digestive disorders. He and his colleagues found that patients with digestive disorders could tolerate dietary proteins and fats fairly well. But complex carbohydrates from grains and starchy vegetables made the problem worse. Sugar, lactose and other double sugars also had to be excluded from the diet. However, certain fruit and vegetables were not only well tolerated by his patients, but improved their physical status. Dr Haas treated over 600 patients with excellent results – after following his dietary regimen for at least a year there was "complete recovery with no relapses, no deaths, no crisis, no pulmonary involvement and no stunting of growth". The results of this research were published in a comprehensive medical textbook *The Management of Celiac Disease*, written by Dr Sidney V. Haas and Merrill P. Haas in 1951. The diet, described in the book, was accepted by the medical community all over the world as a cure for celiac disease and Dr Sidney V. Haas was honoured for his pioneer work in the field of paediatrics.

Unfortunately, "happy end" does not happen in human history too often. In those days celiac disease was not very clearly defined. A great number of various inflammatory conditions of the gut were included in the diagnosis of celiac disease and all those conditions were treatable by the SCD very effectively. In the decades that followed something terrible happened. Celiac disease was eventually defined as a gluten intolerance or gluten enteropathy, which excluded a great number of various other gut problems from this diagnosis. As the "gluten-free diet" was pronounced to be effective for celiac disease, the SCD diet got forgotten as outdated information. And all those other inflammatory gut conditions, which fell out of the sphere of true celiac disease, got forgotten as well. The true celiac disease is fairly rare, so the "forgotten" gut conditions constitute a very large group of patients, which used to be diagnosed as celiac and which do not respond to treatment with the gluten-free diet. Incidentally, a lot of "true" celiac patients do not get better on the gluten-free diet either. All these conditions respond very well to the SCD diet, developed by Dr Haas. GAP Syndrome would fall into this group.

Following the whole controversy about celiac disease, the Specific Carbohydrate Diet would have been completely forgotten if it wasn't for, you guessed it, a parent!

Elaine Gottschall, desperate to help her little daughter, who suffered from severe ulcerative colitis and neurological problems, went to see Dr Haas in 1958. After two years on SCD her daughter was completely free of symptoms, an energetic and thriving little girl. Since the success of SCD with her daughter, Elaine Gottschall over the years has helped thousands of people, suffering from Crohn's disease, ulcerative colitis, celiac disease, diverticulitis and various types of chronic diarrhoea. But the most dramatic and fast recoveries she has reported were in young children who, apart from digestive problems, had serious behavioural abnormalities, such as autism, hyperactivity and night terrors. She has devoted years of research into the biochemical and biological basis of the diet and has published a book, called *Breaking the Vicious Cycle. Intestinal Health Through Diet*. This book has become a true saviour for thousands of children and adults across the world and has been reprinted many times. A number of websites and web groups have been set up to share SCD recipes and experiences.

The diet appropriate for GAPS patients is largely based on the Specific Carbohydrate Diet. Through the years I had to make alterations to the diet in order to adapt it for my patients. As time has passed, my patients have named it the GAPS Diet.

What about dairy?

The Specific Carbohydrate Diet permits lactose-free dairy products. Lactose is a milk sugar with a double molecule. It is present in fresh milk and many commercially available dairy products. According to various sources, from 25% to 90% of the planet's population cannot digest lactose due to the lack of the lactose digesting enzyme, called lactase. Children and adults with GAPS and people with gut problems most certainly cannot digest it and have to avoid it. Well-fermented milk products, such as yoghurt, soured cream and natural cheeses, are largely free of lactose because in the process of fermentation the fermenting bacteria consume lactose as their food.

However, apart from lactose, milk contains other substances which GAPS people have to avoid. The most researched substance is the milk protein casein. In the previous chapters we have discussed casomorphins – peptides with an opiate structure, which are found in the urine of autistic, schizophrenic, depressed and other patients. Casomorphins come from misdigestion of milk protein casein. They absorb through the damaged gut lining into the bloodstream of the GAPS person, cross the blood–brain barrier and affect the functions of the brain. And indeed when dairy products get completely removed from the diet of some (not all) autistic children or schizophrenic patients we observe an improvement in the clinical picture, sometimes quite dramatic. There is a debate about what particular form of casein is the problem. The group of proteins called beta-caseins have received most attention. For example, Cade and other researchers have shown that in an unhealthy digestive system they convert into beta-casomorphin-7, which gets taken up by 32 various areas of the brain, many of which are responsible for vision, hearing and communication.

Another problem with dairy is its great ability to create allergies and intolerances. Real allergy to milk is one of the most common allergies in existence, because dairy products have a wide range of antigens (various immunoglobulins). According to various research papers it is the main reason for infantile colic. Even in breastfed babies, if the mother consumes dairy products, the child may develop colic due to sensitivity to dairy antigens being passed through the mother's milk.

In many cases when the breastfeeding mother stops consuming dairy foods the colic in her baby goes away.

All this information is correct if you do not take into account a wonderful natural process, called fermentation. When milk is properly fermented at home, a large percentage of proteins get pre-digested, immunoglobulins get broken down and lactose consumed by the fermenting microbes. Fermentation makes milk much easier for the human gut to handle. On top of that, fermenting bacteria produce lactic acid, which has a healing and soothing influence on the gut lining, many vitamins (B vitamins, biotin, vitamin K2 and others) and active enzymes. Unfortunately, commercially available fermented dairy products are not fermented long enough to make the milk suitable for GAPS patients. On top of that they are often pasteurised after fermentation, which kills the probiotic microbes, destroys enzymes and many vitamins and changes the structure of proteins, fats and other nutrients in the product. That is why only home-fermented dairy products are recommended for GAPS people (please see the recipe section). In my experience, the majority of GAPS children and adults tolerate homemade yoghurt, sour cream (crème fraiche) and kefir perfectly well as a part of their GAPS Introduction diet. Whether you are sure or not if you belong to this group, I recommend you do the **Sensitivity Test** first to see if there is a real allergy to dairy. Take a drop of your homemade yoghurt, sour cream or kefir and place it on the inside of the wrist of the patient. Do it at bedtime. Let the drop dry on the skin, and let your patient go to sleep. In the morning check the spot: if there is no reaction, then go ahead and introduce dairy as a part of the GAPS Introduction Diet. If there is an angry red reaction, then there is an allergy. In that case you will have to do the Introduction Diet without diary, and later in the diet you can try to follow the *Dairy Introduction Structure*, using the Sensitivity Test at every step.

The good news about dairy products is that for many sensitive patients they do not have to be out of the diet forever. As the gut lining starts to heal many GAPS patients, who used to react to dairy, are able to introduce these products.

Dairy Introduction Structure

This structure is for:

1. those who have shown an allergy to dairy products on the Sensitivity Test, and
2. those who have chosen not to follow the GAPS Introduction Diet, but start with the Full GAPS Diet. The Introduction Diet allows the gut to heal and recover more quickly, that is why we are able to introduce fermented dairy products from the beginning as part of the Introduction Diet. Some people, particularly those without severe digestive problems, decide to implement the Full GAPS Diet straight away. In this case it is advisable to follow this Dairy Introduction Structure.

Milk fat, which contains virtually no milk proteins or lactose, is generally well tolerated by most people, even those who show an allergy to other dairy products. Pure milk fat is called ghee or clarified butter. It is easy to make at home from organic butter (please look in the recipe section). Unfortunately, commercially available ghee often contains preservatives and other additives. To make sure that your ghee is pure it is best to make it at home. Ghee contains a lot of valuable nutrients and is excellent for cooking and baking. Some people with severe dairy allergy cannot tolerate even ghee and have to avoid it. However, in my experience, the majority of GAPS children and adults have no reaction to ghee and can use it in their diet right from the beginning. If your patient has shown a reaction to yoghurt, kefir and sour cream on the Sensitivity Test, you may be able to introduce ghee in the second stage of the Introduction Diet. Do the Sensitivity Test to your ghee first before introducing it.

After ghee the first dairy product to add to the diet is butter. Butter is virtually pure milk fat and contains only very small amounts of whey, which at a certain stage in the diet the patients can usually handle. Butter should be bought organic, because non-organic butter contains a lot of pesticides, hormones and antibiotics, which non-organic cows consume. For sensitive individuals I generally recommend trying to introduce butter after 6 weeks on the diet. Doing the

Sensitivity Test will let you know if your patient is ready for this step. It is preferable to have unsalted butter, as a lot of salt products, which are used to preserve butter, contain flow agents and other additives. I would like to emphasise here that butter and ghee contain a lot of valuable nutrition for children and adults and should not be avoided, unless there is a true allergy. Butter and ghee provide various fatty acids with important health giving benefits, vitamins A, D, E, K2, beta-carotene and other nutritious substances in an easy-to-digest form.

Once ghee and butter are well introduced, in 6–12 weeks time a gradual introduction of protein-containing lactose free milk products is possible: yoghurt, sour cream, kefir and cheeses. As the gut flora gets established and the digestive system heals, many GAPS patients are able to digest milk protein without absorbing it in the opiate-like form of casomorphin. However, all patients are different. Some are ready for this step in a few months, some require much longer. It is critical to proceed very carefully and slowly, introducing milk protein-containing foods one at a time and starting with tiny amounts, watching for any reaction. Any signs of regression in a child or an adult with GAPS would indicate that he/she may not be ready. It may be an increase in self-stimulation and worsening of eye contact, sleep disturbances and an increase in anxiety, mood alterations and hyperactivity, bed-wetting in a potty-trained child, eczema flare-up or worsening allergies. Every patient would have symptoms typical for him or her. Generally, from clinical experience, I can say that the younger the patient is the sooner he or she is ready for this step. Adults, on average, take longer than children. In some cases dairy proteins have to be avoided indefinitely, particularly in long-standing cases of schizophrenia and cases complicated by epilepsy, severe asthma and severe eczema. The first protein-containing milk products that can be introduced are homemade yoghurt and sour cream.

There is a question about what is the best milk to use for making yoghurt – cow's or goat's. There are some other rare milk products on the market, like sheep and deer, which are not researched to any degree yet and are not practical to discuss here. Goat's milk is considered to be more digestible by humans as it contains less casein and different types of fats and proteins. However, when it comes to beta-casein, which is supposed to be the problem for autistic and schizophrenic patients, goat's milk contains more of it compared to cow's milk. Unfortunately, there is not much scientific data on this subject for us to rely on. However, in a clinical setting some patients (not all) do report that goat's milk is much better tolerated than cow's milk. So, initially you may want to try making your kefir or yoghurt from goat's milk rather than cow's milk. If it is not possible to find goat's milk in your area, try to make yoghurt from cow's milk, as indeed Elaine Gottschall used to treat her child and thousands of other patients very effectively. A very important point here is to use only organic milk, as there is a noticeable difference in the clinical observations of the effects of non-organic and organic yoghurt. People who react to non-organic yoghurt often tolerate an organic one perfectly well, because non-organically reared animals have to consume a whole array of chemicals from antibiotics to pesticides, most of which finish up in the milk.

It is important to introduce homemade yoghurt gradually, starting with one teaspoon a day and slowly increasing the daily amount to one or two cups a day. The reason for this is the fact that yoghurt provides alive probiotic bacteria, which can cause a die-off reaction. What is a die-off? As these probiotic bacteria attack and kill pathogens in the gut, those pathogens release toxins. These are the toxins which make the person autistic, hyperactive, asthmatic, etc, In every person the die-off symptoms are very individual. Introducing probiotic foods gradually allows us to control the die-off symptoms (you can learn more on this subject in the chapter on probiotics). As you introduce yoghurt, it can be added to homemade soups and stews, served as a dessert with fruit and honey or mixed with fruit smoothies and drinks. You can drain yoghurt through a cheese cloth to produce thicker yoghurt or cottage cheese. At the same time as yoghurt you can introduce sour cream (cream fermented with yoghurt culture), it will provide excellent nutrition for the GAPS immunity and nervous system. Just as with yoghurt, introduce sour cream gradually, starting with one teaspoon per day. Yoghurt and sour cream will give a nice variety to the diet. However, I would repeat that the patient's digestive system has to be ready for them! So, do not rush with this step!

Once the GAPS patient can tolerate homemade yoghurt and sour cream without any problem, kefir can be introduced. Kefir is similar to yoghurt product but uses a different combination of fermenting bacteria and yeasts. You can get kefir starter from commercial companies or use kefir grains. Kefir usually produces a more pronounced die-off reaction, than yoghurt, that is why I recommend introducing yoghurt first before trying kefir. GAPS patients are affected by pathogenic yeasts, candida in particular. Introducing beneficial yeasts in kefir will help to take pathogenic yeasts under control. You can ferment cream with kefir culture and introduce it at the same time as the kefir made from milk. Just as with yoghurt, start with one teaspoon per day and gradually increase the daily amount of kefir. Continue consuming good amounts of yoghurt and sour cream (fermented with yoghurt) while introducing kefir.

Once yoghurt, sour cream and kefir have been well introduced, natural organic cheese can be tried. It has to be said that cheese is one of the more difficult dairy products to introduce as it provides a very concentrated milk protein. Cheese is also a great breeding ground for yeasts and moulds, which a lot of GAPS people cannot tolerate. Some GAPS patients find that they can have homemade yoghurt without any problem but can never have cheese. However, in the majority of cases, providing that their digestive system had a good chance to heal, GAPS children and adults can enjoy a good variety of natural cheeses, like cheddar and parmesan (for a full list look at the end of this chapter). As with kefir and yoghurt, introduce cheeses one at a time, starting with a very small amount (no more than one mouthful) and watching the patient's reaction.

In a few months after safely introducing cheese many patients find that their digestive system is in a good enough state to handle commercially produced live natural yoghurt (with no additives), sour cream and crème fraiche. At the end of the second year on the diet, fresh cream can be added to the list.

Dairy Introduction Structure – the summary

Step 1. Only homemade ghee is allowed. This stage lasts on average 6 weeks. If your GAPS patient cannot tolerate ghee, you may find that this patient will never tolerate any dairy product. However, it is worth leaving it out for a few months and then trying again to introduce it. Always do the Sensitivity Test beforehand.

Step 2. Organic butter can be added gradually, if the Sensitivity Test is negative. Watch for any reactions. The majority of people are ready for this step in about 6 weeks.

Step 3. Homemade yoghurt and sour cream (fermented with yoghurt culture) can be introduced, starting with one teaspoon a day and gradually increasing the daily amount. If there is any negative reaction, wait for a month and then try again. The majority of GAPS patients are ready for this step in 6–12 weeks after introducing butter.

Step 4. Introduce homemade kefir and kefir-fermented sour cream starting with one teaspoon per day and gradually increasing the daily amount. Use the Sensitivity Test before introducing this step. Continue with already introduced dairy: ghee, butter, yoghurt and sour cream fermented with yoghurt culture.

Step 5. Try a mouthful of organic cheddar cheese with a meal. Watch for any negative reaction for three to five days, as the reaction may be delayed. If there is no negative reaction, gradually increase the amount. Once cheddar cheese is well tolerated, try to introduce another natural cheese (for a full list of allowed cheeses look at the end of the chapter). Introduce this step only after homemade yoghurt is well tolerated.

Step 6. Try some commercially available *live* natural yoghurt, sour cream and crème fraiche. Do not rush with this step. The majority of GAPS people are ready for this step by the end of two years on the diet.

After two years on the diet a lot of GAPS people find that *on an occasional basis* they can have any natural dairy product without any apparent problems, including cream and cheeses off the allowed list. However, I recommend limiting these products to occasional use and staying safe with those milk products which are allowed on the diet. I would only make an exception for alive raw milk.

What is alive (raw) milk? It is milk straight from the cow or goat, milk which has not been pasteurised, homogenised or tampered with in any other way. This milk can be called alive because it is full of life. It is full of enzymes which will digest this milk for you, leaving very little work for your digestive system to do. For example, many people who cannot digest lactose handle raw milk without any problems. Alive milk is full of "alive" vitamins, amino acids, proteins, essential fats and many other nutrients in the biochemical shape and form which our bodies need. When we pasteurise milk we destroy many of these nutrients; we alter their biochemical structure, which makes them difficult for us to digest and assimilate and, as a result, they cause allergies and other problems. For thousands of years people used to give their babies raw milk straight from the cow with great benefits and no problems. We started getting problems only when we started giving our babies processed dead milk. In many countries of the world people still give their babies raw milk with no problems. They know that the baby must not have milk which has been pasteurised, boiled, homogenised or processed in any other way because the baby would get sick from processed milk. Vets in Western countries know very well the harmful effects of pasteurised milk and do not recommend giving it to cats, dogs or any other animals. Incidentally, all these animals thrive beautifully on raw milk. For some reason human health did not receive such detailed attention – we are not told about what harm pasteurised milk can do to our health.

Why do we pasteurise our milk? Because there is a risk of getting some serious infections from raw milk. However, these infections only come from infected cows and goats. If the animal is healthy and is regularly examined by a veterinarian there is no risk of getting any infection from her milk. In fact salmonella, E. coli and many other harmful microbes cannot survive in raw milk, they get destroyed by beneficial bacteria, enzymes and immune complexes naturally present in the milk. If these pathogenic microbes get into pasteurised milk however, they thrive in it because the enzymes and beneficial bacteria have been destroyed by pasteurisation. That is why we still get serious outbreaks of these infections through drinking pasteurised milk. Because most milk in the West gets pasteurised, the farmers are not obliged to look after their cow's health rigorously enough: if the cow is ill and passes any infection into her milk the pasteurisation will destroy that infection. Fortunately there are dairy farmers who are taking a more conscientious approach: they look after the health of their animals and, as a result, are able to provide their consumers with organic raw milk without any risk of infections. For an updated list of these farmers please look at www.westonprice.org and www.realmilk. com. If you are lucky you may be able to find somebody locally who can provide you with organic raw milk from healthy cows or goats. In that case make all your yoghurt, kefir and sour cream from raw milk and cream and buy raw butter. In my clinical experience raw milk is tolerated very well by the majority of people. However, GAPS patients need to go through the *Dairy Introduction Structure* before trying raw milk: once all homemade fermented raw milk products are well tolerated and cheese has been introduced, many GAPS people can start drinking raw organic milk. As with all dairy products, start gradually with a tiny amount. It goes without saying that all milk available in our shops is "dead" and should never be consumed by GAPS people as milk. In order to make it useful for us we have to make it alive again by fermenting it with beneficial bacteria. If you are unable to find raw milk, then buy organic pasteurised milk and ferment it.

One more important point about dairy: adding whey, yoghurt and kefir does miracles for those who are prone to diarrhoea. Different substances in sour milk products, lactic acid in particular, soothe and strengthen the gut lining, slow down food transit through the intestines and the bowel and firm up the stool fairly quickly. So, if your patient is prone to diarrhoea, follow the GAPS Introduction Diet and introduce fermented milk products right from the beginning. Constipation, however, is a different matter. If your patient is prone to chronic constipation introduce sauerkraut juice and juice from fermented vegetables from the start, but be cautious with dairy. In my experience, people with constipation do well with high fat dairy products, such as ghee, butter and sour cream, but not with high protein dairy, such as yoghurt, whey, kefir and cheese: high protein dairy can aggravate constipation. This may not be the case in every constipated person as all of us have a unique gut flora, but in my experience it happens in more than half of the cases.

So, what is for dinner?

In the previous chapter we have talked in detail about the kind of carbohydrates or sugars allowed on the diet: mono-sugars. They are found in fruit and non-starch vegetables. All complex carbohydrates, those found in grains and starchy vegetables, have to be rigorously excluded from the diet. I cannot overemphasise how important it is to make sure that not even a speck of anything made from sugar, grains or starchy vegetables sneaks into the menu. This is the point when I usually see the panic on the parent's faces, particularly parents who went through all the pain of implementing the GFCF diet. No rice! No biscuits! No cakes! No pasta! No bread! Even gluten free! No chips! No crisps! No popcorn! No ice cream! No sweets! But that is all my child will eat! My child is going to starve!

Indeed GAPS children and adults usually limit their diets to processed carbohydrates, which they crave due to their abnormal gut flora. So, the important thing is to find replacements for all those foods which are compatible with the diet. The fact that the GAPS people cannot have grains and sugar does not mean that they have to be deprived of breads, cakes, biscuits, crackers, pancakes, waffles and muffins. This diet provides you with excellent and very nourishing recipes, where you will replace wheat flour with nuts ground into flour consistency or nut flour (the same thing), and instead of sugar you will use unprocessed natural honey and dried fruit. In the recipe section you will find a number of different delicious recipes. Elaine Gottschall's book will provide you with many more wonderful recipes, and, if you have access to the Internet, you will find even more on:

www.gaps.me
www.scdiet.org
www.breakingtheviciouscycle.com
www.geocities.com
www.pecanbread.com
www.uclbs.org

Far from starving, your child will be receiving a most nourishing diet. Let's just have a look at what our GAPS person is going to eat.

Recommended foods

For a full alphabetic list of recommended foods and foods to avoid please look at the end of this chapter.

Meats and fish

All fresh or frozen meats, game, organ meats, poultry, fish and shell-fish.

Meats and fish are an excellent source of nutrition. Contrary to popular belief it is the meats and fish and other animal products that have the highest content of vitamins, amino acids, nourishing fats, many minerals and other nutrients which we humans need on a daily basis. All this nutrition in meats and fish also comes in the most digestible form for us humans. I find it deceptive to see some vitamin tables in some books on nutrition showing that grains provide all our vitamins. First of all the form in which grains contain these vitamins is difficult for us to digest. Secondly, if you compare the amounts of vitamins in meat, fish or other animal products with grains, it is the animal products which are at the top of the list. Let us just have a look at some of them.

Vitamin B1 (thiamin): the richest sources are pork, liver, heart and kidneys.
Vitamin B2 (riboflavin): the richest sources are eggs, meat, milk, poultry and fish.
Vitamin B3 (niacin): the richest sources are meat and poultry.
Vitamin B5 (pantothenic acid): the richest sources are meats and liver.
Vitamin B6 (pyridoxine): the richest sources are meat, poultry, fish and eggs.
Vitamin B12 (cyanocobalamin): the richest sources are meat, poultry, fish, eggs and milk.
Biotin: the richest sources are liver and egg yolks.
Vitamin A: the richest sources are liver, fish, egg yolks and butter. We are talking about the real vitamin A, which is ready for the body to use. You will see in many publications that you can get your vitamin A from fruit and vegetables in the form of carotenoids. The problem is that carotenoids have to be converted into real vitamin A in the body, and a lot of us are unable to do this, because we are too toxic, or because we have an ongoing inflammation in the body. So, if you do not consume animal products with the real vitamin A, then you may develop a deficiency in this vital vitamin despite eating lots of carrots.

Vitamin A deficiency will lead to impaired immunity, eye problems and impaired learning and development. GAPS people cannot convert carotenoids into the real vitamin A and must consume it in a ready made form from animal foods.

Vitamin D: the richest sources are fish liver oils, eggs, fish.

Folic acid: the richest source by far is liver. Green leafy vegetables are considered a good source, though they contain much less folic acid and are more difficult to digest. It is easier for the human digestive system to extract nutrients from animal foods. Folic acid is particularly essential to have in pregnancy in order to prevent neural tube defects in the baby. That is why every traditional culture made sure that pregnant women ate liver regularly in order to provide plenty of folic acid, as well as many other nutrients, in the biochemical form which is easy to digest and assimilate.

Vitamin K2 (menaquinone): the richest sources are organ meats, full fat cheese, good quality butter and cream (yellow and orange from grass-fed animals), animal fats and egg yolks. This vitamin is essential for normal calcium metabolism, its deficiency leads to deposition of calcium in soft tissues and initiation of inflammation, while the bones and teeth do not get enough calcium. Apart from the high fat foods an important source of this vitamin is our own gut flora: the probiotic bacteria in the gut produce and release vitamin K2. Fermented foods are full of vitamin K2 as the bacteria produce it in the process of fermentation; natto (fermented soy beans) is one of the richest plant sources.

The two well-researched vitamins which meats and fish do not provide, as far as we know, are vitamin C and vitamin K1 (phylloquinone); they have to come from vegetables and fruit.

Fruit, apart from avocado, generally interferes with the digestion of meats and should be eaten between meals. Vegetables, however, combine with meats and fish very well and would provide the missing nutrients. There is another important reason for eating meats and fish with vegetables, which is the way we metabolise food. After digesting and utilising meats and fish our body tissues accumulate acids. After digesting most vegetables our body becomes alkaline. By combining the meats and vegetables in one meal we balance the acidity in the body, which is important because both too acid and too alkaline states are not very healthy. Raw vegetables have stronger alkalising ability than cooked. However, make sure that your patient's digestive system is ready for raw vegetables before introducing them.

The majority of GAPS patients are anaemic. It is essential for people with anaemia to have red meats on a regular basis (lamb, beef, game and organ meats in particular) because these foods are the best remedy for anaemia. They not only provide iron in the haem-form: the form which the human body absorbs best, they also provide the B vitamins and other nutrients essential for treating anaemia. Meats also promote better absorption of non-haem iron from vegetables and fruit while vitamin C from vegetables and greens promotes absorption of iron from meat. Large epidemiological studies show that eating red meat is associated with a much lower incidence of iron deficiency in different countries of the world.

An absolute resuscitation for an anaemic person is eating liver. Liver is a true powerhouse of nutrition. Whichever nutrient you take, you will find it in abundance in liver, including all the nutrients which GAPS people are deficient in. Making sure that your GAPS patient eats some liver on a regular basis will do immeasurably more for his or her nutritional status than the best and the most expensive supplements in the world. An anaemic person should eat liver and other organ meats once a week at least. A child needs a small amount: one to two tablespoons of cooked ground liver every other day, which can be mixed with any meat dish, or a full liver meal once a week. For some ideas on how to cook liver, look in the recipe section.

Make sure that you buy meats and fish fresh or frozen, but not preserved, as preserved meats and fish will have a lot of additives (E numbers, preservatives, starches, sugar, too much salt, lactose and other ingredients) which will not allow the digestive system to heal. Ham, bacon, delicatessen meats and all commercially available sausages are preserved meats and should be avoided. Sausages are a popular food, which children in particular like. I recommend finding a local butcher who makes his own sausages and ask him to produce pure meat sausages for you. The only ingredients in these sausages should be full fat minced meat, salt and pepper. If you wish to add some fresh garlic, onion or fresh herbs to the mince, that is fine. It is important to specifically emphasise that no commercial seasoning or sausage mix should be added. Most commercial seasonings for sausages contain a flavour enhancer MSG (monosodium glutamate) which GAPS people must not consume.

Meat, bone and fish stock is a wonderful nutritional and digestive remedy. As you cook meats, bones and fish in water a lot of nutrients get extracted into the water. Use these stocks for making soups, stews and simply as a warming therapeutic drink with and between meals. In the recipe section you will find detailed instructions on how to make meat, bone and fish stocks. It goes without saying that all commercially available stock granules and cubes are to be avoided. They do not possess any of the healing properties of a homemade meat stock and are full of detrimental ingredients. Meats cooked in water are easier to digest for a person with a sensitive digestive system. Avoid lean meats; our physiology can only use meat fibres when they come with the fat, collagen and other substances that a proper piece of meat will provide. GAPS people need plenty of animal fats, so cook pieces with a good fat covering for them. When we eat poultry it is important to eat the skin and the fats, as well as the meat. When we eat fish it is essential to eat the skin as well as the meat; that is why fish must always be descaled before cooking.

Eggs

Eggs are one the most nourishing and easy-to-digest foods on this planet. Raw egg yolk has been compared with human breast milk because it can be absorbed almost 100% without needing digestion. Egg yolks will provide you with most essential amino acids, many vitamins (B1, B2, B6, B12, A, D, biotin), essential fatty acids, a lot of zinc, magnesium and many other nutrients which GAPS children and adults are deficient in. Eggs are particularly rich in vitamin B12, which is vital for normal development of the nervous system and immunity. The large majority of GAPS patients are deficient in B12 and hence anaemic.

Egg yolks are very rich in cholin – an amino acid essential for the nervous system and the liver to function. Cholin is a building block of a neurotransmitter called acethylcholin, which the brain uses for

cognitive or learning processes and memory amongst its many functions. Cholin supplementation is recommended for people with neurological damage, memory loss and poor learning ability. Cholin is also
prescribed to people with liver problems. GAPS patients almost invariably have cognitive problems and an over stressed liver and benefit
from extra cholin in their diet. Egg yolks, particularly uncooked, would
provide the best food source of cholin.

Sadly, based on some faulty "science" and commercial publicity,
eggs have been made unpopular despite their wonderful nutritional
value. This happened because eggs contain cholesterol. In the last
decade there have been a number of clinical studies confirming that
consuming eggs has nothing to do with heart disease or atherosclerosis. In fact people who consume eggs show a lower risk of these health
problems. The majority of people do not know that 85% of blood
cholesterol does not come from food but is produced by the liver in
response to consumption of processed carbohydrates and sugar. So,
these are the foods to avoid in order to protect your heart, not the eggs.
To learn more on the subject, please read my book *"Put your heart in
your mouth"*.

I suggest getting your eggs from a source you trust. Free-range
organic eggs are the best because the hens have much better nutrition,
are not fed antibiotics and agricultural chemicals and are exposed to
sun and fresh air. Free-range organic eggs are also better from another
important point of view – the concern about *Salmonella*. According to
the National Egg Marketing Board around one in 7000 eggs may
harbour *Salmonella*. These are the numbers for battery eggs laid by hens
in cages. Salmonella-infected eggs come from an infected hen. Free-
range organically reared hens are much less likely to have *Salmonella*,
as they possess much healthier immune systems. Raw egg yolks are
more nourishing than cooked. However, if you feel unsure about raw
egg yolks, then cook the eggs whichever way you prefer. *Salmonella*
gets destroyed when eggs are cooked thoroughly.

Egg whites are usually cooked well, simply because most of us don't
like the taste of raw whites. Though one case of biotin deficiency was
described in the literature where a person lived on a self-fashioned diet
of raw egg whites, there is no conclusive evidence as to why we should
not eat them raw as well. However, when it comes to egg allergy whites

are usually the part of the egg which the majority of sufferers react to, because the whites contain very complex proteins and antigens. Egg yolks contain single amino acids, which virtually do not need digestion. That is why a lot of people with egg allergy can tolerate the egg yolks if carefully separated from the whites.

If you suspect a real allergy to egg, which can be dangerous, before introducing it do the **Sensitivity Test**. You need to test egg yolks and egg whites separately. Take a drop of raw egg yolk (carefully separated from the white, so there is no contamination with the white) and place it on the inside of the wrist of the patient. Do it at bedtime. Let the drop dry on the skin, then let your patient go to sleep. In the morning check the spot: if there is an angry, itchy red reaction, avoid egg yolks for a few weeks, and then do the test again. If there is no reaction, then go ahead and introduce egg yolks gradually, starting with a small amount. Do the Sensitivity Test with the raw egg white the same way on a separate night.

If a GAPS child or adult has a true allergy to eggs and must avoid them, you will find a lot of delicious egg-free recipes in the recipe section of the book. If there is no allergy eggs should be a regular part of your GAPS patient's diet. I generally recommend for a GAPS child to consume 2–6 uncooked or lightly cooked egg yolks per day (with or without the whites), for an adult 4–8 egg yolks per day with or without the whites.

Non-starch fresh vegetables

French artichoke, beets, asparagus, broccoli, Brussels sprouts, cabbage, cauliflower, carrots, cucumber, celery, green beans, marrow, courgette (zucchini), aubergine (eggplant), garlic, onions, kale, lettuce, mushrooms, parsley, green peas, peppers of all colours, pumpkin, runner beans, squash, spinach, tomatoes, turnips, watercress.

Frozen vegetables can be used, as long as they are not coated with starch, sugar or anything else. All vegetables should be peeled, deseeded and cooked until diarrhoea has completely cleared. After that raw vegetables can be slowly introduced with meals or as snacks.

There is a plethora of publications on the virtues of eating vegetables, so we will not concentrate on this subject here. However, one point is important: organic vegetables are better than non-organic. I had patients who were getting persistent diarrhoea from eating particular vegetables until they switched to organic ones. A GAPS patient's sensitive digestive system would undoubtedly react to pesticides and other chemicals in non-organic vegetables.

If you are sensitive to nightshade foods (tomatoes, aubergine/ eggplant and peppers), then initially avoid them. As you complete the Introduction Diet, you may find that you do not react to them anymore. Introduce them gradually and one at a time.

All fruit, including berries

Fruit can be fresh, cooked or raw, dried (no sorbates, no sulphites, sugar, starch or anything else added), and frozen (providing there is nothing added to the fruit). If the patient has diarrhoea, avoid fruit initially. As the diarrhoea settles, start introducing cooked fruit (peeled and deseeded prior to cooking). When the stool becomes consistently normal then you can slowly introduce raw fruit as a snack between meals. It is not a good idea to have raw fruit with the meals as the fruit may interfere with the digestion of meats. The fruits that do combine with meats fairly well are lemons, fresh lemon juice, avocado and sour-tasting varieties of apple.

Fruit should be ripe, as unripe fruit has too much starch. For example, bananas have to have brown spots on their skins.

Avocado is a wonderfully nutritious fruit and combines with meats well. It is easy to digest and is particularly rich in nourishing oils. Make sure it is ripe and serve it with meats, fish, shellfish and salads. Great drinking smoothies for children can be made with avocado (please look in the recipe section).

Berries are wonderful powerhouses of nutrition. They are very rich in vitamins, minerals and a whole host of anti-cancer and detoxifying substances. All sorts of edible berries are allowed on the diet: strawberries, blueberries, raspberries, blackcurrants, redcurrants, whitecurrants, blackberries, elderberries, etc. However, do not give them to a person with diarrhoea. When the diarrhoea has cleared completely, introduce berries gradually starting from cooking them or baking in pies and muffins. If cooked berries are well tolerated then go ahead with raw berries. In some cases, when the digestive tract is too sensitive, you have to remove the seeds by putting your cooked berries through a sieve.

Nuts and seeds

Walnuts, almonds, brazil nuts, pecans, hazelnuts, cashew nuts, peanuts, sunflower seeds, pumpkin seeds and sesame seeds. Nuts and seeds should be bought in their shells or freshly shelled. They should not be roasted, salted, coated or processed in any other way. Peanut butter with just peanuts and salt is allowed, providing the person is not allergic to peanuts. A lot of peanut allergy is due to contamination with moulds and their toxins, so make sure to get good quality peanuts. Blanched ground almonds (nut flour) can be purchased for baking in health food shops.

Nuts and seeds are highly nourishing. They are very rich sources of some vital minerals, amino acids and fats: magnesium, selenium, zinc, omega-6 and omega-3 oils. Epidemiological studies show that people who regularly consume nuts and seeds have lower rates of heart disease, cancer and many other degenerative diseases.

This diet uses nuts and seeds extensively. However, they are fibrous and should not be introduced until the diarrhoea is settled. After the diarrhoea is cleared baking with nuts, ground into flour consistency, can be introduced. When baked products with ground nuts (nut flour) are well tolerated, then raw nuts can be gradually and slowly introduced as snacks between meals. If for any reason ground almonds are not well tolerated, you can try to bake with ground pecans, cashews or walnuts, which you will have to grind yourself.

Seeds also should not be used until the diarrhoea has settled. Sunflower seeds, pumpkin seeds and sesame seeds are best soaked in water for about 12 hours or slightly sprouted. This way they are much easier to digest and are more nourishing. Sprinkle your soaked or sprouted seeds on salads and ready-made dishes. You can add them to your baking mixtures and grind to use as flour. You can use tahini (creamed sesame seeds), almond butter, hazelnut butter, peanut butter and pumpkin seed butter in your baking, providing they are pure without any additives.

Some people find it difficult to digest nuts and seeds, as they contain enzyme inhibitors, phytic acid and other substances to protect them from being digested. It is not a problem for everybody, but if you feel that it may be a problem for your patient, as soon as you buy your nuts to make them more digestible I recommend the following: soak the nuts (shelled) in salty water for 24 hours (1 tablespoon of sea salt per litre of water), drain them, rinse the salt off and dry in your oven at 50∞C for 3–24 hours (keep checking them as different nuts take different times to dry). You can also eat nuts and seeds straight after soaking without drying them or grind them wet to use in your baking. Once they are dried keep them in an airtight container or well-sealed plastic bag. They become nice and crunchy and make an excellent snack food together with dried fruit. Fermenting nuts and seeds with some whey in water will also help to make them more digestible: cover the nuts with water and add half a cup of whey, keep in a warm place for 24 hours, drain, rinse and use for baking wet or dry them in the oven.

Beans and pulses

Dried white (navy) or haricot beans, lima beans (dried and fresh), string beans as well as lentils and split peas. Apart from the ones mentioned, all other beans are too starchy to give to GAPS patients and should be avoided. With dried beans, lentils and peas it is very important to soak them in water for at least 12 hours, then drain and rinse well under running water to remove some harmful substances (lectins and some starches) before cooking. Do not use commercially available bean flours, as the beans are not usually presoaked before grinding them into flour. In cases of nut allergy cooked and mashed white (navy) beans can be used instead of nuts in baking. Beans, lentils and peas should be avoided until the diarrhoea and other digestive symptoms have cleared completely.

Beans, lentils and other legumes are generally very hard to digest, as they contain many anti-nutrients, such as phytic acid, lectins, enzyme inhibitors and starches. That is why it is important not to rush with introducing this group of foods into your patient's menu. When you feel that you are ready to try them, introduce them first in a fermented form: after soaking for 12 hours minimum and rinsing, cover the beans with water and whey (half a cup of whey per litre of water) and leave to ferment at a room temperature for 4–5 days. After rinsing, your beans will be ready to cook (please, see the recipe of *baked beans* in the recipe section).

Honey

All natural honey is allowed. Cold-expressed honey is preferable because many honey producers heat it in order to speed up the process of extraction from the honeycomb, which damages some micro-elements in the honey. Try to buy your honey as unprocessed as possible. Honey is sweeter than table sugar and contains two monosaccharides: fructose and glucose, which the GAPS digestive system can handle. Use honey as a sweetener. In the initial stages of the diet try to limit all sweet things, including honey, because they may encourage growth of *Candida albicans* in the gut.

Before the introduction of sugar in the 17th century honey was the only sweetener which humans used in their diet. At the end of the 17th century sugar, being cheaper and more available, replaced honey in people's diet, starting an era of sugar-related health problems.

Honey is far more natural for our bodies and, far from damaging health, has a lot of health-giving properties. It has been used as food and medicine for thousands of years. In Greek mythology honey was considered a "food fit for the gods". There are dozens of books written about the health-giving properties of natural honey. It works as an antiseptic and provides vitamins, minerals, amino acids and many other bio-active substances. Depending on the variety of flowers which a particular honey has been collected from, different flavours and compositions of nutrients and bio-active substances can be found in the honey. Traditionally it has been used to treat digestive disorders, chest and throat infections, arthritis, anaemia, insomnia, headaches, debility and cancer. It can be applied therapeutically to open wounds, eczema patches, skin rashes, skin and mouth ulcers and erosions.

Beverages

A GAPS child or adult should drink water, freshly pressed juices and meat/fish stock.

For an adult weak tea and coffee without milk is allowed. Tea and coffee must be freshly made, not instant. A slice of lemon in tea is beneficial. Herbal teas are allowed as long as they are made from fresh single herbs and not from commercially available herbal tea bags. Freshly made ginger tea is a good digestive.

Some milk replacements are allowed: homemade almond milk and homemade coconut milk. Please look in the recipe section for how to make them.

Drinking water is a very healthy habit. Children should be encouraged to develop this habit. An adult on average should drink 1.5 litres of water a day. It is not advisable to drink tap water unless it is filtered. Tap water is chlorinated and damages the gut flora balance. It is best to drink bottled mineral water or filtered water. A GAPS person's day should always start with a glass of still mineral or filtered water, cold or warm to personal preference. A slice of lemon or a teaspoon of apple cider vinegar in the water is beneficial. The same should be drunk between meals. Drinking a lot of water with meals is not advisable, as it may interfere with digestion. It is better to drink warm homemade meat stock with meals, which stimulates production of digestive juices in the stomach.

Freshly pressed fruit and vegetable juices are highly recommended. They will speed up the detoxification processes in the body and support the liver. You will need to have a good juicer at home to make these juices. A good juicer often comes with a recipe book, but you can experiment with your own mixtures and combinations (look in the recipe section). For more on juicing look in the chapter *Detoxification for People with GAPS.*

Apart from freshly pressed juices I do not recommend any commercially available juices for a number of reasons. Commercial juices get pasteurised, which destroys a lot of nutrition in the juice and turns it into a source of processed sugar. Some commercial juices can be mislabelled by not mentioning added preservatives, sweeteners and other substances. Most commercially available juices are prone to having moulds and fungi in them, which GAPS people very often react to. It goes without saying that all cordials and other soft drinks have to be out of the diet.

˘Alcoholic beverages are best avoided by people with GAP Syndrome as they add more toxicity for the liver to deal with. However, on rare occasions a small amount of dry wine, gin, Scotch whisky, bourbon and vodka are permissible. Beer has to be completely avoided as it has a high starch content.

Fats and oils

All natural fats on meats – lamb, pork, beef, poultry, etc. – are the best fats for GAPS people. They provide all the right nutrients for restoring immunity, gut and nervous system. GAPS people need to consume them in ample amounts. In fact the more fresh animal fats your patient consumes, the quicker you will see recovery.

Animal fats are the best fats to cook with because they do not change their chemical structure, when heated. All cooking oils or vegetable oils are full of harmful trans fatty acids and should be avoided. Cooking should be done with butter, ghee, pork dripping, beef fat (lard), lamb fat, goose fat, duck fat or chicken fat. If you roast a duck, collect the fat from the baking tray, put it through a sieve or a cheese cloth and you will have a large jar of excellent cooking fat. If you roast a goose you will have enough for half a year. You can bake with these fats too if you have any concerns about using butter and ghee in your baking. If you can find natural non-hydrogenated coconut oil, you can use it for cooking and baking. Unfortunately many brands of coconut oil available in the West are hydrogenated and best avoided.

Avoid all commercially available oils apart from *virgin cold-pressed* olive oil. You should not cook with it, as heating will destroy a lot of nutrients and change unsaturated fatty acids into trans fats. Use it as a dressing on your ready to serve meals, salads and vegetables in ample amounts. Other cold-pressed oils, like flaxseed oil, evening primrose oil, avocado oil, etc., are very beneficial but, again, should never be heated.

Avoid all artificial fats like margarine and butter replacements. Avoid all foods cooked with these fats.

For a detailed explanation about fats and oils please look at the chapter: *Fats, the Good and the Bad.*

Salt

Only a small percentage of all salt production goes for human consumption. More than 90% of all salt produced is used for industrial applications: the making of soaps, detergents, plastics, agricultural chemicals, PVC, etc, etc. These industrial applications require pure sodium chloride. However, salt in Nature contains many other elements: in fact natural crystal salt and whole sea salt contain all the minerals and trace elements, which the human body is made of. In this natural state salt is not only good for us, but essential. Because the industry requires pure sodium chloride, all the other elements and minerals get removed from the natural salt. We consume it under the name of "table salt" and of course all our processed foods contain plenty of it.

This kind of salt comes into the body like a villain, upsetting our homeostasis on the most basic level. Our bodies have been designed to receive sodium chloride in combination with all the other minerals and trace elements which a natural salt would provide. Pure sodium chloride draws water to itself and causes water retention with many consequences, such as high blood pressure, tissue oedema and poor circulation. As the body tries to deal with the excess of sodium chloride, various harmful acids and gall bladder and kidney stones are formed. As sodium in the body works in a team with many other minerals and trace elements (potassium, calcium, magnesium, copper, zinc, manganese, etc.), the levels of those substances get out of normal balance. The harmful results of table salt consumption can be numerous and very serious. That is why most medical practitioners, including the mainstream doctors, tell us not to consume table salt.

Our planet has plenty of good quality salt for us to consume. Throughout human history, salt was highly valued: it used to be called "the white gold", the Roman Empire paid its soldiers with salt (hence the word "salary"). Natural salt is just as fundamental to our physiology as water is. We need to consume salt in its natural state: as a crystal salt (such as Himalayan crystal salt) or as a whole unprocessed sea salt (such as Celtic salt). There are a number of companies around the world who can provide you with good quality salt.

Implementing the diet

GAPS diet is structured in three major parts:

1.   Introduction Diet
2.   The Full GAPS Diet
3.   Coming off the GAPS Diet

Part 1: The GAPS Introduction Diet

The Introduction Diet is designed to heal and seal the gut lining quickly. It achieves this aim by providing three factors:

1.   Large amounts of nourishing substances for the gut lining: amino acids, gelatine, glucosamines, fats, vitamins, minerals, etc. – all the substances which the gut lining is made from. As we have discussed in the previous chapters, the gut lining renews itself all the time by shedding off old and worn out enterocytes and giving birth to the new ones. In order to produce healthy enterocytes, your patient's gut lining needs very special nourishment.
2.   The majority of GAPS people have inflammation and ulcerations in their gut lining, which they may not be aware of, as they do not always produce particular symptoms. Your patient's gut lining may be sore and very sensitive. GAPS Introduction Diet removes fibre and any other substances which may irritate the gut and interfere with the healing process.
3.   The cell regeneration process in the gut lining is ruled and orchestrated by the beneficial bacteria, which normally live on its surface. Without their presence there cannot be any healing! GAPS Introduction Diet provides probiotic bacteria in a food form right from the start.

I recommend that most GAPS patients follow the Introduction Diet before going into the Full GAPS Diet. Depending on the severity of your patient's condition you can move through this programme as fast or as slow as the symptoms will permit: for example you may move through the First Stage in one or two days and then spend longer on the Second Stage.

Following the Introduction Diet fully is absolutely essential for people with serious digestive symptoms: reflux, diarrhoea, abdominal pain, bloating, severe constipation, etc. This diet will reduce the symptoms quickly and initiate the healing process in the digestive system. Even for healthy people, if you or your child get a 'tummy bug' or any other form of diarrhoea, following the Introduction Diet for a few days will clear the symptoms quickly and permanently, usually without needing any medication.

People with **food allergies and intolerances** should go through the Introduction Diet in order to heal and seal their gut lining. The reason for allergies and food intolerances is a so-called "leaky gut", when the gut lining is damaged by abnormal micro flora. Foods do not get the chance to be digested properly before they get absorbed through this damaged wall and cause the immune system to react to them. Many people try to identify which foods they react to. However, with damaged gut wall they are likely to absorb most of their foods partially digested, which may cause an immediate reaction or a delayed reaction (a day, a few days or even a couple of weeks later). As these reactions overlap with each other, you can never be sure what exactly you are reacting to on any given day. Testing for food allergies is notoriously unreliable: if they had enough resources to test twice a day for two weeks, they would find that they are "allergic" to everything they eat. As long as the gut wall is damaged and stays damaged, you can be juggling your diet forever, removing different foods and never getting anywhere. From my clinical experience, it is best to concentrate on healing the gut wall with the Introduction Diet. Once the gut wall is healed, the foods will be digested properly before being absorbed, which will remove many food intolerances and allergies.

If you suspect a real allergy (which can be dangerous) to any particular food, before introducing it do the **Sensitivity Test**. Take a drop of the food in question (if the food is solid, mash and mix with a bit of water) and place it on the inside of your patient's wrist. Do it at bedtime. Let the drop dry on the skin and let your patient go to sleep.

In the morning check the spot: if there is an angry red or itchy reaction, avoid that food for a few weeks, and then try again. If there is no reaction, then go ahead and introduce the food gradually starting with a tiny amount. Always test the food in the state you are planning to introduce it: for example, if you are planning to introduce raw egg yolks, test the raw egg yolk and not the whole egg or cooked egg.

Those without serious digestive problems and food intolerances can move through the Introduction Diet quite quickly. However, try not to be tempted to skip the Introduction Diet and go straight into the Full GAPS Diet, because the Introduction Diet will give you the best chance to optimise the healing process in the gut and the rest of the body. I see cases where skipping the Introduction Diet leads to long-term lingering problems, difficult to deal with.

If you have decided to go straight into the Full GAPS Diet, keep in mind that about 85% of everything your patient eats daily should consist of meats, fish, eggs, fermented dairy and vegetables (some well-cooked, some fermented and some raw). Baking and fruit should be kept out of the diet for a few weeks, and then be limited to snacks between meals and should not replace the main meals. Homemade meat stock, soups, stews and natural fats are not optional – they should be your patient's staples. Please, read the chapter on dairy to learn how to introduce dairy products safely one by one. Despite the decision not to follow the Introduction Diet, please study it thoroughly and make sure to introduce fermented foods gradually.

Start the day with a cup of still mineral or filtered water. Give your patient the probiotic. Make sure that the water is warm or at least at room temperature, not cold, as cold will send a wave of contractions along the digestive tract and may aggravate your patient's condition. Only foods listed are allowed: you must not give your patient anything else. On the First Stage the most drastic symptoms of abdominal pain and diarrhoea will quickly subside. If, when you introduce a new food, your patient gets diarrhoea again, abdominal pain or any other symptoms which started going in the previous stage, then he or she is not ready for that food to be introduced. Wait for a week and try again.

First stage:

- Homemade meat or fish stock. Meat and fish stocks provide building blocks for the rapidly growing cells of the gut lining and they have a soothing effect on any areas of inflammation in the gut. That is why they aid digestion and have been known for centuries as healing folk remedies for the digestive tract. Do not use commercially available soup stock granules or bullion cubes, as they do not heal the gut, are highly processed and are full of detrimental ingredients. Chicken stock is particularly gentle on the stomach and is very good to start with. To make good meat stock you need joints, bones, a piece of meat on the bone, a whole chicken, giblets from chicken, goose or duck, whole pigeons, pheasants or other inexpensive meats. It is essential to use bones and joints, as they provide the healing substances, not so much the muscle meats. Ask the butcher to cut the large tubular bones in half, so you can get the bone marrow out of them after cooking. Put the bones, joints and meats into a large pan and fill it up with water, add natural unprocessed salt to your taste at the beginning of cooking and about a teaspoon of black peppercorns, roughly crushed. Bring to the boil, cover and simmer on a low heat for $2\frac{1}{2}$–$3\frac{1}{2}$ hours (if using a slow cooker, cook overnight). You can make fish stock the same way using a whole fish or fish fins, bones and heads; fish stock takes about 1–$1\frac{1}{2}$ hours. After cooking take the bones and meats out and sieve the stock to remove small bones and peppercorns. Strip off all the soft tissues from the bones as best as you can to add later to soups. It is important to eat all the soft tissues on the bones. Extract the bone marrow out of large tubular bones while they are still warm: to do that bang the bone on a thick wooden chopping board. The gelatinous soft tissues around the bones and the bone marrow provide some of the best healing remedies for the gut lining and the immune system; your patient needs to consume them with every meal. Take off all the soft tissues from fish bones and heads and reserve for adding to soups later. The meat or fish stock will keep well in the fridge for at least 7 days, or it can be frozen. Your patient should keep drinking warm meat stock all day with meals and between meals. Do not use microwaves for warming up the stock, use a conventional stove (microwaves destroy food). It is very important to consume all the fat in the stock and off the bones as these fats are essential for the healing process. Add some probiotic food into every cup of stock (the details about introducing probiotic foods follow).

- Homemade soup made with your homemade meat or fish stock. Please look for some recipe ideas in the recipe section. Here we will go through some details, specific for the Introduction Diet. Bring some of the meat stock to the boil, add chopped or sliced vegetables: onions, carrots, broccoli, leeks, cauliflower, courgettes, marrow (zucchini), squash, pumpkin, etc. Simmer for 25–35 minutes. You can choose any combination of available vegetables avoiding very fibrous ones, such as all varieties of cabbage and celery. All particularly fibrous parts of vegetables need to be removed, such as skin and seeds on pumpkins, marrows and squashes, stalks of broccoli and cauliflower and any other parts that look too fibrous. Cook the vegetables well, so they are really soft. When vegetables are well cooked, add 1–2 tablespoons of chopped garlic, bring to the boil and turn the heat off. Let your patient eat this soup with the bone marrow and meats and other soft tissues which you took off the bones. You can blend the soup using a soup blender or have it as it is. Add some probiotic food into every bowl of soup (the details about introducing probiotic foods follow). Your patient should eat these soups with boiled meat and other soft tissues off the bones as often as he or she wants to all day. Once you have made a large pot of soup, it will keep in the fridge for 5–8 days, so you can warm up some of it any time.
- **Probiotic foods** are essential to introduce right from the beginning. These can be dairy-based or vegetable-based. To avoid any reactions, introduce probiotic foods gradually, starting with 1–2 teaspoons a day for 1–5 days, then 3–4 teaspoons a day for 1–5 days and so on until you can add a few teaspoons of the probiotic food into every cup of meat stock and every bowl of soup. Start by adding juice from your homemade sauerkraut, fermented vegetables or vegetable medley into the cups of meat stock and bowls of soup. Do not add the vegetables themselves yet, as they are too fibrous. Please look in the recipe section for how to ferment vegeta-

bles. Apart from providing probiotic bacteria, these juices from fermented vegetables will help you to restore normal stomach acid production. Make sure that the food is not too hot when adding the probiotic foods, as the heat would destroy the beneficial probiotic bacteria. Apart from some rare exceptions, juice from fermented vegetables is well tolerated by GAPS people. Dairy-based fermented foods are a different matter. In my experience large percent of GAPS children and adults can tolerate well-fermented homemade whey, yoghurt or sour cream right from the beginning. However, some cannot. So, before introducing dairy, always do the sensitivity test. For those who clearly react to dairy, please look at the chapter on dairy.

Adding whey, sour cream, yoghurt and kefir does miracles for those who are prone to diarrhoea. Different substances in sour milk products, lactic acid in particular, soothe and strengthen the gut lining, slow down food transit through the intestines and the bowel and firm up the stool fairly quickly. So, if your patient is prone to diarrhoea, introduce fermented milk products right from the beginning (in parallel with the juices from sauerkraut and other fermented vegetables), starting with whey and sour cream. Constipation, however, is a different matter. If your patient is prone to chronic severe constipation introduce sauerkraut juice and juice from fermented vegetables from the start, but be cautious with dairy. In my experience, people with constipation do well with high fat dairy products, such as sour cream, ghee and butter, but not with high protein dairy, such as yoghurt, whey, kefir and cheese: high protein dairy can aggravate constipation. This may not be the case in every constipated person, as all of us have a unique gut flora, but in my experience it happens in more than half of the cases.

So, *for people who are predominantly prone to diarrhoea,* in parallel with juices from sauerkraut and other fermented vegetables introduce whey from dripping your homemade yoghurt (dripping will remove many proteins). Do the sensitivity test with whey first. If there is no reaction on the sensitivity test, start with one teaspoon of whey added to the soup or meat stock. After 1–5 days on one teaspoon of whey per day, increase to two teaspoons a day and so on, until your patient is having about half a cup to a cup of whey per day with meals. In parallel with the whey you can try to introduce homemade sour cream (fermented with yoghurt culture); it has a beautiful fatty acid profile for your patient's immune system and gut lining. When you feel that your patient is tolerating whey and sour cream well enough, try to add one teaspoon per day of homemade yoghurt (without dripping it), gradually increasing the daily amount. After yoghurt, introduce homemade kefir. Kefir is far more aggressive than yoghurt and usually creates a more pronounced "die-off reaction". That is why I recommend introducing yoghurt first before starting on kefir. In parallel with kefir you can introduce sour cream made with kefir culture.

In cases of chronic severe constipation, start with juices of sauerkraut and other fermented vegetables and work on increasing daily amounts of these juices. When the stools start getting more or less regular and happen more or less daily, try to introduce sour cream (fermented with yoghurt culture), starting from one teaspoon per day and gradually increasing. Once your patient is having about a cup of sour cream fermented with yoghurt culture per day, try to introduce sour cream fermented with kefir culture.

- Ginger tea, mint or camomile tea with a little honey between meals. To make ginger tea, grate some fresh or frozen ginger root (about a teaspoonful) into your teapot and add boiling water, cover and leave for 3–5 minutes. Pour through a small sieve.

__In extreme cases of profuse watery diarrhoea,__ exclude vegetables. Let your patient drink warm meat stock with probiotic foods every hour (preferably whey, sour cream or yoghurt; if dairy is not tolerated yet, then juice from fermented vegetables), eat well-cooked gelatinous meats and fish (which you made the stock with) and consider adding raw egg yolks gradually. Do not introduce vegetables until the diarrhoea starts settling down. When the gut wall is severely inflamed, no amount of fibre can be tolerated. That is why you should not rush to introduce vegetables (even when very well cooked).

Second stage:

- Keep giving your patient the soups with bone marrow, boiled meats or fish and other soft tissues off the bones. He or she should keep drinking the meat stock and ginger tea. Keep adding some probiotic food into every cup of meat stock and every bowl of soup: juices from sauerkraut, fermented vegetables or vegetable medley, or homemade dairy products.

- Add raw organic egg yolks carefully separated from the egg white. It is best to have raw egg yolks added to every bowl of soup and every cup of meat stock. Start with one egg yolk a day and gradually increase until your patient has an egg yolk with every bowl of soup. When egg yolks are well tolerated add soft-boiled eggs to the soups (the whites cooked and the yolks still runny). If you have any concerns about egg allergy, do the sensitivity test first. There is no need to limit the number of egg yolks per day, as they absorb quickly, almost without needing any digestion, and will provide your patient with wonderful and most needed nutrition. Get your eggs from the source you trust: fresh, free range and organic.

- Add stews and casseroles made with meats and vegetables. Avoid spices at this stage, just make the stew with salt and fresh herbs (look for a recipe for Italian Casserole in the recipe section). The fat content of these meals must be quite high: the more fresh animal fats your patient consumes, the quicker he or she will recover. Add some probiotic food into every serving.

- Keep increasing daily amount of homemade whey, sour cream, yoghurt or kefir, if introduced. Keep increasing the amount of juice from sauerkraut, fermented vegetables or vegetable medley.

- Introduce fermented fish or Swedish gravlax, starting with one small piece a day and gradually increasing. Look for the recipes in the recipe section.

- Introduce homemade ghee, starting with one teaspoon a day and gradually increasing. Ghee is usually well tolerated by most GAPS people, regardless of diarrhoea or constipation and regardless of reactions to other dairy products. So, I recommend that all GAPS people try to introduce it, even if other dairy products have not been introduced yet.

Third stage:

- Carry on with the previous foods.
- Add ripe avocado mashed into soups, starting with 1–3 teaspoons per day and gradually increasing the amount.
- Add pancakes, starting with one pancake a day and gradually increasing the amount. Make these pancakes with three ingredients: 1) organic nut butter (almond, walnut, peanut, etc); 2) eggs; 3) a piece of fresh winter squash, marrow or courgette (peeled, deseeded and well blended in a food processor). Fry small thin pancakes using ghee, goose fat or duck fat, making sure not to burn them.
- Egg scrambled with plenty of ghee, goose fat, pork fat or duck fat. Serve it with avocado (if well tolerated) and cooked vegetables. Cooked onion is particularly good for the digestive system and the immune system: melt 4–5 tablespoons of any animal fat (goose, duck, pork, etc.) or ghee in the pan, add sliced large white onion, cover and cook for 20–30 minutes on low heat until soft, sweet and translucent.
- Introduce the sauerkraut and your fermented vegetables (your patient has been drinking the juices from them for a while now). Start with a small amount, gradually increasing to 1–4 teaspoons of sauerkraut or fermented vegetables with every meal.

Fourth stage:

- Carry on with the previous foods.
- Gradually add meats cooked by roasting and grilling (but not barbecued or fried yet). Avoid bits which are burned or too brown. Let your patient eat the meat with cooked vegetables and sauerkraut (or other fermented vegetables).
- Start adding cold-pressed olive oil to the meals, starting with a few drops per meal and gradually increasing the amount to 1–2 tablespoons per meal.
- Introduce freshly pressed juices, starting with a few spoonfuls of carrot juice. Make sure that the juice is clear, filter it well. Let your patient drink it as it is, diluted with warm water or mixed with

some homemade yoghurt or whey. These juices need to be consumed slowly, "chewing" every mouthful. If well tolerated gradually increase to a full cup a day. When a full cup of carrot juice is well tolerated, try to add to it juice from celery, cabbage, lettuce and fresh mint leaves. Your patient should drink the juice on an empty stomach, so first thing in the morning and the middle of afternoon are good times.

- Try to bake bread with ground almonds or any other nuts and seeds ground into flour. The recipe (please look in the recipe section) requires only four ingredients: 1) nut flour; 2) eggs; 3) piece of fresh winter squash, marrow or courgette (peeled, deseeded and finely sliced or grated); 4) some natural fat (ghee, butter, coconut oil, goose or duck fat) and some salt to taste. Your patient should start with a small piece of bread per day and gradually increase the amount.

Fifth stage:

- If all the previous foods are well tolerated, try to add cooked apple as an apple puree: peel and core ripe cooking apples and stew them with a bit of water until soft. When cooked add a generous amount of ghee to it and mash with a potato masher. If ghee has not been introduced yet, add any animal fat (duck, pork, beef, lamb or goose). If the apples are too sour, add a little honey to taste. Start with a few spoonfuls a day. Watch for any reaction. If there is none, gradually increase the amount.
- Add raw vegetables starting with softer parts of lettuce and peeled cucumber. Again start from a small amount and gradually increase if well tolerated. After those two vegetables are well tolerated, gradually add other raw vegetables: carrot, tomato (if there is no reaction to nightshades), onion, cabbage, etc. Make sure that your patient chews raw vegetables well and watch his or her stool: if diarrhoea returns then he or she is not ready for this step.
- If the juice made from carrot, celery, cabbage, lettuce and mint is well tolerated, start adding fruit to it: apple, pineapple and mango. Avoid citrus fruit at this stage.

Sixth stage:

- If all the introduced foods are well tolerated, try some peeled raw apple. Make sure the apple is ripe. Gradually introduce raw fruit and more honey.
- Gradually introduce baked cakes and other sweet things allowed on the diet. Use dried fruit as a sweetener in the baking.

Your patient may be able to move through the Introduction Diet faster or slower depending on his or her individual symptoms: some people complete the whole Introduction Diet in a few weeks, for others it may take a year slowly moving through the stages. Most indicative are abdominal pain and the stool changes: let the pain and diarrhoea start clearing before moving to the next stage. You may have to introduce some foods later than in this programme depending on your patient's personal sensitivities. Make sure that you carry on with the soups and meat stock at least once a day after your patient completes the Introduction Diet.

As we remove fibre from the diet some people go through a stage of being constipated. Using regular enemas or colonic irrigation will not only manage this situation, but allow your patient's body to detoxify sooner through removing old stale matter from the bowel. Please, look at the chapter on constipation.

After the Introduction Diet is completed and when your patient's main digestive problems are gone, move into the Full GAPS Diet.

Part 2: The Full GAPS Diet

Having completed the GAPS Introduction Diet, you will be quite experienced in the whole concept of GAPS cooking and eating. You will also have become an expert on how your patient's body responds to food in its own individual way. This is a unique and very valuable knowledge, which can serve your patient well for the rest of his or her life. That is why it is a very good idea to keep a diary through the Introduction Diet and further, where you record the whole process of food introduction and your patient's individual symptoms and reactions.

The Full GAPS Diet needs to be followed for about two years. Some people with milder conditions can start introducing non-allowed foods in about a year, others have to adhere to the diet strictly for many years.

A typical menu

Start the day with a glass of still mineral or filtered water with a slice of lemon or a teaspoon of apple cider vinegar. It can be warm or cold to personal preference. If you have a juicer your patient can start the day with a glass of freshly pressed fruit/vegetable juice.

A good juice to start the day is 40% apple + 55% carrot + 5% beetroot (all raw of course). You can make all sorts of juice mixes, but generally try to have 50% of therapeutic ingredients: carrot, small amount of beetroot (no more than 5% of the juice mixture), celery, cabbage, lettuce, greens (spinach, parsley, dill, basil, fresh nettle leaves, beet tops, carrot tops), white and red cabbage, and 50% of some tasty ingredients to disguise the taste of therapeutic ingredients: pineapple, apple, orange, grapefruit, grapes, mango, etc. Your patient can have these juices straight or diluted with water.

Every day our bodies go through a 24-hour cycle of activity and rest, feeding and cleaning up (detoxifying). From about 4 a.m. till about 10 a.m. the body is in the cleaning up or detoxification mode. Eating fresh fruit, drinking water and freshly pressed juices and having probiotic foods will assist in this process. Loading the body with food at that time interferes with the detoxification. That is why many of us do not feel hungry first thing in the morning. It is better to have breakfast around 10am when your body has completed the detox stage and is ready for feeding. At that stage we usually start feeling hungry. Children may be ready for their breakfast earlier than adults.

Breakfast choices

* Eggs cooked to personal liking and served with sausages and vegetables, some cooked, some fresh as a salad (tomato, cucumber, onions, celery, any fresh salad greens, etc.) and/or avocado and/or meat. The yolks are best uncooked and the whites cooked. Use

plenty of cold-pressed olive oil as a dressing on the salad and eggs. Mix a tablespoon of pre-soaked or sprouted sunflower and/or sesame and/or pumpkin seeds with the salad. Sausages (full fat) should be made of pure minced meat with only salt and pepper added (you can also add chopped onion, garlic or fresh herbs). Make sure that there is no commercial seasoning or MSG (Monosodium Glutamate) in the sausages. I recommend finding a local butcher who would make pure meat sausages for you to order. If diarrhoea is present then the vegetables should be well cooked and the person should not have seeds at this stage. Serve a cup of warm homemade meat stock as a drink.

- Avocado with meat, fish or shellfish, vegetables raw and cooked, lemon and cold-pressed olive oil. Serve a cup of warm meat stock as a drink with food.
- Homemade soup with sour cream and meat.
- Pancakes made with ground nuts. These pancakes are delicious with some butter and honey, or as a savoury snack. If you blend some fresh or defrosted berries with honey, it will make a delicious jam to have with pancakes. Weak tea with lemon, ginger tea or mint tea.
- Any of the home baked goods: muffins, fruit cake or bread.

Lunch

Homemade soup or stew with sour cream and meat/fish.

Avocado with meat, fish, shellfish and raw or cooked vegetables. Use olive oil with some lemon squeezed over it as a dressing. Serve a cup of warm homemade meat stock as a drink.

Any meat/fish dish made with vegetables and probiotic foods.

Dinner

One of the dishes from the lunch or breakfast choice.

For snacks between meals your patient can have fruit, nuts and home-baked products. If your patient wants something before bed serve a cup of homemade yoghurt, kefir or sour cream with a bit of honey or Russian custard (please see the recipe section).

Part 3: Coming off the GAPS diet

The strict GAPS diet should be adhered to for at least 1½–2 years. Depending on the severity of the condition, some people recover more quickly while others take much longer. Your patient needs to have at least 6 months of normal digestion before you start introducing foods not allowed on the GAPS diet. Do not rush with this step.

The first foods you will be able to introduce are new potatoes and fermented gluten-free grains (buckwheat, millet and quinoa). The recipe section will explain how to ferment grains. Don't forget that potato is a nightshade plant, so if your patient is sensitive to this group of foods, then you need to try introducing tomato, aubergine (eggplant) and peppers first before trying potato.

Introduce one food at a time and always start with a small amount: give your patient a small portion of the new food and watch for any reaction for 2–3 days. If there are no digestive problems returning, or any other typical-for-your-patient symptoms, then in a few days try another portion. If there are no reactions, gradually increase the amount of the food. These are starchy foods, so do not forget to serve them with good amounts of fat (butter, ghee, olive oil, any animal fat, coconut oil, etc.) to slow down the digestion of starch. Do not rush with the introduction of these new foods, it may take several months to do it properly.

Once new potatoes and fermented grains are introduced, try to make sourdough with good quality wheat or rye flour. You can make pancakes or bread with the sourdough. I would recommend a wonderful book by Sally Fallon *Nourishing Traditions* for a wealth of recipes. Once sourdough is well tolerated you may be able to buy commercially available good quality sourdough breads.

At that stage you may find that your patient can digest buckwheat, millet and quinoa without fermenting them prior to cooking. Gradually you will find that you can introduce various starchy vegetables, grains and beans.

YOUR PATIENT WILL NEVER BE ABLE TO GO BACK TO THE TYPICAL MODERN DIET FULL OF SUGAR, ARTIFICIAL AND PROCESSED INGREDIENTS AND OTHER HARMFUL "FOODS". USE THE YEARS OF

FOLLOWING GAPS NUTRITIONAL PROTOCOL FOR DEVELOPING HEALTHY EATING HABITS FOR LIFE !

In conclusion: at first glance the GAPS diet appears to be very hard work. However, it is a very wholesome and healthy diet and will allow your patient to heal and seal the gut lining and lay a strong foundation for good health for life. It means that the majority of GAPS people do not have to adhere to a special diet for the rest of their lives: once the digestive system starts functioning normally, they can gradually introduce most wholesome foods commonly eaten around the world. Some people achieve this target in two years, some take longer – it depends on the severity of the condition and the age of the person: children generally recover more quickly than adults.

Once introduced, the GAPS diet is no more difficult than any normal cooking and feeding the family. And shopping is very simple: just buy everything fresh and unprocessed.

A few words about vegetarianism

I had a few families where parents were dedicated vegetarians and wanted their children to be vegetarians as well. These cases are the most difficult to treat because after eliminating all grains, sugar and starchy vegetables from the diet there is not much left to eat. What these parents need to know is some statistics:

1.   Vegetarian children are more prone to health problems than children who eat meat, particularly to psychomotor impairment and diseases of the blood.
2.   Vegetarians are prone to muscle loss and bone damage. They, on average, have lower muscle strength.
3.   According to census data vegetarians die younger than people who eat meat.

From my clinical observations I have yet to meet a healthy vegetarian. In the process of evolution we humans have evolved to be omnivores, eating everything we can find in the environment: plants, eggs and meats. Our physiology is designed to work on these foods. To be healthy and full of energy we require a substantial amount of protein every day. GAPS people are particularly in need of high-quality proteins from meats, fish and eggs because their digestive systems are not in a fit state to handle hard-to-digest proteins from plants. Imposing vegetarianism on your GAPS child will undermine his or her chance of recovery.

Vegetarians have every right to follow their beliefs and to make decisions about their personal eating habits. But I strongly advise not imposing these beliefs on your GAPS child! Get your child healthy and well first through using GAPS Nutritional Protocol! Then allow your child grow and be mature enough to make his/her own decision whether to be a vegetarian or an omnivore. After all our children have a right to choose for themselves!

The decision to become a vegetarian has to be taken very seriously. One must study nutritional values of foods, learn to cook properly and plan meals carefully in order to obtain all the necessary nutrition from vegetarian foods. Unfortunately, in many cases this does not happen. For example, I see case after case of anorexia nervosa in teenage girls developing after a period of irresponsible vegetarianism.

This story of an18-year-old girl Sara (the name has been changed) would represent a typical example.

When Sara was 10 she decided to become a vegetarian because she felt sorry for animals. As typically happens in this sort of situation, Sara's vegetarianism translated into living largely on pasta and cheese, bread and cakes, chocolate bars and vegetarian sandwiches. After 1–2 years of her vegetarianism she developed digestive problems and became very susceptible to any cold or virus going around. She had developed a typical picture of IBS (Irritable Bowel Syndrome) with bloating, constipation and abdominal pain. A chain of chest infections were treated by numerous courses of antibiotics. At the age of 15 she was diagnosed with anorexia nervosa. After one year of hospital treatment her anorexia flipped into bulimia. Sara became depressed and had very low levels of energy. She found it difficult to study, work or participate in any social activity. She developed suicidal thoughts and a desire to hurt herself. After a few suicidal attempts she ended up being sectioned in a psychiatric hospital under the control of neuroleptic drugs.

If your child (teenaged or younger) suddenly decides to become a vegetarian, this has to be taken extremely seriously. Misguided vegetarianism is rapidly becoming a major cause of mental illness in our young people. What these young people do not know is that plant foods are generally hard to digest and they are low in useful nutrition. Foods from animal origin are easy for the human gut to digest and assimilate and animal foods provide concentrated amounts of all essential nutrients for human physiology. As plant foods are hard to digest and as they contain a list of anti-nutrients, which can damage the gut, digestive problems are the first symptoms which appear in those beginner vegetarians. They usually develop IBS symptoms, such as bloating, indigestion, constipation, diarrhoea and flatulence. If the person already has a weak digestion, moving to a plant-based diet is positively dangerous. As the digestive system becomes more and more damaged, it is less able to nourish the person, and so nutritional deficiencies develop quite soon. Vitamins B12, B6, B1, B2, niacin, essential amino acids, zinc and proteins are the first nutritional deficiencies a beginner vegetarian usually develops. As malnutrition sets in, the immune system cannot function well, leading to endless infections and courses of antibiotics. Every course of antibiotics damages the gut and the immune system even further.

Apart from causing malnutrition though the damage to the digestive system, plant foods are a very poor source of nutrients to start with. But what about all those tables published in popular nutrition books, which show that plants are full of nourishment, you would ask? All those B vitamins, proteins and carotenoids? Yes, when we analyse different plant foods in a laboratory, they show good amounts of various nutrients. This information is then published in common nutritional literature, luring vegetarians into a false sense of security. Unfortunately, these tables of the nutrient content of plants are deceptive. Why? Because, in a laboratory we can use all sorts of methods and chemicals for extracting nutrients from plants: methods which our human digestive system does not possess. Human gut has a very limited ability to digest plants and to extract anything useful from them. Nature has created herbivorous animals (ruminants) to eat plants and in order for them to be able to digest these plants, Nature has equipped them with a very special digestive system: it is very long with several stomachs full of special plant-breaking bacteria. The human digestive system is similar to the gut of predatory animals, such as wolves and lions: our digestive system is fairly short and we have only one stomach with virtually no bacteria in it. In fact our human stomach is designed to produce acid and pepsin, which are only able to break down meat, fish and eggs. In short, our digestive systems have been designed to cope best with animal foods. People knew this fact for millennia. They knew that the best foods for them come from animals; they would only eat plants as a supplement to meat or when animal foods were in short supply. People knew that plant foods are hard for humans to digest, that is why all traditional cultures have developed methods of food preparation to extract more nutrition from plants and to make them more digestible, such as fermentation, malting, sprouting and special ways of cooking. Unfortunately, in our modern world these methods are largely forgotten.

Of course, your youngster is not going to be familiar with this information when he or she decides to become a vegetarian. We live in a world full of misinformation about food. Vegetarian diets have been touted as "healthy" and "planet saving" and "kind to animals" for decades. Every one of these statements is not only wrong, but downright deceptive. Do not allow your child to become a vegetarian until he or she has thoroughly studied the subject and can provide you with all the information to justify such a fundamental life-changing decision. An excellent book to read on this subject is *The Vegetarian Myth* by Lierre Keith.

Recommended foods

Almonds, including almond butter and oil
Apples
Apricots, fresh or dried
Artichoke, French
Asiago cheese
Asparagus
Aubergine (eggplant)
Avocados, including avocado oil
Bananas (ripe only with brown spots on the skin)

Beans, dried white (navy) or haricot, string beans and lima beans, properly prepared

Beef, fresh or frozen

Beetroot (beets)

Berries, all kinds

Black, white and red pepper: ground and peppercorns

Black radish

Blue cheese

Bok choy

Brazil nuts

Brick cheese

Brie cheese

Broccoli

Brussels sprouts

Butter

Cabbage

Camembert cheese

Canned fish in oil or water only

Capers

Carrots

Cashew nuts, fresh only

Cauliflower

Cayenne pepper

Celeriac

Celery

Cellulose in supplements

Cheddar cheese

Cherimoya (custard apple or sharifa)

Cherries

Chicken, fresh or frozen

Cinnamon

Citric acid

Coconut, fresh or dried (shredded) without any additives

Coconut milk

Coconut oil

Coffee, weak and freshly made, not instant

Collard greens

Colby cheese
Courgette (zucchini)
Coriander, fresh or dried
Cucumber
Dates, fresh or dried without any additives (not soaked in syrup)
Dill, fresh or dried
Duck, fresh or frozen
Edam cheese
Eggplant (aubergine)
Eggs, fresh
Filberts
Fish, fresh or frozen, canned in its juice or oil
Game, fresh or frozen
Garlic
Ghee, homemade
Gin, occasionally
Ginger root, fresh
Goose, fresh or frozen
Gorgonzola cheese
Gouda cheese
Grapefruit
Grapes
Haricot beans, properly prepared
Havarti cheese
Hazelnuts
Herbal teas
Herbs, fresh or dried without additives
Honey, natural
Juices freshly pressed from permitted fruit and vegetables
Kale
Kiwi fruit
Kumquats
Lamb, fresh or frozen
Lemons
Lentils
Lettuce, all kinds
Lima beans (dried and fresh)

Limburger cheese
Limes
Mangoes
Meats, fresh or frozen
Melons
Monterey (Jack) cheese
Muenster cheese
Mushrooms
Mustard seeds, pure powder and gourmet types without any non-allowed ingredients
Nectarines
Nut flour or ground nuts (usually ground blanched almonds)
Nutmeg
Nuts, all kinds freshly shelled, not roasted, salted or coated
Olive oil, virgin cold-pressed
Olives preserved without sugar or any other non-allowed ingredients
Onions
Oranges
Papayas
Parmesan cheese
Parsley
Peaches
Peanut butter, without additives
Peanuts, fresh or roasted in their shells
Pears
Peas, dried split and fresh green
Pecans
Peppers (green, yellow, red and orange)
Pheasant, fresh or frozen
Pickles, without sugar or any other non-allowed ingredients
Pigeon, fresh or frozen
Pineapples, fresh
Pork, fresh or frozen
Port du Salut cheese
Poultry, fresh or frozen
Prunes, dried without any additives or in their own juice
Pumpkin

Quail, fresh or frozen
Raisins
Rhubarb
Roquefort cheese
Romano cheese
Satsumas
Scotch, occasionally
Seaweed fresh and dried, once the Introduction Diet has been
completed
Shellfish, fresh or frozen
Spices, single and pure without any additives
Spinach
Squash (summer and winter)
Stilton cheese
String beans
Swedes
Swiss cheese
Tangerines
Tea, weak, freshly made, not instant
Tomato puree, pure without any additives apart from salt
Tomato juice, without any additives apart from salt
Tomatoes
Turkey, fresh or frozen
Turnips
Ugly fruit
Uncreamed cottage cheese (dry curd)
Vinegar (cider or white); make sure there is no allergy
Vodka, very occasionally
Walnuts
Watercress
White navy beans, properly prepared
Wine dry: red or white
Yoghurt, homemade
Zucchini (courgette)

Foods to avoid

Acesulphame
Acidophilus milk
Agar-agar
Agave syrup
Algae
Aloe vera, once digestive symptoms are gone, you can introduce it
Amaranth
Apple juice
Arrowroot
Aspartame
Astragalus
Baked beans
Baker's yeast
Baking powder and raising agents of all kind apart from pure bi-carbonate of soda
Balsamic vinegar
Barley
Bean flour and sprouts
Bee pollen
Beer
Bhindi or okra
Bitter gourd
Black-eye beans
Bologna
Bouillon cubes or granules
Brandy
Buckwheat
Bulgur
Burdock root
Butter beans
Buttermilk
Canellini beans
Canned vegetables and fruit
Carob
Carrageenan

Cellulose gum
Cereals, including all breakfast cereals
Cheeses, processed and cheese spreads
Chestnuts and chestnut flour
Chevre cheese
Chewing gum
Chickpeas
Chickory root
Chocolate
Cocoa powder
Coffee, instant and coffee substitutes
Cooking oils
Cordials
Corn
Cornstarch
Corn syrup
Cottage cheese
Cottonseed
Couscous
Cream
Cream of tartar
Cream cheese
Dextrose
Drinks, soft
Faba beans
Feta cheese
Fish, preserved, smoked, salted, breaded and canned with sauces
Flour, made out of grains
FOS (fructooligosaccharides)
Fructose
Fruit, canned or preserved
Garbanzo beans
Gjetost cheese
Grains, all
Gruyere cheese
Ham
Hot dogs

Ice cream, commercial
Jams
Jellies
Jerusalem artichoke
Ketchup, commercially available
Lactose
Liqueurs
Margarines and butter replacements
Meats, processed, preserved, smoked and salted
Millet
Milk from any animal, soy, rice, canned coconut milk
Milk, dried
Molasses
Mozzarella cheese
Mungbeans
Neufchatel cheese
Nutra-sweet (aspartame)
Nuts, salted, roasted and coated
Oats
Okra
Parsnips
Pasta, of any kind
Pectin
Postum
Potato, white
Potato, sweet
Primost cheese
Quinoa
Rice
Ricotta cheese
Rye
Saccharin
Sago
Sausages, commercially available
Semolina
Sherry
Soda soft drinks

Sour cream, commercial
Soy
Spelt
Starch
Sugar or sucrose of any kind
Tapioca
Tea, instant
Triticale
Turkey loaf
Vegetables, canned or preserved
Wheat
Wheat germ
Whey, powder or liquid
Yams
Yoghurt, commercial

3. Recipes

You can find many more recipes in Elaine Gottschall's book *Breaking the vicious cycle* and on the following websites on the Internet:

www.gaps.me
www.scdiet.org

www.breakingtheviciouscycle.com
www.geocities.com
www.pecanbread.com
www.uclbs.org

1. Condiments

Most fresh salads can be dressed with olive oil and fresh lemon juice. When homemade yoghurt is well tolerated it can also be used as a salad dressing.

Ketchup

2 cups tomato juice
1–3 tablespoons white vinegar
honey to taste
bay leaf (optional)
salt and pepper to taste

Mix all the ingredients except the honey and simmer on the stove until thick, stirring often to prevent sticking. When almost the desired thickness, add honey to taste and complete cooking. Ladle into sterilised jars and seal immediately or place in small containers and freeze. (Recipe courtesy of Elaine Gottschall)

Guacamole

2 ripe avocados
juice of 1 orange
1 clove of crushed garlic
small amount of water

In the food processor blend together all the ingredients. Reduce the amount of garlic, if the guacamole is too hot. Use as a dip for vegetables and a spread for homemade bread.

Mayonnaise

1 whole egg
1 cup olive oil or slightly more
1 tablespoon white vinegar or fresh lemon juice
¼ teaspoon dry mustard powder
salt and pepper to taste
a little honey to taste

Blend in your food processor for a few seconds: egg, lemon juice (or vinegar), mustard, salt, pepper and honey. While the machine is running, add the oil in a fine stream. Do not add oil quickly; it should take at least 60 seconds. As mayonnaise thickens, the sound of the machine will deepen.

Suggestions:

Use to thicken gravy: add 2 tablespoons of mayonnaise to about 1 cup of meat stock and heat gently for about 1–2 minutes, stirring constantly.

Use as a base for tartar sauce by adding ½ cup chopped dill pickles (unsweetened) and ¼ cup of chopped onion.

Use as mock Hollandaise sauce by adding grated cheddar cheese (if well tolerated). Spread over vegetables such as cooked cauliflower or broccoli. Cover and heat in oven.

Mix with homemade yoghurt (1 part mayonnaise, 1 part yoghurt) and use as salad dressing.

(Recipe courtesy of Elaine Gottschall)

Salsa

4 medium-size tomatoes
half a pepper (green, red, orange or yellow)
1 medium onion (white or red)
1–3 cloves of garlic
dill and parsley
olive oil
salt and pepper to taste

Put all ingredients into the food processor and chop coarsely. Can be served with meats and vegetables. You can also use it for cooking meats. To do that bring salsa to simmer, add diced meat (beef, pork, lamb or chicken) and generous amount of butter (or any animal fat), cover and simmer for 30 minutes.

Aubergine dip

2 aubergines (eggplants)
salt
3 medium-size tomatoes
3–4 cloves of garlic
$^1/_3$ cup olive oil
fresh dill or parsley

Cut the aubergines into 1 cm-thick slices, rub well with salt and any animal fat. Place on a baking tray and bake at 150∞C for 30–40 minutes or until soft. Cool down.

In the food processor blend together the baked aubergines, tomatoes, garlic, herbs and olive oil. Serve with meats and fish and as a dip with vegetables.

Fruit chutney

1 kg of cooking apples
$^1/_2$ kg of plums
1kg of dried dates without stones (or/and dried figs)
3 peppers (green, red or yellow)
3–4 medium-size onions
2 cups apple cider vinegar
1 teaspoon black/green/red peppercorns, crushed
1–2 teaspoons of aromatic seeds: cumin, coriander, dill, fennel, etc.
$^1/_2$ teaspoon cayenne pepper or chilli pepper powder
1 teaspoon of natural salt

In a large pan slowly bring to the boil the dates with $^1/_2$ cup of water. When soft, mash the dates with a potato masher or a soup blender.

Then add apples, cored and cut into large pieces, plums without stones, peppers and onions finely chopped, vinegar and the rest of the ingredients. Mix well and put on a very low heat. Cook for 1–1½ hours mixing occasionally or in a slow cooker for a few hours. As apples and plums get well cooked, they will fall apart and mix into a rough paste with the rest of the ingredients. While the chutney is cooking, sterilise glass jars and their lids (metal or glass) by placing them in the cold oven and heating it up to about 120∞C (250∞F) for 30–40 minutes. Do not put the lids on the jars while sterilising, keep them separate.

Ladle hot chutney into the jars and close the lids. When cooled down, place the jars with the chutney into a refrigerator. Keep refrigerated and serve with meats and fish.

Basic liver pate

100g liver
1 large onion, finely chopped
3 cloves of garlic, finely chopped

Fry the liver, onion and garlic in ghee (butter, any animal fat) until well cooked through. Blend in a food processor with mayonnaise or sour cream.

To make variations you can add one of the following when blending:

- 1 raw tomato
- 4–5 cooked prunes (unsweetened and without stones)
- raw garlic
- greens (dill, parsley, basil)
- raw onion
- peeled, cored and grated apple

2. Salads

Salads should be served when diarrhoea is no longer present.

To increase the nutritional value of your salads it is good to sprinkle coarsely chopped walnuts or seeds on top. Seeds: sunflower seeds, pumpkin and sesame should be soaked in water overnight. It makes them more nourishing and easier to digest.

Beetroot salad

8 small beetroots
$^1/_3$ cup of shelled walnuts
2 cloves of garlic
8 dried prunes without stones
mayonnaise
$^1/_3$ teaspoon of salt

Wash the beetroots and cut all tops and ends off. Cook the beetroot by steaming until a knife goes through easily. Alternatively you can buy already cooked beetroots (in water, not in vinegar!). Grate the beetroot through a coarse grater. In the food processor chop together the walnuts, garlic and prunes. Mix well with the grated beetroot. Add salt, mayonnaise and mix. Enjoy with meats and vegetables.

Tuna salad

200g canned tuna in its own juice or water
1 large onion
2 large carrots
2 hard-boiled eggs
mayonnaise

Drain the tuna and mash with a fork. Chop the onion finely. Cook the carrots. Peel and chop the hard-boiled eggs.

On a flat dish put a layer of tuna (use half the tuna) and top it up with half of the chopped onion. Cover with mayonnaise. Grate one carrot on top and cover with mayonnaise. Make a layer of one chopped hard-boiled egg and cover with mayonnaise. Repeat with the same layers of tuna, onion, carrot and egg. Decorate on the top with some dill or parsley. Make sure that every layer is well covered with mayonnaise.

Salad with cabbage and apple

100g of white cabbage
1 large apple
$1/2$ cup of homemade yoghurt or crème fraiche
1 teaspoon of honey
a pinch of salt
2 tablespoons of raisins

Grate the cabbage. Peel, core and grate the apple. Slightly fry the raisins in butter to make them soft. Mix honey and salt with yoghurt. Mix all ingredients together.

Salad with tomatoes and cucumber

2 tomatoes
$1/3$ of a long cucumber
1 stick of celery
spring onion
dill or parsley
salt

Cut cucumber into $1/2$ cm thick slices. Cut tomato into bite-size pieces and slice the celery into small pieces. Sprinkle with salt. Chop the spring onions, dill and parsley. Mix all ingredients and dress with cold-pressed olive oil.

Russian salad

$1/2$ long cucumber
1 large carrot, cooked (steamed)
100g cooked meat or sausages (leftovers are good)
1 onion
2 hard-boiled eggs
2 tablespoons of sauerkraut (optional)
fresh dill and/or parsley
$1/3$ teaspoon salt

mayonnaise
yoghurt or crème fraiche

Cut cucumber and carrot into small cubes. Cut the meat and/or sausages into small cubes. Finely chop the onion. Peel and cut the eggs into small cubes. Finely chop dill and parsley. In a separate pot mix mayonnaise and yoghurt in equal proportions and add salt. Mix all ingredients together.

Carrot salad

1 large carrot
1 tablespoon of raisins
1 tablespoon of coarsely chopped walnuts
yoghurt

Slightly fry the raisins in butter to make them soft. Finely grate the carrot. Mix the carrot, raisins, walnuts and yoghurt.

3. Soups

I strongly recommend making your soups based on a homemade meat stock. Meat stock aids digestion and has been known for centuries as a healing folk remedy for the digestive tract. Also homemade meat stock is extremely nourishing; it is full of minerals, vitamins, amino-acids and various other nutrients in a very bio-available form. Do not use commercially available soup stock granules or bouillon cubes, as they are highly processed and are full of detrimental ingredients.

Once you have made your meat stock, it can be frozen or it will keep well in a refrigerator for at least a week. You can make soups, gravies and stews with this meat stock or warm up a cup of it to give your GAPS patient as a drink with meals or between meals. If you make sure that you always have some meat stock in your fridge, you will find that it is very easy and quick to make nourishing meals for your GAPS child or adult and the rest of the family. Do not take fat out of the stock; it is important for your GAPS patient to consume the fat together with the stock.

You need meat and bones to make a good meat stock. Beef, lamb, pork, game, poultry and fish are all highly suitable and will make stocks with different flavours and different nutritional compositions. So, make sure that you alternate between different meats to provide a whole spectrum of nourishment. Bones and joints are particularly important as they enrich the stock with the kind of nourishing substances which meat alone cannot provide. In fact it can be very inexpensive to make a good quality meat stock as you use the parts of the animal which butchers usually give away almost free. The meat and bones can be fresh or frozen and there is no need to defrost them prior to cooking. Apart from bones and meat all you need is a large pot full of water and a bit of salt and pepper.

How to make a meat stock

Lamb, pork, beef or game
Put the joints, bones and meat into a large pot, add 5–10 peppercorns, add salt to taste and fill it up with water. Heat up to a boiling point. Cover the pan, reduce the heat to a minimum and simmer for 3 hours at least. The longer you cook the meat and bones, the more they will "give out" to the stock and the more nourishing the stock will be. Take the bones and meat out and pour the stock through a sieve into a separate pan to remove any small bones and peppercorns.

Chicken stock
Put a whole or half a chicken into a large pot, fill it up with water, add salt and heat it up to the boiling point. Simmer for 1½–2 hours. Take the chicken out and put the stock through a sieve. Keep in the refrigerator. The chicken, cooked this way, is delicious and can be served for dinner with vegetables and a hot cup of your freshly made chicken stock.

Fish stock
To make a good fish stock you need bones, fins, skins and heads of the fish, not the meat. So buy your fish whole, cut the meat off to cook as a separate meal and use the rest of the fish to make your fish stock. Your fishmonger can do all the trimming for you. Put the heads,

bones, fins and skin of the fish into a large pan, add 8–10 peppercorns and fill the pan with water. Bring up to the boil, reduce the heat to a minimum and simmer for 1–1½ hours. Add salt to taste at the end of cooking. Take the fish out and sieve the stock. Take the meat off the fish skeleton to use for soup making.

The basic soup recipe

To make a soup bring some of your homemade meat stock to the boil, add chopped or sliced vegetables and simmer for another 20–25 minutes. You can choose any combination of available vegetables: onion, cabbage, carrot, broccoli, cauliflower, pumpkin, courgettes, marrow, squash, leeks, etc. If you are planning to blend your soup, then you can cut vegetables roughly into any size pieces. If you prefer to have your soup without blending, then make sure that you cut or dice your vegetables into nice small pieces before cooking. If your meat stock was made with lamb, pork or beef you can add a handful of dried French or Italian mushrooms for a wonderful flavour. It is customary to crush the dried mushrooms by hand before adding to the soup. At the end of cooking add 1–2 tablespoons of chopped garlic, bring to the boil and turn the heat off. Blend with a soup blender until smooth unless you planned to have it without blending.

You can serve your soup with any combination of the following:

- some chopped parsley, coriander or dill
- hard-boiled egg cut into pieces
- a spoonful of your homemade yoghurt or crème fraiche (sour cream)
- cooked meat cut into small pieces
- red onion cut into very small pieces
- spring onion cut into small pieces
- a spoon of cooked and ground liver

From this basic recipe you can improvise and develop your own recipes. Here I will just provide a few ideas.

A spring nettle soup

$1^1/_2$ l of homemade meat stock
large bunch of spring nettles
2 tablespoons of dried French or Italian mushrooms
1 medium onion
1 medium carrot
2 courgettes or $^1/_2$ of a marrow or squash
4 eggs, hard boiled

Young shoots of stinging nettles appearing in spring are full of wonderful nourishment. They are high in iron, magnesium, copper, zinc, vitamin C, carotenoids and other useful substances. For this recipe collect a large bunch of spring nettles. You will have to wear gloves and a long-sleeved shirt to do this. Rinse the nettles and shake the excess water off. Using scissors cut the leaves and tender shoots of the nettles into small pieces, discarding the hard stems. Reserve for the recipe.

Cut the marrow, squash or courgettes into small cubes, thinly slice the carrot and chop the onion. Bring the homemade meat stock to a boil. Add all the vegetables and the French or Italian dried mushrooms, crumbling them with your hands before adding to the meat stock. Simmer under a tight lid for 15–20 minutes. Add your prepared nettles, mix and immediately take off the heat. Serve with 1–2 tablespoons of hard-boiled egg, cut into small pieces, and a spoonful of homemade yoghurt (if well tolerated).

Russian borsch

$1^1/_2$ l of homemade meat stock
1 medium onion, finely chopped
1 medium carrot, finely sliced
$^1/_2$ of a medium-size white cabbage, finely sliced
2 medium-size beetroots, or 4 small beetroots, raw or cooked
3 cloves of garlic
1 finely chopped tomato

If the beetroot is cooked (in water, not in vinegar):
Bring the meat stock to the boil and add the onion, carrot and cabbage. Cover and simmer for 20 minutes. In the meantime slice the cooked beetroots into long thin strips. Add into the soup, mix well and simmer for another 5 minutes. Take off the heat. Crush the 3 cloves of garlic and add to the soup together with the chopped tomato. Serve with a large spoon of crème fraiche (sour cream) or homemade yoghurt (if well tolerated) and some chopped parsley and/or a thick slice of hard-boiled egg.

If the beetroot is raw:
Wash and peel the beetroot. Slice into long thin strips by hand or using your food processor. Bring the meat stock to the boil and add the beetroot. Simmer for 10–15 minutes, then add the rest of the vegetables (onion, carrot and cabbage). Simmer for a further 20 minutes or until the cabbage is cooked. Take off the heat. Crush the 3 cloves of garlic and add to the soup together with the chopped tomato. Serve with a large spoon of crème fraiche or homemade yoghurt (if well tolerated), some chopped parsley and/or a thick slice of hard-boiled egg.

Fish soup

1 l of homemade fish stock
1 large onion, finely chopped
1 carrot, thinly sliced
1 courgette or an equivalent amount of marrow or squash, cut into small cubes

Bring the fish stock to the boil and add the onion, carrot and squash, marrow or courgette. Simmer under a lid for 10–15 minutes and take off the heat. Add the cooked fish meat which you took off the bones when you made the fish stock. Serve with a spoonful of homemade yoghurt (if well tolerated) and/or with a hard-boiled egg (sliced or chopped).

If there is no meat left on the bones you can use the meat (skinless and boneless) of any available fish. Cut the meat into small cubes and add into the boiling soup in the last 5–8 minutes of cooking.

Meatball soup

400 g of minced meat (mixture of pork and beef is best)
1 large onion, finely chopped
1 large carrot, thinly sliced
1 cup winter squash or courgette, cut into small cubes
1 cup of cabbage, finely chopped (optional)
2 tablespoons of chopped garlic
salt and cayenne pepper to taste
2–3 tablespoons of homemade sauerkraut

In a pan bring 2 litres of water or meat stock up to the boil. Add salt and cayenne pepper to taste. With your hands shape meatballs about 2 cm in diameter and add them, one at a time, into the boiling water. Cover and simmer on low heat for 30 minutes. Add all the vegetables apart from garlic, cover and simmer for another 20 minutes. Add the garlic and switch the heat off. Let it sit for 5–10 minutes then add 2–3 tablespoons of sauerkraut. Serve with a spoonful of homemade yoghurt and finely chopped dill.

The beautiful winter squash soup

1½ l of homemade meat stock (turkey or chicken stock work best for this recipe)
1 leek, washed and sliced
broccoli, 3–4 medium-sized rosettes
1 medium-size carrot, sliced
½ of a medium-size buttercup squash or a 1/3 of a butternut squash or any winter squash with sweet orange flesh
3 garlic cloves, peeled

Peel and deseed the squash and cut it into chunks. Wash and cut into pieces all the vegetables. Put them into your soup pan, add the meat stock and bring to the boil. Reduce the heat to a minimum, cover with the lid and simmer for about 30 minutes. Blend with a soup blender. If your family is at the stage of tolerating homemade goat's yoghurt, then add ½ cup into the soup. Serve warm. It is particularly soothing if the child has a tummy ache or diarrhoea.

Meat jelly

2–4 pig trotters (pig's feet) or a pig's head
1 large carrot
garlic
salt and black peppercorns

Put pig trotters (or pig's head) into a large pan, fill it up with water, add salt and a teaspoon of black peppercorns. Bring up to the boil, reduce heat to a minimum, cover with a lid and let it simmer for 3 hours.

In the meantime cook a large carrot by steaming, cool it down and cut into thin slices. You can cut it into decorative slices if you have the tools for doing that.

When the cooking is complete take the pig trotters (or pig's head) out and pour the stock through a sieve into a separate pan. Let the trotters or head cool down completely. Take all the meat off (including the skin and other soft tissues) completely stripping the bones. Cut the meat into small pieces.

Lay the pieces of meat, the carrot pieces and thin slices of garlic in a large deep tray. You can add more or less garlic to your family's taste. Pour the meat stock in to fill the tray to ³/₄. Place it in the refrigerator for the jelly to set. You can also set this jelly in different jelly shapes and dishes as individual servings.

This dish is wonderful to have on a hot summer's day. It contains a lot of nourishing substances, including gelatine, glucosamine, glyco-proteins and phospholipids, and is considered to be a folk remedy for digestive problems.

4. Fats for cooking

Cooking (roasting, frying, baking, etc.) should be done with stable natural fats, because these fats do not alter their chemical structure when heated. These fats are: pork dripping, goose fat, duck fat, natural beef lard, lamb fat, coconut oil, butter and ghee. You can purchase many of these fats in shops. It is also easy to make many of these fats at home, which has an advantage: you know exactly what is in it. I would like to repeat here that animal fats are vital for a GAPS person to have in generous amounts daily. The more animal fats your patient consumes with breakfast, lunch and dinner, the quicker will be the recovery. For more information on this subject please look in the chapter: *Fats: the Good and the Bad.*

Ghee

Ghee is a clarified butter. It is traditionally used in many cultures around the world for cooking and baking. Butter can be used for cooking very effectively. However, small amounts of whey in the butter often burn. Also whey contains lactose and some milk proteins, which many GAPS patients have to avoid in the initial stages of the diet. Ghee on the other hand does not contain any whey, milk protein or lactose at all, just milk fat, and does not burn.

Preheat your oven to around 60–120°C (140–250°F). Put a large block of organic, preferably unsalted butter into a metal dish or pan. Leave it in the oven for 45–60 minutes. Take it out and carefully pour the golden fat from the top (ghee), making sure that the white liquid at the bottom stays in the pan. Discard the white liquid. Keep in glass jars and refrigerate. With some varieties of butter the white liquid accumulates at the top. In that case put the dish in the fridge. As it cools down the ghee will become solid, and you will be able to pour the liquid off and wipe the rest of it with a paper towel.

Goose or duck fat

Roast a goose or a duck in the oven in the usual way. Take the bird out and pour the fat through cheesecloth or a fine metal sieve. Keep in glass jars and refrigerate. These fats can be used for all cooking, baking and frying; they give a nice flavour to roasted meats and vegetables in particular. Use in liberal amounts.

Pork, lamb or beef fat (lard)

You can collect these fats in much the same way as the duck and goose fats. You need any bits of fat from the animal. It is particularly good to use the internal fat layer from the animal, which the butcher often gives away almost free. You will be amazed by how much cooking fat you will collect from a fairly small piece. It is wise to use organic animals for this purpose, as fat is a natural body storage for various toxins. Investing in a small piece of organic fat once or twice a year will not cost you much and will last for many months.

Roast the fat on a fairly low heat (120–130°C, 250–260°F) for 2–3 hours depending on the size of the piece. Pour the fat through the cheesecloth or a fine metal sieve. Store in glass jars and refrigerate. Use for all cooking, baking and frying in liberal amounts.

Coconut oil is very good for cooking. It contains largely saturated fats and hence does not change its chemical structure when heated. However, make sure that you buy good quality natural coconut oil, as a lot of brands sold in the West have been hydrogenated to increase shelf life.

5. Main dishes

An Italian meat casserole

This is an alternative way of making an excellent meat stock, as well as preparing a meal for the whole family. You can use any of the following: a leg or a shoulder of lamb, a joint of pork, a joint of beef, a pheasant, 2–4 pigeons, 2 quails, a joint of venison, a whole chicken, turkey legs. You need a large casserole with a lid for this dish. Put your meat joint or a whole bird(s) into the casserole, add water to fill 2/3 of the casserole, add some salt, peppercorns, dried herbs to taste, bay leaves and a sprig of rosemary. Cover with the lid and put into the oven for 5–6 hours on low heat (140–160°C, 285–320°F). Add various vegetables 40–50 minutes before your dinner time: rosettes of broccoli and cauliflower, whole peeled small red or white onions, Brussels sprouts, pieces of swede or turnip and large pieces of carrot. When ready take the meat and vegetables out and serve to your family. Put the meat stock through a sieve and serve it in bouillon cups with the dinner. Meat stock left from this dinner will keep well in the refrigerator and can be used for making soups or warming up as a nourishing drink.

Stuffed peppers

6 large peppers (a combination of green, red, yellow and orange)
$\frac{1}{2}$ kg of full fat minced meat (a mixture of $\frac{1}{2}$ pork and $\frac{1}{2}$ beef is best)
2 medium-size carrots
1 large onion
salt and pepper

Grind the carrots and chop the onion. Mix them well together with the minced meat, adding salt and pepper to taste.

Cut off the tops of the peppers and take out the seeds. Fill the peppers with the mixture of the meat and vegetables. Place the stuffed peppers upright into a pan. You will need the correct size pan to fit all the peppers, so they stand upright and support each other. Add 3–4 cups of water to the bottom of the pan and cover it with the lid. Bring up to the boil, reduce the heat to a minimum and simmer for an hour. Serve a pepper per person with a ladle of the stock from the bottom (best to serve in a soup bowl). Put a tablespoon of your homemade yoghurt (if well tolerated) with a clove of crushed garlic mixed into it. Garnish with chopped parsley.

Meatballs

500g of full fat minced meat (a mixture of pork and beef is best)
1 large onion
$\frac{1}{2}$ red pepper
1 courgette
2 tablespoons of chopped fresh garlic
1 tablespoon tomato puree
salt, pepper, 2–3 bay leaves

To make the sauce cover the bottom of the pan with 3–4 cm of water. Mix into the water tomato puree, salt and pepper. Bring to the boil. With your hands shape balls out of the mincemeat about 4 cm in diameter. Put the balls one at a time into the boiling sauce. Make sure that you use a large enough pan to fit all the balls in one layer. Cover with the lid and simmer on low heat for 30 minutes.

In the meantime prepare the vegetables. Finely chop the onion and red pepper. Cut the courgette into small cubes. Chop the garlic.

After cooking the meatballs for 30 minutes add the chopped onion, pepper and courgette, and mix with the sauce gently in order to preserve the shape of the meatballs. Cover and cook for another 25 minutes. Add the bay leaves and garlic. Cover and turn the heat off. Let it sit for 10 minutes before serving. Sprinkle with finely chopped coriander and serve with cooked vegetables.

Meat cutlets

500g of full fat minced pork
500g of full fat minced beef or lamb
1 large onion, finely chopped
salt and pepper

Mix all the ingredients well with your hands and make oval shaped cutlets about 4–5 cm thick. Place the cutlets on a greased baking tray and bake in a preheated oven for about an hour at 160–180°C (320–355°F). Serve with cooked vegetables and a salad.

Fish cutlets

2–3 fairly large freshwater or sea fish (a mixture of different fish works very well)
1 egg
3–5 tablespoons of butter (ghee, goose fat, duck fat, pork dripping or coconut oil)
1–2 cups of shredded coconut
salt and pepper

Cut all the meat off the fish, remove skin and large bones. Use the bones, heads and skin for making a very nourishing fish stock (recipe in the *soup* section). Alternatively you can buy fish fillets already without skin and large bones.

In the food processor put the meat of the fish, one egg, butter, salt and pepper to your taste and grind it to make mince. If you have a meat mincer it will do the same job for you. With your hands make oval-shaped flat cutlets about 2 cm thick, roll them in shredded coconut and slightly fry them on both sides. Use coconut oil (or butter, ghee, pork dripping, lard, goose fat or duck fat) for frying. Place the cutlets on a large oven tray, greased with any of the mentioned fats. Add half a cup of water and put into preheated oven. Bake for 20–30 minutes at 150°C (300°F).

Swedish gravlax – the best way to eat fresh salmon

skinless and boneless salmon fillet
1 l water at room temperature
1¹/₂ tablespoons of salt
1 tablespoon of honey
fresh dill and coarsely ground black pepper

The fish has to be very fresh. Cut the fish into 0.5cm thick slices and place in a dip tray (any baking tray will do). Sprinkle with finely chopped dill and black pepper. Dissolve the salt and the honey in the water to make a brine. Cover the fish with the brine and leave at room temperature for 1–1¹/₂ hours. Pour the water out and serve the fish with some lettuce and mayonnaise.

This dish works particularly well with wild salmon. Because the fish is not cooked, all the essential fatty acids and other nutrients are preserved. Refrigerate and consume within two days.

Marinated wild salmon

6 boneless wild salmon fillets with the skin on (each fillet is the serving size for one person)
3–4 large lemons
1 heaped teaspoon of natural sea salt
1 heaped teaspoon of grainy mild mustard
¹/₂ teaspoon of dill seeds or some fresh dill, chopped
coarsely ground black pepper to taste

The fish has to be very fresh. In a glass or glazed baking tray of suitable size lay three of the salmon fillets skin down. The fillets should fill the tray completely fitted in tightly together. In a separate bowl make the marinade: cut the lemons in half and squeeze the juice and scoop the flesh out of them into the bowl. Add the rest of the ingredients and mix well. Don't worry if the lemon flesh is in chunks. Cover the layer of fish in the tray with all the marinade and lay the other three fish fillets on top flesh down (skin on the top). Press the two layers of fish together with a heavy object so the marinade covers the fish completely. For a heavy object you can use another baking tray with something heavy in it or a slab of clean stone/granite. Leave in the fridge for 24 hours to marinade. Take the fish out and peel the skin off: it comes off fairly easily. Using scissors cut the fish into bite-size pieces and serve with avocado and some lettuce, using the marinade as a dressing. This dish is delicious and easy to digest. Because the fish is not cooked, all the essential fatty acids and other nutrients are preserved.

Fermented fish – the best way to eat cold water oily fish

3–4 very fresh large herrings or mackerel
1 small white onion
1–2 tablespoons of salt per litre of the brine
1 tablespoon of peppercorns
5–7 bay leaves
1 teaspoon of coriander seeds
fresh dill or some dill seeds
1 cup of kefir whey
a suitable glass jar

Skin the fish and remove large bones, cut into bite-size pieces. Peel and slice the onion. Put the pieces of the fish into the glass jar mixing with peppercorns, slices of white onion (optional), coriander seeds, bay leaves and dill seeds or dill herb. In a separate jug dissolve 1 tablespoon of sea salt in some water and add half a cup of the kefir whey. Pour this brine into the jar until the fish is completely covered. If the fish is not covered just add more water. Close the jar tightly and leave to ferment for 3–5 days at room temperature, then store in the fridge. Serve with vegetables, fresh dill, spring onion and some mayonnaise. Consume within 1–3 weeks.

Fermented sardines

5–7 very fresh sardines
1–2 tablespoons of salt
1 tablespoon of peppercorns
5–7 bay leaves
1 teaspoon of coriander seeds
fresh dill or some dill seeds
1 cup of kefir whey
a suitable glass jar

Descale the fish, cut the heads off and clean the belly out. Put into a suitable size glass jar or a glazed pan. Add all the other ingredients. Top up with water so the fish is completely covered, float a small plate on top of the fish to keep it submerged in the brine. Cover the pan or put the lid on the jar and let it ferment for 3–5 days at room temperature. When the fish is ready take the meat off the bones, cut into bite-size pieces and serve with fresh dill and some chopped red onion.

Baked beans or French cassoulet

500g white (navy) beans
1 duck
1 tablespoon cider vinegar
1 teaspoon sea salt
2 tablespoons tomato puree
cayenne pepper and black pepper
5–6 bay leaves, a sprig of rosemary, a teaspoon of thyme

Soak the beans in water for 12–24 hours, drain, rinse well in cold water and drain again. Soaking and rinsing removes some harmful substances from the beans (lectins and phytates). Cover the beans with water again and add 4–5 tablespoons of your homemade whey, kefir or kefir starter. Leave to ferment for a week at a room temperature. Beans and other legumes are generally hard to digest, as they contain many anti-nutrients. Fermenting will make the beans more digestible. After rinsing your beans are ready to be cooked.

Cut all the meat from the duck: the legs, wings, breasts and all the fat. Cut the meat into chunks and the fat into small pieces. You can use the carcass of the duck and the giblets for making meat stock later. In a large pan put 2 litres of water, cider vinegar, sea salt, tomato puree, a pinch each of cayenne pepper and black pepper, bay leaves, rosemary and thyme. Mix in the beans and the duck pieces (the meat and the fat). Cover the pan with a lid and put it into an oven. Cook at 140–160°C (285–320°F) for 4–5 hours. Check occasionally. If the beans are getting dry, add more water.

Serve hot. The baked beans left from this meal will keep in the fridge for a long time and can be served with other dishes.

You can make this dish without the meat, in that case add plenty of animal fat (duck, pork, goose, beef, lamb, ghee, etc.). You can preserve this dish for about a year if you ladle it hot into sterilised glass jars and keep them refrigerated. To sterilise glass jars and their lids (metal or glass) place them in the cold oven and heat it up to about 120°C (250°F) for 30–40 minutes. Do not put the lids on the jars for sterilising, keep them separate.

Casserole with turkey

turkey legs, wings, carcass and other pieces with the skin on
1 l of water
1 heaped tablespoon of tomato puree
1 teaspoon of salt
6–10 peppercorns
a pinch of cayenne pepper
fresh or dried herbs: oregano, rosemary, bay leaves
a combination of available vegetables: choose from carrots, winter squash, pumpkin, courgette, marrow, peeled small/medium onions, cauliflower, broccoli, peppers, aubergine and Brussels sprouts

In a large oval casserole put the water, salt, tomato puree, peppercorns, cayenne pepper and herbs. Mix well. Add the turkey pieces. Brush the parts of the turkey pieces which are not covered with the water with some goose fat (or duck fat, ghee, pork dripping or lard). Do not cover the casserole with the lid, leave it open. Cook in the oven at 160°C (320°F) for 2–2½ hours. About 50 minutes before the end of cooking add available vegetables, cut into large chunks. Mix them well into the sauce and leave cooking. When the vegetables are cooked so a sharp knife goes through them easily, take the casserole out. Serve the meat and the vegetables with some freshly chopped parsley and garlic.

Liver pudding

100g liver (calf or lamb)
1 egg
2 tablespoons of butter (or ghee, goose/duck fat)
1 medium-size onion
salt
parsley

Soak the liver in water with some lemon juice or homemade yoghurt for a few hours to remove any bitter taste. You can also soak the liver in whey – liquid left from draining your homemade yoghurt. Wash the liver, dry with a paper towel and blend into a pulp in the food processor. Put through a sieve to remove any hard bits. Add salt, egg yolk, butter, finely chopped parsley and finely chopped onion. Whip the egg white stiff and fold into the mixture. Put the mixture into a suitable dish, cover with a sheet of baking paper and cook with steam. You can use a steamer or a large pan. To steam in a pan put some water at the bottom of the pan and place the dish in it. Make sure that you don't have too much water in the pan, so it does not get into the dish with the liver. Cover the pan with a lid and put it on the stove. Steam for about one hour. Serve with cooked vegetables or vegetable "risotto".

Liver in a clay pot

100g liver (calf or lamb)
100g lamb's hearts

1 large onion
10 dried prunes with stones
1 large pot of natural yoghurt or soured cream (you can use your
homemade yoghurt or replace with ¹/₂ cup of butter/ghee)
a pinch of allspice, salt, pepper

Soak the liver in water with some lemon juice or homemade yoghurt
for a few hours to remove any bitter taste. You can also soak the liver
in whey – the liquid left from draining your homemade yoghurt.
Wash, dry and cut into small pieces using scissors. Cut lamb's hearts
into small pieces using scissors. In a suitable size clay pot put the liver
and lamb's hearts, finely chopped onion and prunes. Into the yoghurt
add salt, pepper, allspice and mix well. Add to the clay pot and mix
with the meats. Cover the pot with the lid or foil. Bake in the oven for
about 1 hour at 160–180°C (320–355°F).

Quick liver recipe

100g liver
1 large onion
6–7 cloves of garlic
¹/₂ cup of butter/ghee (use any animal fat if avoiding butter)
fresh parsley or dill
salt and pepper to taste

Soak the liver in water with some lemon juice or homemade yoghurt for
a few hours to remove any bitter taste. You can also soak the liver in the
liquid left from draining your homemade yoghurt. Wash and dry the
liver and cut into small pieces using scissors. In a frying pan melt the
butter/ghee, add the sliced onion and finely chopped garlic. Fry slightly
until the onion and garlic start turning golden. Add the liver, salt and
pepper and stir-fry for about 4–5 minutes. Sprinkle chopped parsley or
dill on top and drizzle with olive oil. Serve immediately.

Fermented grains

After about two years on the diet and when all digestive problems are gone, your patient may be ready to have some gluten-free grains: buckwheat, millet and quinoa. First try them fermented as the fermentation process will predigest them. To ferment buckwheat, millet or quinoa wash the grain, cover with water and add $\frac{1}{2}$ cup of whey. Leave to ferment at room temperature for a few days: quinoa for 1–2 days, buckwheat for 2–3 days, millet for 4–5 days. When the fermentation is complete, drain the liquid out and cook the grain in your homemade meat stock or water with some salt (for 1 cup of grain 2 cups of meat stock or water). Bring the meat stock to the boil and add the grain, mix well, bring to the boil, cover and reduce heat to the minimum. Simmer for 20–30 minutes, stirring occasionally. When the grain is cooked all the liquid should be completely absorbed and the grain should be soft and fluffy. Serve it with meats and vegetables or bake with it, using it instead of flour. Introduce gradually, starting from 1–2 spoonfuls a day and watching for any reaction. Do not forget to serve grains with plenty of natural fat: butter, ghee, olive oil, coconut oil or any animal fat; the fats will slow down the digestion of the grains and help to control the blood sugar level.

6. Vegetables

Cooked vegetables are nourishing, warming and easy to digest, they are gentle on the gut lining and should be a regular part of the diet. You can cook your vegetables by steaming, stir-frying, stewing, roasting, grilling or as a soup. Instead of boiling vegetables I recommend steaming them, as boiling removes a lot of nutrients into the water, which then gets thrown away. The best vegetables to steam are broccoli, cauliflower, Brussels sprouts, fresh green beans (runner beans, string beans, etc.) carrots, asparagus, French artichokes and beetroot.

If diarrhoea is not present raw vegetables should also be a normal part of every meal. They provide a lot of active enzymes, which will help you to digest your food. Carrots, cucumber, tomato, greens, cabbage, onion, garlic, lettuce, baby spinach, celery, cauliflower can all be served as salads or cut into rosettes and sticks to eat with a dip (mayonnaise, guacamole, liver pate, aubergine dip, etc).

Sauerkraut

Sauerkraut is a fermented white and/or red cabbage, commonly consumed in Germany, Russia and Eastern Europe. It is a wonderful healing remedy for the digestive tract full of digestive enzymes, probiotic bacteria, vitamins and minerals. Eating it with meats will improve digestion as it has a strong ability to stimulate stomach acid production. For people with low stomach acidity I recommend having a few tablespoons of sauerkraut (or juice from it) 10–15 minutes before meals. For children, initially add 1–3 tablespoons of the juice from the sauerkraut into their meals. You do not need to add any starter to the sauerkraut, as fresh cabbage has natural bacteria living on it, which will do the fermentation for you.

Slice thinly a medium-size white cabbage and add two shredded carrots. You can use red cabbage or a mixture of white and red. Add 1–2 tablespoons of salt. Salt is essential as it will draw the juice from the cabbage during kneading. In addition salt will stifle the putrefactive microbes in the initial stages of fermentation until the fermenting bacteria produce enough lactic acid to kill the pathogens. Knead the mixture well with your hands until a lot of juice comes out. If the cabbage is not juicy enough add a little water. Pack this mixture into a suitable glass or enamelled bowl, pressing it firmly so there is no air trapped and the cabbage is drowned in its own juice. Fermentation is an anaerobic process: if the cabbage is exposed to air, it will rot instead of fermenting. Place a plate on top of the cabbage, which is about 1cm smaller in diameter than the bowl. The gap will allow the fermentation gases to escape. On top of the plate place something heavy enough to keep the cabbage constantly submerged in its juice. Cover the whole thing with a kitchen towel to keep it in the dark. It should take 5–7 days inside the house for the sauerkraut to be ready, (it will take two weeks in a cool place, like a garage). Alternatively you can pack the cabbage into glass jars for fermentation, making sure that the cabbage is submerged in its own juice. Don't forget to leave at least $2\frac{1}{2}$ cm of space in the jar at the top, as the cabbage will expand during fermentation. Sauerkraut is delicious with any meal and it can be added to your homemade soups and stews.

Vegetables fermented with kefir culture

Using yoghurt/kefir whey or the yoghurt/kefir starter you can ferment vegetables. Take some cabbage (white, red or any other variety), beetroot, garlic, cauliflower and carrot, slice them into nice bite-size pieces or shred them roughly, add some salt to taste and pack into a one litre glass jar. Take ½ litre of cold water and dissolve the contents of a kefir sachet in it. Alternatively add half a cup of your kefir whey to the water. Add this water to the jar until it completely covers the vegetables. It is important that the vegetables are completely covered by the water because if they are left dry at the top they will get mouldy. Don't forget to leave at least 2½ cm of space in the jar at the top, as the vegetables will expand during fermentation. Cover tightly with the lid and leave to ferment at room temperature for a week. Introduce the vegetables gradually starting with a small amount. These vegetables, and the liquid which they ferment in, are an excellent probiotic food and will assist digestion.

Vegetable medley

This probiotic food will provide you with delicious fermented vegetables and a wonderful beverage to drink, full of great nutrition and beneficial bacteria. In a 5-litre enamelled pan or a large glass jar put a whole cabbage, roughly cut, a medium-size beetroot, sliced, a teaspoon of dill seeds or dill herb (fresh or dried) and a handful of peeled garlic cloves (the pan should be half filled with the vegetables). Add 2 tablespoons of good quality sea salt, a cup of kefir whey and top up with water until the pan is full. Float a small plate on top of the brine to keep the vegetables completely submerged in the brine, because if the vegetables are dry at the top they will get mouldy. Leave to ferment for 1–2 weeks at room temperature. When ready, the vegetables will be soft and tangy. To stop the fermentation move, the pan into the refrigerator. You can add these vegetables to your soups and stews, drink the brine diluted with water with your meals or between meals and eat the vegetables with meat. When the brine and the vegetables start getting low, add fresh cabbage, beetroot and garlic, some salt to taste, top up with water and ferment at room temperature again. To this vegetable medley you can add a few rosettes of cauliflower, sliced carrot, Brussels sprouts and broccoli. You can have this vegetable medley going forever, as long as you keep feeding it with more fresh vegetables. The brine from this medley is an excellent remedy for any tummy upset, sore gums and sore throat.

A nice way to cook cabbage

$^1/_2$ cabbage, finely sliced
1 large carrot, finely sliced
$^1/_2$ onion, finely chopped
1 tomato, finely chopped
1 tablespoon of chopped garlic
salt and pepper to taste

Cover the bottom of the pan with homemade meat stock, add 3–5 tablespoons of any animal fat and bring to the boil. Add cabbage, carrot, onion, salt and pepper. Cover and cook on a low heat for 30 minutes. Add the chopped tomato and garlic, mix, cook for another 3 minutes and take off the heat. Mix in $^1/_2$ cup of homemade kefir, yoghurt or soured cream. Serve with meat.

Quick vegetable "risotto"

2 courgettes or $^1/_2$ of a medium-size marrow (zucchini)
1 large onion
10 cloves of garlic
1 pepper (red, yellow or green or a combination of different coloured peppers)
1 tablespoon of tomato puree
salt and pepper

In a frying pan melt about 50–100g of butter or any animal fat. Mix in sliced courgettes or marrow, onion, garlic, sliced peppers, tomato puree, season to taste with salt and pepper. Cover with a lid and leave for 10 minutes on minimum heat. Alternatively you can stir-fry it on a low heat. Mix well and serve with plenty of cold-pressed virgin olive oil and freshly chopped dill or parsley. Enjoy with meat and fish.

Cauliflower "potatoes"

1 large cauliflower cut into pieces
$\frac{1}{4}$ cup butter or $\frac{1}{4}$ cup homemade yoghurt
salt and pepper to taste
parsley and paprika garnish

Cook cauliflower until just tender. Drain.

Puree in blender or food processor. Add butter or yoghurt, salt and pepper and blend thoroughly. Reheat and serve. Garnish with parsley and paprika.

The pureed cauliflower may be placed in a baking dish, sprinkled with grated cheddar cheese and heated in the oven until the cheese melts.

(Recipe courtesy of Elaine Gottschall)

Baked vegetables

You can bake any combination of the following vegetables:

onions, white or red, or shallots
peppers, red, yellow, orange or green
Brussels sprouts
courgettes or marrow
pumpkin
winter squashes
large mushrooms
turnips and/or swedes
aubergines (eggplant)

Peel the onion and cut into halves or quarters. Shallots do not need to be peeled, just bake them in their skins.

Cut the peppers into quarters, remove seeds.

Peel the outer leaves from Brussels sprouts.

Peel and cut into large chunks courgettes, marrow and pumpkin. Remove the seeds from the pumpkin and the marrow. Rub courgettes and marrow with salt.

Peel and slice winter squash, remove the seeds.

Peel the turnips and cut like potato chips.

Cut the aubergine into chunks and rub with salt.

Rub plenty of any animal fat on the vegetables, place them in a baking tray and bake at 160–180°C (320–355°F) for 20–40 minutes or until a sharp knife goes through easily. Serve with meat or fish.

7. Baking at home

The basic bread/cake/muffin recipe

2$\frac{1}{2}$ cups of ground almonds
$\frac{1}{4}$ cup of softened butter (or coconut oil, goose fat, duck fat or homemade yoghurt or crème fraiche)
3 eggs

You can buy ground almonds in most health food shops. Instead of ground almonds you can use walnuts, pecans, hazelnuts, peanuts, pine nuts, sunflower seeds and pumpkin seeds or a mixture of all of the above, which you can grind in your food processor to a flour consistency.

Mix all the ingredients well. You may want to add more or less ground almonds to reach porridge-like consistency. Grease your baking pan with butter or ghee, line it with greased baking paper and put the mixture into it. Bake in the oven at 150°C (300°F) for about an hour. Check occasionally with a dry clean knife. If the knife comes out dry then the bread is ready.

To make variations of this bread you can add some salt, pepper, dried herbs, tomato puree, grated cheddar cheese (if well tolerated), nuts, seeds, dried fruit, fresh or frozen berries, chunks of cooking apple, grated carrot, chunks of pumpkin (without the skin and seeds). If you want to sweeten the mixture add $\frac{1}{2}$ cup of honey into it and/or 1$\frac{1}{2}$ cups of dried fruit (dates, apricots, raisins, figs) and/or 2 ripe bananas. If the dried fruit is too hard, soak it in water for a few hours to soften or bring up to the boil in a little water.

Improvise to make your own variations. You can bake this mixture as a bread or cake or in small paper cups as muffins or make a pizza base. It really is very easy and manageable, even for the most inexperienced cooks.

If, after your first attempt, you find that your patient cannot tolerate this recipe (gets abdominal pain or diarrhoea), try to ferment the nut flour or the mixture of nuts and seeds before grinding them into the flour. Nuts and seeds have substances in them (phytates, phenols, oxalates, fibre, etc.) which can make them difficult to digest for some people. Cover the nuts or the nut flour with a little whey and leave to ferment at room temperature for 24 hours, drain and use in baking. If none of the nuts are tolerated, try to sprout sunflower seeds and grind them into flour consistency for baking.

Pizza

Make a pastry following the previous recipe. Spread it on a baking tray covered with greased baking paper in a layer about 2 cm thick. Bake in the oven at 150°C (300°F) for about 30 minutes. Check with a dry knife to see if it is ready.

Cool down. Spread tomato puree on the top and sprinkle with salt.

On top of the tomato puree you can put your choice of filling: slices of red/yellow/green pepper, mushrooms, pieces of cooked meat or sausages, slices of tomato, chopped greens, anchovies, fish, prawns and pineapple, etc.

Put grated hard cheese (cheddar and/or parmesan) on top of your filling if your patient is at the stage when he or she can tolerate cheese. If the cheese is not tolerated then you can use homemade mayonnaise instead.

8. Desserts

Baked apples

With a sharp knife scoop out the cores with the seeds from large cooking apples. Fill each apple with a teaspoon of honey, a teaspoon of butter, ground or coarsely chopped apricot kernels (or walnuts, or any other available nuts, or desiccated coconut). Add a dried apricot per apple (optional) cut into small pieces. Bake in the oven at 160–180°C (320–360°F) for 20–25 minutes.

Crème caramel

For one person you need:
1 egg
3 tablespoons of water
1 teaspoon of honey
ground cinnamon

Multiply the ingredients per number of people you want to serve.

Mix all the ingredients well. Pour into shallow ramekin dishes (or any other small terracotta dishes): you need one ramekin dish per person. Sprinkle some cinnamon on top. Preheat the oven to 150°C (300°F). Bake for 30–40 minutes.

Apple crumble

4 cooking apples
2 eggs
carrot pulp from juicing 1 kg of carrots or $^1/_2$ kg carrots, very finely chopped
10 dried apricots
$^1/_2$ cup of honey
$^1/_2$ cup of unsalted butter

Cut the apples into pieces and place on the bottom of your baking dish. Chop dried apricots into small pieces.

Mix together eggs, butter, carrot pulp, chopped dried apricots and honey. Put the mixture on top of the apples and mix slightly. Bake in the oven at 160°C (320°F) for approximately 40 minutes.

Apple pie

4 large cooking apples
a handful of raisins
$^1/_2$ cup of honey
1 cup of fresh or frozen blackcurrants
2–3 cups fresh pumpkin, peeled and finely chopped

2 cups pitted dried dates
1 cup of hazelnuts
$^1/_2$ cup of ground almonds

Soak hazelnuts in whey overnight, drain. Soak the dates in 2 cups of water for 2–3 hours or overnight. Drain the dates and put the soaking water into your baking dish. Add cored and sliced apples, raisins and blackcurrants. Spread them evenly and sprinkle with the ground almonds. Pour honey on top, spreading evenly.

In a food processor blend the dates, pumpkin and hazelnuts. Spoon this mixture on top of the pie, spreading evenly. Slightly press and smooth with a spoon or a knife so that the top looks like the top of a pie. Bake at 150–170°C (300–350°F) for an hour.

Winter squash cake

6 eggs
2 cups of grated (packed tightly) winter squash with sweet orange flesh (buttercup, butternut or other)
$^1/_2$ cup of honey
$^1/_3$ cup of butter (or ghee, coconut fat, goose fat or duck fat)
3 cups of ground almonds
3 medium-size apples

Grease your baking dish and cover the bottom with apples, cored and cut into slices. If your patient's digestive system is sensitive, then peel the apples. Otherwise you can leave the skins on.

Blend the rest of the ingredients in your blender and put the mixture on top of the apples. Smooth the top and bake at 150–70°C (300–340°F) for 40–50 minutes.

Cake Pinocchio

2 cups of shelled hazelnuts
1 cup of honey (250ml)
4 eggs
150g unsalted butter, preferably organic
4 tangerines to decorate

Preheat the oven to 175–200°C (350–400°F).

Roast the hazelnuts in the oven and rub their skins off. Reserve 1 cup of the nuts for the cream and grind the rest into a coarse flour.

Make 4 circles out of baking paper large enough to fit on a large cake dish and grease them with butter. Separate the whites of the eggs from the yolks. Whip the egg whites stiff with half of the honey. Carefully fold in the ground hazelnuts. Spread the mixture on the four baking paper circles and bake for 5–10 minutes. Cool down and remove the baking paper.

Cream Soften the butter by leaving it in the room for a few hours. Whip the 4 egg yolks with the rest of the honey until they increase in volume and become pale whitish in colour. Beat in the butter gradually, adding it in small amounts.

Coarsely chop the rest of the hazelnuts, reserving 10–15 whole nuts for decorating.

Layer the meringue circles with the cream, sprinkling every cream layer with the coarsely chopped hazelnuts. Cover the top with a thin layer of the cream. Peel the tangerines and separate them into segments. Decorate the top with the segments of tangerines and the 10–15 whole hazelnuts. Refrigerate.

Peanut butter pie

6 eggs
2 tablespoons of butter
1 cup of peanut butter
2 cups of carrot pulp left after juicing carrots (you can use winter squash as a substitute, peel it and chop very finely in a food processor)
$^1/_2$ cup of honey
1 cup of ground almonds
2 large cooking apples
a handful of raisins

Peel the apples, cut them into small pieces and place them in a greased baking dish. Sprinkle the raisins on top of the apples.

Put the rest of the ingredients in a blender and blend well. Put the mixture on top of the apples. Smooth the top and bake at 150–170°C (300–340°F) for 40–50 minutes.

Russian custard

for one person:
2 egg yolks
$\frac{1}{2}$–1 teaspoon of honey
multiply the ingredients for the number of people to be served

Russian custard can be used instead of cream on fruit or you can serve it on its own with some chopped nuts on the top or pieces of fruit. It can also be used instead of cream in making cakes. Separate the egg yolks from the whites, add the honey and whip the mixture until it goes thick and almost white. As well as being a delicious desert, it provides very good nutrition. Get your eggs from a source you trust. Free-range organic eggs are the best.

Apple sauce

5–6 large cooking apples
$\frac{1}{2}$ cup butter
1–2 cups water
honey to sweeten

Peel and core the apples, cut them into pieces and cook in a pan with the water until soft. Take off the heat and add butter. Cool down, mash and sweeten with honey to your taste.

You can make pear sauce the same way, though you may not need to add honey, as pears are naturally very sweet.

This sauce will keep well in the refrigerator and can be served with some yoghurt, chopped nuts, Russian custard or on its own.

Birthday cake

Make an apple sauce from 5–6 large cooking apples and cool it down. Make it quite sweet as the pastry of the cake is not going to be sweetened. You can make a pear sauce instead of apple. If sour cream has been introduced, use it instead of the apple sauce. Whip about 750g of sour cream with honey to taste, making it very sweet. If the sour cream is too thick, add a bit of whey to it before whipping.

Separate yolks and whites of 6 eggs into two large bowls. Whip the yolks until thick and light in colour. Whip the whites until firm and no longer runny. Combine the two and add 2 cups of ground almonds. Mix well. Bake in a cake tin lined with greased baking paper for 40–60 minutes at a temperature of 150°C (300°F). Test with a dry knife whether it is cooked inside (the knife will come out dry if the cake is ready). Depending on the oven the baking time may vary. When ready allow the cake to cool down.

Now the fun part starts. With a long knife cut off the top of the cake, making sure that this layer is no more than 1 cm thick. Put it aside for using as the top of your cake later. Using a tablespoon carefully spoon out the inside of the cake in medium-sized chunks into a separate dish leaving just an outside shell, which will look like a dish ready to be filled. Fill it up with layers of your apple sauce (or whipped sour cream), frozen raspberries, chopped nuts and the chunks of cake which you spooned out before. Here you can really improvise by using different berries, stoned cherries, pieces of soft fresh fruit, chopped nuts and seeds (sesame, poppy, and sunflower). When the "cake dish" is filled, cover it with the top layer you removed earlier. Spread the remaining apple sauce (or whipped sour cream) on and decorate. To decorate you can use fresh fruit, berries, nuts and desiccated coconut. After decorating put the cake into the refrigerator. It is best to make this cake the day before the party so it has the time to "mature" overnight.

This is the basic recipe. You can improvise by adding seeds, chopped nuts, grated carrot or pumpkin into the pastry before baking, filling it with different combinations of fruit and berries, and decorating it any way you like. Children like to be involved in decorating. Any of the decorating ingredients which I have mentioned before are optional, depending on your family's sensitivities. These are fruit, berries, nuts, seeds, fresh mint leaves and coconut.

Banana ice cream

Buy in advance some very ripe bananas (with brown spots on the skin), peel them and put in the freezer. On a day when you want to make the ice cream, get these frozen bananas out and leave them in the room for about 30 minutes to slightly defrost. Blend them in a food processor. Add a little bit of water to make a good creamy consistency. You can blend some fresh or frozen berries, pieces of fruit, desiccated or fresh coconut into the mixture and some coarsely chopped nuts to make different flavours.

Dairy ice cream

You can start making this ice cream when homemade sour cream has been introduced into the diet. Whip ¹/₂ litre of your sour cream with honey to taste. Separate 2 egg yolks from the whites and whip them separately until the whites are stiff and the yolks are pale yellow and thick. Mix the whipped cream with the whipped yolks and add any fruit, berries, nuts, seeds and spices of your choice. Mix well, then gently fold in the whipped egg whites. Put into a plastic container and freeze immediately.

Fresh coconut

When you are buying a coconut, make sure that the shell has no cracks or any other damage to it. Put the nut close to your ear and shake it. If the coconut is healthy, you will hear its juice splashing inside. When a coconut is damaged and its juice has leaked out, it will be rancid and unsuitable to eat.

When you bring your coconut home, the fun bit starts. You will need a screwdriver and a hammer. At the top of the coconut there are three round dots. Push your screwdriver through two of those dots to make two holes. Drain the juice through one of the holes allowing the air to get inside through the other hole. The juice is very nourishing and can be used in cooking or drunk as it is. It should have a fresh sweet taste. If the juice tastes rancid, then there is no point in cracking your coconut, as it will be unsuitable to eat. After draining the juice crack the shell with the hammer and separate the pulp from the shell. Rinse the pulp with the water to wash off any small bits of shell. There are a number of ways to eat it:

- Cut the pulp into small pieces and eat it as it is. It has a very pleasant sweet taste.
- Grind it in your food processor to make sweets (next recipe).
- Put the pulp through your juicer to produce a thick coconut cream, which can be diluted with water to make a delicious coconut milk. The cream and milk can be added to your cooking, used as a dressing for fruit and vegetable salads, as a cream for cakes or a replacement for custard.
- Mince the coconut pulp to use in your baking, homemade ice cream and other desserts, soups, stews, salads and sauces.

A word of caution for children and adults with diarrhoea. Coconut is very fibrous and may make the diarrhoea worse, so initially I suggest putting the coconut through a juicer, which would separate the fibre from the rest of it. This way you can enjoy the freshly made coconut milk and cream, getting all the good nutrition from them without the fibre.

Coconut sweets

1 medium-size coconut
1 cup of dried fruit (any of the following: dried apricots, figs, dates or raisins, or a mixture of them. Make sure they are not sorbated or coated in starch)
1 cup of sesame seeds or ground almonds

Soak the dried fruit for 6–8 hours. Drain.

Make two holes in the coconut and drain the liquid. Put the liquid through a fine sieve and reserve for the recipe.

Shell the coconut and rinse the pulp to wash away small bits of shell. Cut the coconut pulp into pieces small enough to put through your grinder or juicer.

Grind the coconut pulp with the dried fruit. Mix well in your food processor or by hand. If the mixture is too dry, add some liquid from the coconut, which you have reserved.

With your hands roll small balls from the mixture and coat them in sesame seeds or ground almonds. Place on a large plate and refrigerate or freeze.

9. Egg-free recipes

Eggs are used in baking as a binder to keep all the other ingredients together. Some children have a true allergy to eggs and have to avoid them. The following ingredients will act as a binder in your baking instead of eggs.

- Gelatine, well dissolved in a small amount of hot water;
- Pumpkin, baked and mashed;
- Butternut squash and other winter squashes (acorn, turban, hubbard, spaghetti), baked and mashed;
- Banana, mashed;
- Apple, baked and mashed or made into an apple sauce;
- Pear, baked and mashed or made into a sauce;
- Zucchini (marrow or courgettes), baked, mashed and drained of excess liquid.

Egg-free bread/cake/muffin mixture

2 cups of ground nuts (almonds, cashews, walnuts, hazels, etc.)
3 tablespoons of butter (or coconut oil, ghee, goose fat, duck fat)
2 cups of cooked and mashed squash (butternut squash, pumpkin or other less watery squashes, apple sauce, pear sauce)

To prepare the squash (pumpkin), cut it into halves and remove the seeds. Place on a baking tray with the cut surface down and bake in the oven until very soft (a knife should go through it very easily). Cool, scoop out all the inside and mash with a fork.

You can improvise on this recipe by adding to the mixture honey, dried fruit, coarsely chopped nuts, shredded coconut, berries and fruit pieces.

Mix all the ingredients well. Put into a well-buttered baking dish and bake in the oven at 150–175°C (300–350°F) for 45–60 minutes. Occasionally check with a dry knife if it is ready (the knife has to come out dry).

If you add 2 tablespoons of pure tomato puree (with a single ingredient: tomato) and some salt and pepper in the same mixture, you can bake a pizza base. Just spread the mixture on a baking paper, shaping it with a spoon.

Experiment with your own versions, using ingredients available to you from the allowed list. Here are a few examples of egg-free recipes you can make.

Egg-free banana muffins

2 cups of cashew nuts or any other nuts
2 ripe bananas
4 teaspoons of honey
4 teaspoons of gelatine powder or crystals
4–8 tablespoons of coconut oil or butter

Grind the nuts into a flour (you can use ground almonds instead). Mash the banana. Dissolve gelatine powder in half a cup of hot water.

Mix all the ingredients together. Fill paper muffin cases with the mixture and bake at 150–170°C (290–380°F) for 15–20 minutes.

You can vary this recipe by folding different berries into the mixture, small pieces of fruit, coarsely chopped nuts or seeds (sunflower, sesame or pumpkin).

Egg-free Easter eggs

2 cups of pecans
a handful of coconut flakes
4 tablespoons of butter or ghee
2 tablespoons of honey

Blend all the ingredient into a fine paste in the food processor. With your hands roll out small eggs. Put them in the freezer until ready to eat.

With this mixture you can make different biscuits, using children's biscuit shapes. Roll the mixture on a well-buttered surface until 1 cm thick. Put it into a freezer for 2 hours or longer, take out and cut into shapes (squares, animals, tractors, etc.). You can let your children do the cutting out.

Egg-free crackers/biscuits

2 tablespoons of butter (coconut oil or duck fat/goose fat)
2 cups of ground nuts (almonds, hazels, walnuts, etc.)
2–3 tablespoons of water (or almond milk or coconut milk)

You can improvise by adding to this mixture herbs, cinnamon, paprika, cayenne pepper, black pepper, salt, grated cheddar cheese (if well tolerated) or peanut butter.

Mix the ingredients well. Roll out thinly on a board, sprinkled with some ground nuts. Cut into squares or any other shapes. Sprinkle some coarse salt, poppy seeds, caraway seeds or coriander seeds on top. Bake in the oven on well-buttered baking paper at 150°C (300°F) for 10–15 minutes.

Egg-free fruit dessert

1. Blend or cut into small pieces available berries and fruit and cover the bottom of your baking tin with the mixture. Nice combinations are plums and apples, pears and raspberries, cherries and pineapple, apple and blackcurrants.
2. Pour about 3 cups of ground almonds over the fruit.
3. Sprinkle 1½ cups of shredded coconut over the almonds.
4. Spread 1–2 cups of pecan halves over the coconut (you can use any other available nuts, coarsely chopped).
5. Cover the top with 200g of butter, cut into slices (you can use coconut oil or ghee instead of butter).
6. Bake at 160–175°C (320–350°F) for about 40 minutes.

Egg-free apple pie

1. Fill your baking dish halfway up with peeled and chopped cooking apples and plums (take the stones out). Instead of plums you can use blackcurrants, raspberries, blackberries, pears, elderberries, etc.
2. Pour half a cup of honey over the fruit and mix lightly.
3. Soak two handfuls of dried dates in half a cup of hot water to make them softer. Drain and use for the crust. The soaking water is very sweet and can be poured over the fruit.
4. To make the crust blend the dates with 1 cup of ground almonds and 2 tablespoons of butter. With your hands shape the mixture into a ball, put it on a large sheet of baking paper or cling film and roll it out into a round pancake shape large enough to cover the top of your baking dish. Lift up the baking paper with the rolled out pastry and carefully flip it over the fruit. Make sure that the pastry covers the whole of the fruit, trim off any excess and fill any holes with it.
5. Bake in the oven at 130–150°C (265–300°F) for about 40–50 minutes.

Egg-free cookies (biscuits)

2 cups of ground nuts (nut flour)
1 cup of cooked and mashed butternut squash
pear sauce made from 1 large pear
1 tablespoon of butter or any other acceptable fat

Mix all the ingredients well and bake small biscuits on baking paper at 150–160°C (300–320°F) for about 20 minutes.

10. Beverages

Nut/seed milk

You can use almonds, sunflower seeds, sesame seeds, pine nuts, etc. to make milk. Almonds make the best milk. You can add a teaspoon of flaxseeds to make the milk thicker. Soak the nuts/seeds in water for

12–24 hours, drain. Blend in a food processor with water: for 1 cup of nuts/seeds add 2–3 cups of water. A good juicer will crush the nuts/seeds well, making a paste, which you blend with water. Mix well and strain through a cheesecloth or a fine strainer and you have got milk. You can add some soaked dates or raisins when blending, they will make the milk sweet. If you find that the milk is too rich, just add more water. You can add some freshly pressed apple juice or carrot juice to it to make a very tasty and nourishing drink.

Coconut milk

Bring to the boil 1 cup of unsweetened shredded coconut and 1 cup of water. Cool down and blend well in the food processor. Strain through a cheesecloth or a fine strainer.

Ginger tea

1 tablespoon of freshly grated ginger root
water

In your teapot put the grated ginger root and add boiling water. Cover and brew for 5–10 minutes. Pour through a sieve. It is a warming drink and aids digestion.

Freshly squeezed juices

Use only organic fruit and vegetables for making juices. Wash your fruit and vegetables and cut any bad bits off. Do not peel and do not remove seeds.

A good juice to start the day is pineapple + carrot + small amount of beetroot.

The most therapeutic juices do not taste very nice: green and vegetable juices. To make your juices tasty and enjoyable to drink I recommend making mixes of different fruit and vegetables. You can make all sorts of juice mixes, but generally try to have:

- 50% of highly therapeutic ingredients: carrot, small amount of

beetroot (no more than 5% of the juice mixture), celery, white and red cabbage, lettuce, greens (spinach, parsley, dill, basil, fresh nettle leaves, beet tops and carrot tops).
- 50% of some tasty ingredients to disguise the taste of therapeutic ingredients: pineapple, apple, orange, grapefruit, grapes, mango, etc.

Your patient can have these juices as they are or diluted with some water. If throughout the day your GAPS child would not drink just water, you can add some of these freshly squeezed juices to the water to make a tasty drink. Initially start with 1 cup of juice a day. With a small child you may want to start with a very small amount, like 1 teaspoon a day. Increase the daily amount very gradually until your child has 2 cups of freshly squeezed juices a day. These juices should be taken on an empty stomach, so first thing in the morning and middle of the afternoon are good times.

With these juices you can make ice lollies. Just fill ice lolly forms with freshly squeezed juice and freeze.

You can also make ice cubes from these juices, which can be used to make a cold drink in hot weather. Just fill the glass with these ice cubes and add mineral water (still or carbonated).

The carrot pulp left from juicing can be used in your baking mixtures together with ground nuts or as a replacement for ground nuts. You can also use pulp left from other fruit and vegetables depending on your taste preferences.

Fruit smoothies

You can make all sorts of combinations. If you make your own yoghurt and sour cream, then you can use them as well. Here are a few ideas.

Blend a banana with ½ ripe avocado, half a cup of homemade yoghurt or sour cream and a bit of honey to taste.

Half an avocado blended with freshly squeezed apple/carrot juice or freshly squeezed pineapple juice.

Banana blended with freshly squeezed carrot juice (apple juice, pineapple juice, orange juice, etc.) and half a cup of yoghurt or sour cream.

Fermented probiotic beverages

Using whey as a starter you can make delicious fermented beverages for the whole family. They will provide you with beneficial bacteria, enzymes and many nutrients which the fermentation process will release from the fruit and vegetables.

Kefir or yoghurt whey

The clear yellow liquid left after dripping your yoghurt or kefir is called whey. It is a very nourishing beverage and an excellent source of probiotic bacteria. You can add it to freshly pressed juices, soups and stews. You can add some salt and spices to it and drink it as it is or diluted with some water. You can use it as a starter for fermenting vegetables, fruit, fish and grains (when you are ready to introduce them).

Beetroot kvass

Using a knife slice medium-size beetroot finely. Don't grate the beetroot in a food processor as that will make it ferment too quickly, producing alcohol. Put the beetroot into a 2-litre jar, add 1–2 tablespoons of good quality sea salt, 1 cup of whey, 5 cloves of garlic, a teaspoon of freshly grated ginger (optional) and fill up with water. Let it ferment for 2–5 days in a warm place. After that keep in the refrigerator. Drink diluted with water. Keep topping the water up in the jar so your kvass will keep going for a long time. When it starts getting pale then the beetroot is spent, so start again.

Kvass from other fruit and vegetables

You can make kvass from any combination of fruit, berries and vegetables, so try to experiment. Another good recipe is apple, ginger and raspberry kvass. Slice a whole apple including the core, grate ginger root (about a tea spoonful) and get a handful of fresh raspberries. Put them all into a 1-litre jar, add ¹/₂ cup of whey and top up with water. Let it brew for a few days at room temperature, then keep in the refrigerator. Drink diluted with water. Keep topping up your brew with water until the fruit is spent, then start again.

Probiotic tomato juice

Blend well 1 cup of whey, 1 tablespoon of tomato puree, 1 cup of water and some salt to taste.

11. Yoghurt, kefir and crème fraiche (sour cream)

In the initial stages many (not all) GAPS patients tolerate goat's milk products better than cow's. So, try to use goat's milk first. I strongly recommend using only organic milk. If you cannot find organic goat's milk then try cow's. The best milk to use is **raw** organic milk, which has not been pasteurised or processed in any other way. All milk sold in shops has been pasteurised, which changes the structure of the milk and destroys many useful nutrients in it. Please, see the chapter on dairy for a full discussion on raw milk. A lot of milk on the supermarket shelves, apart from being pasteurised, has been subjected to a process called homogenisation in order to stop milk from separating in the bottle (a purely cosmetic purpose). This process breaks down the fat globules and changes the structure of milk even further, making it harmful for the body. Try to buy organic milk which has not been processed at all. If it is not possible to buy unpasteurised milk, try to buy milk which, apart from pasteurisation, has not been subjected to any other processing. If that is not possible then do your best to buy any organic milk labelled "fresh". Despite the fact that it has been pasteurised and homogenised, the fermentation process will do a lot to restore its nutritional value.

Goat's yoghurt is quite a lot more liquid than cow's yoghurt. You can use it as a drink, or if you want to thicken it you can drip it through cheesecloth. Sometimes cow's yoghurt turns out to be quite liquid as well, so you can drip it through cheesecloth to make it thicker or to make cottage cheese and whey.

To make yoghurt you need to introduce bacteria into the milk. You can buy commercially available yoghurt starters from many health food shops or small-holding suppliers. Alternatively you can use commercially available *live* yoghurt as a starter. After making their first yoghurt many people successfully perpetuate their own yoghurt by using it as a starter for the next batch. You can also keep the liquid left from dripping your yoghurt, called whey, in a clean dry jar in your refrigerator to use as a starter for making the next batch of yoghurt. If, at any point, your own yoghurt or the whey do not work, you need to start again with a commercial starter or commercial live yoghurt.

After yoghurt has been introduced I recommend introducing a variety of yoghurt called kefir. Kefir produces a more pronounced die-off reaction, which is why I recommend introducing it after the yoghurt, which is quite a bit milder. Apart from good bacteria a healthy body is populated by beneficial yeasts which normally protect the person from pathogenic (bad) yeasts, such as *candida albicans*. Kefir contains these beneficial yeasts (as well as the beneficial bacteria) which help to take pathogenic yeasts under control.

Instructions for making kefir and yoghurt
1. If you are using pasteurised milk bring 1 litre of milk (goat's or cow's) close to the boil in a pan, stirring occasionally. You need to bring the milk close to the boiling point in order to destroy any bacteria, which may linger in the milk and interfere with the fermentation. However, do not boil the milk, as it will change its structure and taste. Take the pan off the heat. Cover the pan with the lid and cool down by placing the pan in cold water until the temperature of the milk is around 40–45°C (105–113°F). If you do not have a suitable thermometer use your own hand to determine the right temperature. To do that take a teaspoon of milk from the pan (using a clean dry spoon) and put the milk on the inside of your wrist. If it feels just slightly warm then the temperature is right.

    If you are using raw organic milk, which has not been pasteurised or processed in any other way, you don't need to heat it, so you can just skip this step. Keep in mind though that raw milk has got its own bacterial population, so the fermentation is not going to be as controlled as with using heated milk. That means that your yoghurt may turn out to be more liquid or lumpy or sour, than you expect. If you are dealing with a fussy patient who would only accept a certain consistency of yoghurt, then heat the raw milk close to the boiling point to make the fermentation more predictable. Gentle heating at home is not as destructive for the milk as commercial pasteurisation: it will kill the bacteria and change some things in the milk, but not as badly as commercial treatment.

2. If you are using a commercial kefir or yoghurt starter in a powder form you need to dissolve the powder in a little milk first before adding it to the pan. If you are using your own kefir, yoghurt or commercial live kefir or yoghurt add 1/3 cup to the milk. Stir well, cover with the lid and put in a warm place at 40–45°C (105–113°F). You can use a clean dry thermos for this purpose, a yoghurt maker, an electric plate, the top of your boiler or your airing cabinet (if it is warm enough). Ferment the kefir or yoghurt for at least 24 hours or longer.

3. After the fermentation is complete, move your kefir or yoghurt to a clean, dry glass jar, cover and refrigerate.

4. To drip the kefir or yoghurt, line a large colander with cheese-cloth. Place the colander into a large bowl and pour your yoghurt into the lined colander. Cover with a tea towel and let it drip for a few hours. Whey is a clear yellow liquid which drips out through the cloth. Diluted with water or any freshly pressed juice it makes an excellent probiotic beverage, and you can use it as a starter for fermenting other foods. Put it in a clean, dry glass jar and keep it refrigerated. Depending on how long you leave your yoghurt dripping you can make a soft cottage cheese or thicker yoghurt. Both soft cottage cheese and the yoghurt or kefir can be used for baking, adding to salads and soups and as desserts with honey and fruit.

Instructions for making crème fraiche (sour cream)
By using cream instead of milk you can make crème fraiche or sour cream. For 1litre of cream use one sachet of commercial starter or ¹/₂ cup of live kefir or yoghurt.

1. Constantly stirring, bring the cream to the boil but do not let it boil. Skip this step if you are using organic raw cream (not pasteurised or processed in any other way). Fermenting raw cream without heating it produces a more predictable consistency, than fermenting milk. So, there really isn't a need to heat it.

2. Cool down by placing the pan in cold water. Keep the pan covered at all times.
3. Test the temperature – it should be 40–45°C (105–113°F).
4. Add the starter and ferment for 24 hours minimum.

This sour cream or crème fraiche is very nice to use in salads, soups, stews, in baking or as a dessert with some honey and berries. You can blend it with a little honey and frozen fruit or berries to make an instant ice cream. Sour cream has a wonderful profile of fatty acids, nourishing for the immune system and the brain, so use it liberally in your GAPS patient's diet.

4. It's Feeding Time! Oh, no!

Grown-ups never understand anything for themselves,
and it is tiresome for children to be always
and forever explaining things to them.
Antoine de Saint-Exupery
Le Petit Prince, 1943

It is very rare to meet a GAPS child who is not a finicky eater. The same can be said about many GAPS adults as well. This problem is particularly pronounced in autism. The majority of autistic children and adults have feeding problems, sometimes very severe. Some are very fussy and accept only a very limited range of foods. Some cannot chew properly and hold food in their mouth for a long time or try to swallow it in a lump. Some can only suck from a bottle and will not drink from anything else. Feeding time is a nightmare for many parents of autistic children.

There are number of possible reasons why GAPS patients have these problems.

First is a distorted sensory input. The taste buds in their mouth receive the information about food, which gets passed to the brain. A GAPS brain is clogged with toxicity and cannot process this information properly. As a result, to these people the food can taste completely different to what it should taste like. Add to that a distorted feeling of food texture and temperature and we start appreciating why an autistic child, for example, does not accept many foods. The taste, texture and feeling of food can be quite offensive to them.

Second is a craving for sweet and starchy foods that is typical for all people with abnormal bodily flora, particularly with *Candida albicans* overgrowth. No matter how finicky a GAPS child or adult might be, most of them would accept sugary drinks, biscuits, cakes, sweets, sugar-laden breakfast cereals, chocolates, chips, crisps, pasta and white bread. In fact these are the foods to which many GAPS people limit their diet thus feeding the vicious circle of abnormal flora and toxicity in their bodies.

Third is the state of the mouth itself. A human mouth is home for a large population of microbes which normally protect the mouth from pathogenic bacteria, viruses and fungi, and maintain the healthy state of the mucous membranes and various structures in the mouth. GAPS children and adults often have a very abnormal bacterial flora in their mouths, often with an overgrowth of *Candida* and other pathogenic microbes. The activity of this abnormal flora produces a lot of toxins, which are stored in the mucous membranes of the mouth and alter the functioning of taste buds, saliva glands and other structures. Apart from contributing to the distortion of taste, this process causes a chronic inflammation in the mucous membranes of the mouth, making it a target for the immune system. As a result of microbial activity and inflammation, many GAPS patients have bad breath, very red lips and mouth, various spots and ulcers on the mucosa of the cheeks and a coated furry tongue. Many foods, like raw fruit and vegetables, herbs, uncooked nuts and seeds, cold-pressed oils and some other foods have strong detoxifying substances, which bind to the toxins in the mouth trying to remove them. This can feel far from nice, ranging from stinging, itching and burning to simply an unpleasant taste. And indeed, these are the foods that GAPS people commonly will not accept.

There are some contributory factors. For example, any secretion from the body is a way of eliminating toxins. Saliva is one of them. GAPS patients have very toxic bodies and some of these toxins get excreted through saliva. This contributes to the toxic load in the mouth, altering the taste and feel of foods.

In some cases of autism and other GAPS disorders another contributory factor comes into play – an inability of the toxic brain to orchestrate normal movements of the muscles in the mouth, tongue and other structures involved in chewing and swallowing. These are the patients who cannot chew and swallow properly. Foods have to be very soft for them and they very often vomit. Such severe abnormality is fairly rare, but this problem exists in many GAPS children and adults to a milder degree.

So, what are we to do with these feeding problems?

It is the appropriate nutritional management aimed at normalising bodily flora and detoxifying the person that would eventually make foods taste properly to him/her. Generally it is not much of a problem to persuade adults to change their diet, though it can be difficult to get them to stick to it. But how on Earth can we apply any nutritional management to a child who will not eat anything? Indeed, this is the hardest point for many parents in managing their child's condition.

I generally don't believe in hopeless situations. Where there is a will there is a way! There is a way, a very efficient way of introducing foods into your child's diet. It requires a lot of determination from the parents but it brings a huge relief and quite a bit of normality into your family's life. This way is ABA (Applied Behaviour Analysis) or behaviour modification. The main principle of this method is based on the common sense used by parents for centuries. I am sure you all recall your parents telling you "First you have to do your homework, than you can go and play!", or "If you want to go to the zoo on Saturday, you have to...." So, the formula is – if you want something, you have to work for it!

When you first introduce this method into your child's life, he or she is not going to like it, so expect a lot of resistance until your child learns the rules of the game. If you do not give up in those first difficult days, your child will understand pretty quickly that to get what he or she wants your child has to do something for you. As soon as he or she understands that, your life will become much easier. If you already are doing an ABA programme with your child at home, you can make feeding a separate drill for your therapists to work on in the sessions. All you will have to do is to cook the food and bring it into the therapy room.

So, how do we apply this method to children?

Let us start from the more severe end of the spectrum – a non-verbal autistic child.

1. Introducing new foods to a child with severe language problems

Initially use preferred foods as rewards for eating the good food. Show your child the food he/she likes the most (a piece of chocolate, a couple of crisps, a piece of biscuit, etc.). Put it out of his/her reach but in clear view. Offer your child one mouthful of the food you want to introduce. Ignore tantrums, screaming, crying and all other misbehaviours. Do not give him what he wants until he has had that one mouthful of the good food and do not let him leave the table. When he has had only one mouthful of the good food or literally just tasted it, give him the preferred food as a reward with lavish praise, hugs, kisses, tickles (whatever your child would most appreciate) and let him go. In a few minutes repeat the whole procedure again. Only work on one mouthful at a time, reward and let him/her go. In a few minutes repeat again. Give your child only a small amount of the reward food: one or two crisps, a little piece of chocolate, etc. If he comes back for more, get him to eat another mouthful before rewarding him with another crisp, small piece of chocolate, etc. These foods will have to be available only as rewards for eating the good foods, they must not be given to your child at other times, otherwise your child will wait for that time when he/she can get it without any effort. Keep the whole procedure positive and as happy as possible. After your child starts to take one mouthful of a particular food without any trouble, start demanding two mouthfuls of the same food for the same reward. You may spend a few days, a week or even more on the one mouthful stage. In different children it takes different effort. After you have conquered the two mouthfuls, move to three mouthfuls for the same reward. Slowly increase the number of mouthfuls until your child eats the whole meal.

The examples of reward foods which I have given here (chocolate, crisps) are foods which are not allowed on the GAPS Nutritional Programme. However, in the initial stages when you are trying to teach your child the whole ABA concept use whatever works. Once your child has understood the rules of the game move to rewards allowed on the diet. If your autistic child can be motivated by any dessert ideas allowed on the diet, then – hooray! – forget about chocolate and crisps. Apart from favourite foods you can use anything else your child likes as a reward for getting him/her to eat the new food. For example, if your child likes to watch a particular video: put that video on, let it play for 5 minutes, then pause it. Offer your child a mouthful of the food you want to introduce into his diet. Do not switch the video back on again until that mouthful is eaten. Do not give in to tantrums, screaming, crying, etc. When your child has the mouthful, give him/her lavish enthusiastic praise with hugs and kisses and switch the video back on. In a few minutes repeat the procedure again. If your child is not particularly interested in videos, use whatever he/she is interested in – toys, books, games. Obsessive behaviours and self-stimulation generally should not be encouraged in autistic children. However, if that is the only thing that would motivate your child, use them as rewards for eating the right foods.

It is important to work on one food at a time. Do not try to introduce several foods at the same time. Decide for yourself what food is the most important to introduce first into your child's nutrition and work on it. It is sensible to start with foods which you think would be easiest for your child to accept. When you have conquered one or two foods and your child's menu starts growing you will find that introducing consecutive foods becomes easier and easier. In no time at all your child will be having a very nourishing and varied diet.

The important thing is not to get disheartened by the initial resistance from your child, but persevere. Hundreds of parents who have implemented the ABA programme with their children had to go through the initial stage of tantrums to get their children to do anything, from simple "Come here" to more complex things. Nobody can teach a child who does not comply with anything you tell him or her to do. But once you have won that first battle, you have gained your child's compliance, which means that now you have a child whom you can teach!

2. Introducing new foods to GAPS children without language problems

With GAPS children who do not have problems with communication the procedure is similar but much easier. The child has to eat the good food first in order to get what he/she wants: a preferred food, a game, a toy, etc. With these children I would not use non-allowed foods, like chocolate or crisps for rewards. You can use your homemade desserts, allowed on the diet. I am sure that most parents are familiar with the timeless mother's motto: Have your meal first, then you will get your pudding! Apart from that, use more sophisticated rewards like games, toys, trips to the cinema, etc. rather than food rewards.

Just as with autistic children, with other GAPS children it is important to start with small achievable targets, like one mouthful or a small piece of the food. If you try to suddenly introduce a large plateful of food which your child hates, you are going to fail. Once your child will accept a small piece for a reward, slowly move to larger and larger portions. Be patient and consistent! Do not give in to whining, complaining or tantrums! If he/she does not eat the good food, he/she does not get the pudding (or any other reward)! As simple as that! You have to be firm. Once you have asked your child to have the one mouthful of food you cannot back off or allow any negotiations or manipulations. If you allow your child to win on the food issue, you have lost on many other issues!

If your child refused the one mouthful of the good food and does not seem to care that he/she did not get the reward, it means that you have chosen *the wrong reward*! Choose a reward which your child cares enough about to do anything to get it. However, no matter how motivating the reward, never forget to add to it your lavish enthusiastic praise and a hug! Your child has to feel that he/she has done something really good when they had that mouthful of the good food!

In the majority of cases, once the children have had a good taste of a food which they did not touch before they actually start liking it. As their bodily flora starts to improve, a lot of cravings go away and the normal sense of taste returns, so your child will start developing a new liking for different foods. But to start this process off your child needs your help. On his/her own your child is not capable of breaking the vicious cycle of cravings, toxicity and abnormalities in taste. Once your child has a good balanced diet, you can allow him/her not to eat a small number of foods which they particularly dislike. We all have these likes and dislikes. However, make sure that it is within normal proportions.

It is very important to keep the whole process positive! Talk to your child, explain why you want him or her to eat this food, what good it will do in their bodies. Try to talk on this subject at every mealtime using language and phraseology on your child's level and making it fun, a game and a laugh. And when your child complies do not put any limits on your praise or expression of delight! Let your child really feel how happy he or she has made you by eating the good food! Your enthusiasm, combined with the reward, given at the same time, will make this experience something for your child to look forward to, to anticipate with pleasure at the next mealtime.

In conclusion I would say that about 60–70% of parents who come to see me with their children say up front that any idea of introducing any diet into their child's life is impossible! "My child will not eat it!" However, having implemented the ABA principles, which I have described here, most of these parents soon forget just how fussy with food their child used to be. Sitting down to a meal with your family becomes a normal and pleasurable procedure, as it is supposed to be!

5. Failure to Thrive

Failure to thrive is a common phenomenon in GAPS families. An infant with abnormal gut flora can thrive on breast milk. However, when solids are introduced the child instinctively learns that food (apart from breast milk) makes him/her ill. As the unhealthy digestive system cannot handle solids well and absorbs them partially digested, the child may experience many unpleasant symptoms: a tummy ache, muscle ache, itchy skin, headache, drop in energy, etc. So, quite rightly, the infant refuses solids. It is very rare for a child older than six months to get enough nourishment just from breast milk, so without solids the child does not gain weight appropriately or starts losing weight. The diagnosis *failure to thrive* usually follows.

The typical weaning foods (based on grains) are completely inappropriate for these children and must not be given to them. Please, look at the chapter *New Baby* and follow the structured diet for introducing foods described in that chapter. Start with warm homemade meat stock mixed with some probiotic food. Make sure to give the breast only as a reward/top up after your infant had some meat stock with probiotic food from a bottle or a beaker. Your child has to learn that he/she has to eat something before the breast is given. Start with a small achievable target, such as 1–2 teaspoons of the meat stock before the breast is given; gradually increase the amount of the meat stock. Feed every 1–2 hours and choose times when you and your child are calm and happy. Obviously, if your child is distressed for whatever reason, you have to give the breast as a comfort without placing any demands – this is not a good time to try and introduce new foods. The whole experience needs to be calm and happy. As your baby starts consuming good amounts of meat stock with some probiotic food added, gradually introduce all other foods described in the chapter *New Baby*. Keep using your breast milk as a reward for another year or so. It is not common in the Western culture to breastfeed longer than one year. However, these children benefit greatly from breastfeeding for longer: till the age of 18–24 months at least.

6. Eating disorders

If you do not change direction,
you may end up where you are heading!
Lao Tzu,   570–490 BC

Eating disorders are responsible for more loss of life than any other type of mental illness. Both women and men suffer, though undoubtedly women are in a majority: about 90% of eating disorders sufferers are girls between the age of 12 and 25. The statistics vary but generally about 1% of the population is thought to suffer form an eating disorder. Many cases of eating disorders are thought to be unreported and undiagnosed, possibly due to the shame, secrecy and denial associated with these conditions. The incidence is much higher in affluent Western countries than in the rest of the world. There are a number of diagnoses a person with an eating disorder may receive: anorexia nervosa, bulimia nervosa, binge eating disorder, compulsive overeating, etc. But in a majority of patients these different forms can blend into each other, a person can be anorexic for some time then flip into bulimia or have periods of binging. Eating disorders often overlap with other mental problems or can lead to them: ADHD/ADD, obsessive-compulsive disorder, bi-polar disorder, panic attacks, anxiety, substance abuse, alcoholism, schizophrenia, etc.

The official position is that eating disorders are largely psychological in their origin, so treatment focuses on psychotherapy, cognitive therapy, behavioural therapy, family therapy and nutritional counselling. Psychotropic drugs are often used. Support groups, exercise, massage and other therapies are also employed. Nevertheless, the relapse rate is very high: by different estimations it is at least 50%. Many patients believe that they cannot recover from an eating disorder, they can only control it and live in its shadow for the rest of their lives. There is no doubt that psychological factors play a role in developing eating disorders. However, the official position that it is "all in the mind" and that all you have to do is "re-educate the person to eat" without any regard to *what* the person is given to eat, is probably the main reason for relapsing.

To understand the whole picture let us have a look at a case history of a girl, called Hanna (the name has been changed). Her story is very typical.

Hanna was a healthy child until the age of 13: she did well at school, played sports, had friends and was almost never ill. She had never had antibiotics in her life and was breastfed as a baby for a year. At the age of 13 she decided to become a vegetarian, which her parents did not object to. From that point on her diet consisted of breakfast cereals, pasta, rice and a lot of bread and potatoes. However, she was OK because she ate eggs, full cream dairy and peanut butter and was not concerned how much fat was in her food. Around 16 years of age she went to a dancing school, where she was put under pressure to lose weight. In order to lose weight she decided to become a vegan and stopped eating anything with any fat in it. In a matter of few weeks she got glandular fever, which was treated with a long course of antibiotics. The glandular fever lasted a year and Hanna still feels that she has not recovered from this infection fully. From 17 she went through almost constant throat and chest infections, treated with antibiotics. At 18 she went to university, where she decided to become a model, so she had to lose weight again. In order to do that she started taking laxatives and slimming pills. This went on for two years, she became painfully thin, grew very weak physically, was constantly ill with infections and colds, her menstruations stopped, her digestive system was in a poor shape (she developed constipation alternating with diarrhoea, nausea, vomiting, bloating, abdominal pain and indigestion) and she became depressed. The diagnosis of anorexia nervosa followed, Hanna had psychotherapy and counselling. Her problems led to a conflict with her parents, who were desperate to help her, but all their efforts were sabotaged by Hanna. She continued with her very poor diet, laxatives and all sorts of slimming pills. By 19 she felt suicidal and took an overdose of paracetamol. This led to regular hospitalisations in psychiatric facilities, psychiatric medications and repeated suicidal attempts. I first met Hanna at the age of 21 when she had just been released from an anorexia clinic, where she spent 2 months receiving the typical treatment for this condition. At that point she had normal body weight, but looked pale and had a poor complexion. She was taking an antidepressant and an antipsychotic medication. She was still intent on losing weight and was taking laxatives. Her diet was vegetarian and low fat.

Let us discuss this case. In my clinical experience (and I am sure many other health practitioners would agree) a large percentage of girls and boys who develop an eating disorder start from a vegetarian or a vegan type diet. I have no doubt that the fashion for vegetarian and vegan diets is a major cause of mental illness in our young people! Due to all the misinformation about food published relentlessly in popular media, the population at large has been convinced that vegetarianism is healthy. So, when a young girl in the family announces that she has decided to become a vegetarian, the parents usually do not object. As the child stops eating meat and often other animal products, she or he develops serious nutritional deficiencies. The first deficiency is in proteins, as plant foods are very poor sources of protein and whatever protein they do contain is virtually indigestible for the human gut. The best quality and the easiest-to-digest proteins for humans come from animal foods: meats, fish, eggs and dairy products. Protein malnutrition is a very serious matter: the body cannot produce hormones, enzymes, neurotransmitters and a myriad of other active substances, so the functions these substances accomplish suffer. All this is happening in a growing child, who requires a lot of protein in order to build new tissues and new cells. In parallel with protein deficiency the child develops severe deficiency in zinc, because zinc in human diet comes largely from meat, red meat in particular. This mineral is involved in some 200 enzymatic reactions in the body, all of which suffer. There is so much data accumulated now to show that people with eating disorders are severely deficient in zinc, that even our nutrition-dismissive mainstream medicine is considering supplementing it to this group of patients! Low fat diet leads to deficiency in fat-soluble vitamins: A, D, E and K, which means a disaster for all sorts of metabolic functions in the body, particularly for the immune system. Vitamin B group is another deficiency these children develop very quickly, as meats, eggs and other animal products are the main food sources of these nutrients. Vegetarian diets are largely based on carbohydrates, which require a lot of magnesium to be digested and metabolised, so deficiency in magnesium follows. As carbohydrates alter hormonal balance in the body towards too much insulin production, the whole metabolism shifts to a fat-storing mode; losing weight in this mode is very difficult. In fact people who switch to vegetarian diets usually put weight on. Vegan diet is a more extreme form of vegetarianism. As Hanna did initially, at least a vegetarian child eats dairy and eggs, which provide some essential nutrition. A vegan does not eat anything that comes from an animal. Vegan diets in children have been pronounced to be a form of child abuse by some specialists in this area, as indeed they deprive a growing child of most of essential nutrition. I would go further: in my professional opinion a vegan diet is a form of disguised starvation. Due to amounts of carbohydrates consumed the child may not look thin, but its body is starved of all the essential nutrients: the child enters a slippery slide of malnutrition.

What is the typical scenario that happens in children like Hanna, who was perfectly healthy till the age of 13? Here is what I believe happens:

1. Due to inappropriate diet the child develops multiple nutritional deficiencies. Nutritional deficiencies in protein, zinc, fat-soluble vitamins, magnesium, B vitamins and other nutrients lead to immune system dysfunction. The immune system in these patients becomes malnourished and cannot function properly. The result is constant infections. As infections are treated with antibiotics, the damage to gut flora follows, which impairs immune function even further. The vicious cycle of infections and antibiotics brings more infections and more antibiotics; the result – more damage to the immune system and to the gut flora.

2. GAP Syndrome develops where the abnormal gut flora starts producing toxins, which flow through the damaged gut wall into the blood and get distributed around the body. As these toxins get into the brain, they cause problems with mood, behaviour, learning, concentration, memory and sensory perception. It is the sensory perception, namely self-perception, that goes badly wrong in these children who then go on to develop an eating disorder. When an anorexic girl looks in the mirror, she does not see how painfully thin she looks; all she sees is fat and obesity. She is not pretending and she is not "deceiving herself". The reason for that is her altered sense of perception, caused by toxicity in the brain. In this book we have discussed the altered sensory perception in autism and other learning disabilities; the

same thing happens in these children. Just as in babies with failure to thrive, the brain of the child learns on some level that food makes it ill, so the appetite gets suppressed and the whole attitude to food changes. Toxicity coming from the gut blocks various centres in the brain, so they are unable to handle appropriately the sensory information coming from the eyes, ears, taste buds, tactile nerve endings and other sensory organs. This information gets distorted and misinterpreted by the brain. And not only self-perception suffers in children with eating disorders, but other forms of perception as well: perception of taste and texture of food, sense of smell, tactile perception, sense of danger, reading of social situations, perception of human relationships and emotions, perception of right and wrong, perception of important and trivial, etc., etc.

3. Gut degeneration. Abnormal gut flora damage the gut wall, making it porous and "leaky" and unable to fulfil its functions. Gut lining is the site of active cell regeneration: the cells there are constantly shed off and replaced by newly born young cells. In order to produce new cells the body needs healthy gut flora, nutrients and hormones, none of which are available in these patients. So, the gut lining degenerates and is unable to handle food properly. At the same time the gut cannot produce digestive juices and enzymes essential for food digestion and absorption. As a result the person cannot digest and absorb the food properly, which leads to more nutritional deficiencies. Children and adults with eating disorders suffer from digestive problems, which get worse when they are coaxed to eat (pain, bloating, indigestion, constipation, diarrhoea, flatulence, etc.), as their gut is in no fit state to handle food. The typical carbohydrate-based diet given to these patients harms the gut even further: the food does not get digested properly, instead it feeds the pathogenic microbes in the gut allowing them to produce more toxins. Instead of being a source of nourishment the digestive system in these children becomes a major source of toxicity in the body.

4. Hormonal exhaustion. Hormones are proteins. The body cannot build them without a good supply of protein, zinc, magnesium, fat-soluble vitamins, B vitamins and all the other nutrients these

children are deficient in. As hormones rule our metabolism, growth, repair and a myriad of other functions in the body, the child stops growing, menstruations become irregular or stop altogether, sexual development arrests, the child develops poor muscle tone, osteoporosis, fatigue, emotional and behavioural problems, inability to concentrate or learn, sleep problems, skin problems, etc., etc. As mainstream medicine gives no thought to what particular food these children should eat, in eating disorder clinics these children are largely given carbohydrates. As the child is low in hormones, the body cannot use the calories from these carbohydrates, so they get stored as body fat. That is why these children put weight on very quickly as soon as they start eating, which leads to a relapse of the eating disorder as these girls and boys are frightened of putting weight on. So, the idea of mainstream medicine to "get them to eat anything" is not only wrong, but damaging in the long run.

5. GAPS always comes with a craving for carbohydrates, as these patients have swinging blood sugar levels. The patients with eating disorders, even severely anorexic patients, binge on processed carbohydrates: sweets, chocolates, cakes, soft drinks, etc. When the blood sugar level drops they have an irresistible urge to bring it up again. The processed carbohydrates and sugar feed abnormal gut flora and perpetuate the whole problem further or make it worse in the long run. The only way to take cravings under control is through an appropriate diet! And that, in my opinion, is the only way to deal with an eating disorder, be it anorexia, bulimia, compulsive bingeing or any other form.

We have looked at the typical scenario of a healthy normal child becoming a GAPS patient through poor diet. Indeed many children with eating disorders start that way. However, there are many who have been GAPS children from the start. They suffer all the typical GAPS problems all their lives: ADHD/ADD, dyslexia, dyspraxia, with asthma, eczema, allergies and frequent infections. Because they do not receive appropriate treatment, at some stage in their lives their altered sensory perception leads them to an eating disorder.

GAPS treatment of eating disorders

Trying to help a girl (or a boy) with an eating disorder can be extremely difficult. Due to altered self-perception these patients do not see how ill they are and how extreme their physical degeneration is. They are usually intelligent people and use all their cunning to resist help and to sabotage their recovery. They can be quite good at manipulating people around them and assuming a position of a "poor victim" of forceful parents or carers, setting people against each other. Families of these children often go through a hell of constant conflict and confusion, thanks to their child's disorder.

I believe that patients with eating disorders have to start from the GAPS Introduction Diet. Their gut is in very poor shape and needs slow healing. But before we talk about the diet, we need to get the person to eat. And in order to do that we need to overcome the first hurdle – I call it getting to the "Bingo Day" – the day when more or less normal self-perception returns and your patient suddenly realises just how ill and malnourished she or he is.

The first stage of the treatment programme – getting to the "Bingo Day":

The biggest problem is the calorie counting: these patients are afraid of putting weight on. In order to gain their co-operation we have to start with the "low calorie" approach. We start with the homemade meat stock, vegetable soup and well-chosen supplements.

- Meat stock has very little calories. Also it is a liquid, which people with eating disorders are more likely to accept (it is solid food that they are afraid off). Meat stock will provide amino acids, minerals and other nutrients, badly needed by the starved body of the patient, so make the meat stock really rich (from a good piece of meat with a bone or a whole chicken, add good quality salt at the beginning of cooking and some roughly cut vegetables). Get your patient to drink a cup of warm meat stock every hour all day every day. It can be fat free or with as little fat as the patient will accept. Add a teaspoon of homemade whey or yoghurt into every cup (and/or a teaspoon of sauerkraut juice). This remedy will start the healing process in the gut lining.

- Vegetable soup made with homemade meat stock. Please, look in the Introduction Diet for the list of allowed vegetables. Start with quite a liquid soup with little fat in it: it is low calorie and should be acceptable for your patient. Add a teaspoon of homemade whey or yoghurt into every bowl of soup (and/or a teaspoon of sauerkraut juice). Your patient can eat this soup as many times every day as she or he can be persuaded.
- Supplements are essential at this stage in the programme, as they will allow the immune system and the brain to start functioning on a more or less normal platform. Supplements have virtually no calories in them and as a result are usually accepted by the patients without much trouble. Let us discuss the supplements which I believe to be essential.

1. *Full blend of free-form amino acids*, 15–20 g per day. You can get this product from most well-established multi-supplement companies. Our bodies are made out of proteins and are run by proteins. The majority of symptoms of eating disorders are due to extreme protein starvation. Supplying a full blend of amino acids will allow the body to start building the most urgently needed enzymes, neurotransmitters, hormones and other protein compounds. Another big plus of free-form amino acids is that they do not need digesting, they absorb as they are very easily. This is important, as the gut of your patient may not be in a fit state to digest complex proteins and to break them down into much needed amino acids.

2. *Zinc picolinate*, 45–50 mg per day. Zinc deficiency has almost exactly the same symptoms as anorexia nervosa: weight loss, loss of appetite, amenorrhoea, nausea, skin lesions, malabsorption, altered self-perception, depression, anxiety and impotence in males. There have been a plethora of studies done to show that people with eating disorders are severely deficient in zinc and a number of cases of recovery after supplementing zinc have been recorded.

3. *Three more amino acids: tryptophan, glutamine and asparagine*, 500mg of each three times a day. Tryptophan (or 5HTP) is a precursor to serotonin in the body, a calming neurotransmitter very low in eating disorders. Tryptophan molecules are quite large

and have difficulty competing for absorption with other smaller amino acids, that is why it should be taken at different times from the full blend of free-form amino acids. Glutamine will provide the brain with ready fuel and help the brain to clear out toxins. Asparagine along with glutamine is the most commonly found amino acid in the brain. Most people with emotional and behavioural problems have very low levels of asparagine in the body. These three amino acids should be taken together at a different time from the full blend of amino acids. Taking them with some honey will allow them to reach the brain quicker and improve their function. Your patient can have ginger tea with a little honey at this stage in the diet; this will be a good time to take their supplements of tryptophan, glutamine and asparagine.

4. *Supporting nutrients: full vitamin B blend, vitamin C, calcium, magnesium, iron and iodine*, in standard daily doses. These nutrients act as co-factors for the amino acids and zinc.

This stage of the treatment will start nourishing your patient in the most urgently needed nutrients. As the most severe deficiencies start melting away, the "Bingo Day" will come: your patient will wake up one morning, look in the mirror and suddenly realise just how emaciated she or he looks. That means that normal self-perception has started to return and from this point on you can start really feeding her or him. Move to the second stage.

Second stage:

• Introduce meats immediately, red meats in particular. All meats should be introduced: lamb, beef, game, duck, goose, pork, chicken, turkey, etc. Cooking them very well in water will make them easier for your patient to digest. It is vital to introduce organ meats as soon as possible: liver and hearts in particular. You can grind them after cooking and start adding them in small amount into soups, so your patient is not alarmed too much. Introduce meats gradually and together with soups: as your patient's digestive system starts recovering she or he will be able to digest increasing amounts of meat.

- Start adding a teaspoon of homemade sauerkraut (or fermented vegetables) into every bowl of soup (you have been adding the juice from sauerkraut before now), it will help your patient to digest meat.
- It is a good idea to use digestive enzymes at this stage, as your patient's digestive system may not be in a fit state to digest protein food. Give your patient 1 capsule of Betaine HCl or HCl&Pepsin at the beginning of the meal and a full blend of pancreatic enzymes at the end of the meal, 1–2 capsules.
- Introduce raw egg yolks added to soups and cups of meat stock. Start with one egg yolk a day and quite quickly increase to 6–10 egg yolks per day (the more the better).
- Make the soups thicker and richer with more and more fat left in. Blending the soup will allow you to keep more fat in; the fat will mix with the blended vegetables and will not be visible.
- Introduce good quality cod liver oil, preferably fermented, 2 teaspoons per day with food or after food (or an equivalent in capsules). It is a good idea to start with a few drops of the oil per day and gradually increase the amount.
- Continue with cups of meat stock with some probiotic food added.
- Continue with ginger tea with a little honey. Let your patient take the three amino acids at the same time (tryptophan, glutamine and asparagine).
- Continue with all the supplements from the first stage.

Next stage:

- Please, look at the GAPS Introduction Diet and follow the stages one by one (by now we have reached the third stage).
- When the full dose of cod liver oil is reached (2 teaspoons per day), gradually introduce good quality fish oil with some evening primrose oil added.
- Gradually introduce a good quality probiotic.
- Continue with all the supplements until the end of the GAPS Introduction Diet. When your patient is on the Full GAPS Diet, slowly reduce the dose of the full blend of amino acids to 1–2 g per day, and gradually reduce zinc supplement to 10–15 mg per day.

Continue with the three amino acids and the supporting nutrients for another 3–4 months at the same doses.

- When on the Full GAPS Diet, reduce the daily dose of cod liver oil to one teaspoon per day.
- As your patient recovers you will be able to slowly remove most supplements, apart from cod liver oil and probiotics, which should be taken for a few years.

Continue with the GAPS Nutritional Protocol for a few years. It is possible that your patient will need to adhere to the Full GAPS Diet more or less for most of her or his life, particularly in the case of other mental problems present (such as bi-polar disorder, ADHD, obsessive-compulsive disorder, schizophrenia, epilepsy and chronic anxiety).

The majority of GAPS children are fussy eaters (due to abnormal sensory perception), that is why we use the behaviour modification techniques in introducing foods into their diet, which work very well with small children. In eating disorders we are dealing with teenagers or grown-up children, who are always more difficult to treat. Nevertheless, please read the chapter *It's feeding time. Oh no!*, it may give you an insight into why your daughter or son is behaving the way they do around food and how to go about helping them.

In conclusion:

In my opinion eating disorders are GAPS conditions and should be treated accordingly. As we normalise the gut flora in these patients the flow of toxins from the gut to the brain stops, so the brain is able to function normally again and normal sensory perception returns. At the same time the GAPS diet will heal the gut and nourish the person, so their bodies can start functioning again. It is important to stick to the diet for a few years for this group of patients, because if they start eating processed carbohydrates and junk food again too soon, they are likely to relapse. Once the full recovery has taken place, on an occasional basis they can eat whatever they want, as long as most of the time they make sure to feed their bodies well with the GAPS type diet.

Supplementation for Children and Adults with GAP Syndrome

We all love our small or grown up children very much and we are prepared to do our best for them, no matter how difficult or expensive it might be. That makes us vulnerable to try anything and everything in the hope that it will help our children. I meet family after family who give their child 10, 15, 20 or more of various nutritional supplements without any idea if any of them are doing any good. Nutritional supplements are expensive and the market is full of hundreds of various brands. Many of them have questionable quality and the whole industry is not regulated very well.

I cannot emphasise enough that an appropriate diet has to be the number one intervention in successful nutritional management of the GAPS child or adult. No pill in the world is going to come close to the effect of the diet on your patient's condition. When it comes to digestive disorders in particular, and GAP Syndrome is essentially a digestive disorder, we have to be very careful what we introduce into the gut of the patient. Why? Because a lot of supplements may irritate an already inflamed and damaged gut lining and interfere with the healing process. You do not want to put a lot of effort into implementing the diet and then spoil the whole process by a pill.

However, some supplements can be very beneficial and some are essential. The supplementation protocol has to be very individual and ideally should be worked out by a qualified practitioner. Here we are going to concentrate on absolute essentials. A majority of my patients progress very well with the use of diet and these essential supplements without adding anything else.

The essential supplements for GAPS patients:

1. An effective therapeutic strength probiotic.
2. Essential fatty acids.
3. Cod liver oil.
4. Digestive enzymes.
5. Vitamin and mineral supplements.

Let us have a good look at each of these supplements.

1. Probiotics

Probiotics are the beneficial bacteria in the form of a nutritional supplement or fermented food, which can be taken in an attempt to replace or supplement damaged indigenous flora. Contrary to antibiotic meaning "against life" probiotic means "pro-life" or "for-life".

The use of probiotic bacteria in the form of fermented foods goes back to pre-Christian times. For thousands of years people fermented milk, fruit and vegetables, beans, fish, meats and cereals. Fermenting food improves its taste, makes food more digestible and preserves it. Today many cultures around the world routinely consume beneficial bacteria in fermented foods: sauerkraut – fermented cabbage (Russia, Germany and Eastern Europe), table olives and salami or fermented meat (Mediterranean countries), kefir (Russia), mazun (Armenia), kumiss (Russia and Asia), lassi (India), gioddu (Sardinia), yoghurt and cheese (all over the world), fermented fish (Korea, Sweden, Japan, Russia), fermented grains (Africa) and fermented soy beans (Asia).

A Russian scientist, Ilia Metchnikoff, at the beginning of the 20th century put the subject of probiotics on a scientific basis. Working at the Pasteur Institute in Paris Metchnikoff noticed that country people in Bulgaria regularly consumed fermented milk products and lived to an unusually great age in good health. He isolated a bacterium, which he called "Bulgarian bacillus" and used it in his scientific trials. Today this bacterium is known as *Lactobacillus bulgaricus* and is widely used in yoghurt production. Following his discovery, the use of *Lactobacillus bulgaricus* as a health supplement became very popular in European countries. When antibiotics came along the probiotics were largely forgotten. However, after Metchnikoff's death in 1916 his research was continued in various countries around the world. In Russia, Scandinavia and Japan probiotic bacteria have been in use as a treatment for humans for decades. In the West the probiotics were used mainly in farm animal feed and a lot of scientific data has been collected about their health-giving properties for the animals. In the last couple of decades the use of probiotics for humans has become popular again and we have started to see more and more scientific publications on this subject. The scope of disorders where probiotics have been successfully used as part of treatment is rapidly growing.

Naturally the biggest use of probiotics we have seen is in the treatment of gastro-intestinal disorders:

- viral infections of the digestive tract
- necrotising enterocolitis in infants
- intractable paediatric diarrhoea
- pseudomembranous colitis
- traveller's diarrhoea
- *Clostridium difficile* enterocolitis
- *Helicobacter* infection
- enteropathogenic *E.coli* infection
- inflammatory bowel disorders: Crohn's disease, ulcerative colitis and chronic pouchitis
- irritable bowel syndrome
- lactose intolerance
- prevention of colonic cancer in laboratory studies

In many cases, adding probiotics to the treatment regimen not only improved the clinical picture but also cured the condition.

Apart from digestive problems many other health problems have been shown to respond to treatment with probiotics:

- allergies, including food allergy
- autism
- chronic viral infections
- urogenital infections
- hepatitis, liver cirrhosis and biliary disease
- tuberculosis
- meningitis
- malignancy
- arthritis
- diabetes
- burns of various degree
- perioperative care and intensive care in surgical patients and patients with massive blood loss

- clinical infections
- autoimmune disorders

These are only the conditions about which scientific papers have been published. But, if you talk to any doctor or practitioner with experience in using probiotics, this list becomes much longer.

So, what bacteria do we consider to be probiotic?

1. **Lactobacilli**   This is a large family of bacteria, which produce lactic acid – hence their name. Most commonly known members of this family are *L. acidophilus, L. bulgaricus, L. rhamnosus, L. plantarum, L. salivarius, L. reuteri, L. johnsonii, L. casei* and *L. delbrueskii. Lactobacilli* are normal and essential inhabitants of the human gut, mucous membranes of the mouth, throat, nose and upper respiratory tract, vagina and genital area. They are found in large numbers in human breast milk. *Lactobacilli* get established in the body of a newborn baby in the first few days and form a complex relationship with the host for the rest of his/her life. By producing lactic acid they maintain acidic environment (pH 5.5–5.6) on mucous membranes, which suppresses the growth of pathogenic microbes. Apart from lactic acid they produce a plethora of active substances: hydrogen peroxide – a powerful antiseptic; anti-bacterial, anti-viral and anti-fungal agents, which do not allow pathogens to get a hold in the gut. *Lactobacilli* engage the immune system and stimulate activity of neutrophils, macrophages, synthesis of immuno-globulins, alpha and beta interferons, interleukin-1 and tumour necrosis factor. They are involved in orchestrating the cell renewal process in the gut, keeping the gut lining healthy and intact. They are the most numerous inhabitants of the stomach and intestines and the main protecting agents in those parts of the digestive system. *Lactobacilli* were the first probiotic bacteria to be studied and to be used as a supplement to benefit health. Indeed *Lactobacilli* are the most common bacteria in commercially available probiotics today.

2. **Bifidobacteria**   Most commonly known species are *B. bifidum, B. breve, B. longum and B. infantis*, though there are around 30 different species identified. This is a large family of probiotic bacteria,

which are most numerous in the human bowel, lower intestines, vagina and genital area. 90–98% of all bacteria living in the bowel of a healthy baby are *Bifidobacteria*. In an adult gut they are about seven times more numerous than *Lactobacilli* and fulfil many useful functions. Apart from producing different antibiotic-like substances which protect the gut from pathogens, engaging the immune system, maintaining gut integrity and health, they act as a source of nourishment for the body. *Bifidobacteria* actively synthesise amino acids, proteins, organic acids, vitamin K, pantothenic acid, vitamin B1 (thiamin), Vitamin B2 (riboflavin), vitamin B3 (niacin), folic acid, vitamin B6 (pyridoxine), vitamin B12 (cobalamin), assist absorption of Ca, iron and vitamin D. *Bifidobacteria* are the second most numerous family of bacteria in probiotic supplements available on the market.

3. ***Saccharomyces boulardii***   This is a yeast first discovered by a French scientist, H. Boulard, in 1920. He observed that people in China treated diarrhoea with an extract from lychee fruit. He found the yeast in this extract, which was named *Saccharomyces boulardii*. Supplementing this yeast has been found to be effective in treating various forms of diarrhoea in children and adults. Recently there has been a lot of interest in using *S. boulardii* as an antagonist to a pathogenic yeast – *Candida albicans*.

4. ***Escherichia coli* or *E. coli***   *E. coli* is a large family of bacteria. Pathogenic members of this family can cause serious infections. However, physiological strains of *E. coli* are normal and numerous inhabitants of healthy human gut. They normally occupy particular areas of the digestive system: the bowel and lower parts of the intestines and should not be found anywhere else. If they are found in the mouth, stomach or duodenum that indicates an abnormality in gut ecology – Gut Dysbiosis. Physiological strains of *E. coli* fulfil a number of beneficial functions in the body: they digest lactose, produce vitamins (vitamin K and group B) and amino acids, produce antibiotic-like substances, called colicins, and have a powerful stimulating influence on local and systemic immunity. They are very active against various pathogenic microbes, including pathogenic members of their own family. Indeed having your gut populated by physiological strains of *E.*

coli is the best insurance against succumbing to pathogenic strains of *E. coli*. That is what German physician Alfred Nissle found in 1917 when he was trying to find out why some soldiers in the First World War did not fall prey to typhoid, when most of their comrades were ill. He identified a particular strain of *E. coli* in the stools of these soldiers, which was named the Nissle strain. He grew this bacterium and sealed it in gelatine capsules. After trying this product on himself he started manufacturing it under the name Mutaflor. Mutaflor is still available on the market. Some other physiological strains of *E. coli* have been studied and are used in some commercial probiotic formulas around the world.

5. ***Enterococcus faecium* or *Streptococcus faecalis*** As the name implies these bacteria, as with many other probiotics, were isolated from human stools. They normally live in the bowel where they control pathogens by producing hydrogen peroxide and reducing pH to 5.5. They break down proteins and ferment carbohydrates. There are a number of clinical studies showing that they are effective in treating various forms of diarrhoea. These bacteria are quite common in probiotic formulas on the market.

6. ***Bacillus subtilis* or soil bacteria** *Bacillus subtilis* was first discovered by German microbiologists during the Second World War, which led to the use of this micro-organism in protecting German troops from dysentery and typhoid. After the war *Bacillus subtilis* was extensively studied in Germany, Russia, Italy, Finland, Eastern Europe, China and Vietnam. A number of subspecies were identified: *B. licheniformis, B. cereus, B. brevis, B. mesentericus, B. pumilis*, etc., most of which were shown to be therapeutic in animals and then in humans. This led to the development of a range of products with *B. subtilis* for animal use. For humans there are number of products with *B. subtilis* which have been used by doctors in Russia, Germany, Italy, Eastern Europe, Japan, Vietnam and China for decades. *B. subtilis* is a spore-forming microbe and is resistant to stomach acid, most antibiotics, temperature changes and other influences. It has strong immune-stimulating properties and is considered particularly effective with allergies and autoimmune disorders. It produces a whole host of digestive enzymes, anti-viral, anti-fungal, anti-bacterial and other active substances. Soil bacte-

ria are not indigenous to humans, they are transitional microbes, which do not colonise the gut but go through it doing a lot of work on the way. We humans used to consume soil bacteria in large amounts when we were drinking water from wells and streams. In the process of evolution the human gut has developed a need for these transitional bacteria. One possible need is keeping the gut clean. *B. subtilis* species are used in waste management because they have a great ability to break down rotting matter and to suppress putrefactive microbes. By clearing out old putrefaction in the gut soil bacteria may lay the ground for re-establishment of normal gut flora. In my experience, probiotics which contain soil bacteria are the most effective probiotics on the market.

The market offers a wide range of probiotic products from probiotic drinks to powder, tablet and capsule forms. Unfortunately, many of them are not strong enough or do not contain strong enough species of bacteria to be of therapeutic benefit. There is also a problem of quality control. One of the *Which* magazine reports showed that many brands of probiotics on the market do not have bacterial species listed on the label or do not have a claimed bacterial strength. So, how do we choose a good probiotic?

First of all, it always makes sense to work with a qualified practitioner with experience in using probiotics who will help you to choose good quality supplements. If you are trying to choose a probiotic yourself, then there are some general guidelines to follow.

1. A good probiotic should have as many different species of beneficial bacteria as possible. A human gut contains hundreds of known species of different bacteria. We should try to get as close to that as we can. Different species of probiotic bacteria have different strengths and weaknesses. If we have a mixture of them then we have a better chance of deriving maximum benefit.

2. A mixture of strains from different groups of probiotic bacteria is more beneficial than just one group. For example, many probiotics on the market contain just *Lactobacilli*. A combination of representatives from the three main groups: *Lactobacilli, Bifidobacteria* and soil bacteria usually works best.

3. A good probiotic should have a concentrated amount of bacteria: at least 8 billion of bacterial cells per gram. You need to provide probiotic bacteria in large enough doses to see an improvement.
4. The manufacturer of the probiotic should test every batch for strength and bacterial composition and should be prepared to publish the results of testing.

Once you have found a good probiotic you need to know how to use it. A good therapeutic strength probiotic will always produce a so-called "die-off reaction". What is it? As you introduce probiotic bacteria into a digestive system, they start destroying pathogenic bacteria, viruses and fungi. When these pathogens die they release toxins. These are the toxins which made your patient autistic or schizophrenic or hyperactive. So, whatever characteristic symptoms the patient has may temporarily get worse. Your patient may also feel more tired than usual, generally "off-colour", or develop a skin rash. It is a temporary reaction and usually lasts from a few days to a few weeks in different individuals. To make this reaction as mild as possible, build the dose of your probiotic slowly. Start with a very small amount. Observe the patient for any "die-off" symptoms. If there are none, then increase the dose. When you see a reaction, let your patient settle on this dose until the "die-off" symptoms disappear. Then increase the dose again and let the patient settle on it. Keep on increasing the dose until a therapeutic level is reached. This period of building up the dose can take from a few weeks to a few months in different patients. It is very individual and depends on how much overgrowth of pathogenic microbes the person has in the gut.

The therapeutic dose level of probiotic is individual and your health practitioner should be able to help you with that. Here are general guidelines:

An adult should have around 15–20 billion of bacterial cells per day.
An infant up to 12 months of age can have 1–2 billion of bacterial cells per day.
A toddler from 1 to 2 years of age can have 2–4 billion of bacterial cells per day.
A child from 2 to 4 years of age can handle 4–8 billion of bacterial cells per day.

A child from 4 to 10 years of age can have 8–12 billion of bacterial cells per day.

From the age of 12 to 16 we can increase the dose to 12–15 billion per day.

Once the patient has reached the therapeutic dose level it should be maintained for around six months on average. It takes at least this length of time to remove the pathogenic flora and start re-establishing normal gut flora. Adhering to the diet is absolutely essential in this period. If you carry on feeding your pathogens in the gut with sugar and processed carbohydrates then the probiotic will not have much chance of helping you.

After the therapeutic period is over the dose of the probiotic can be reduced to a maintenance dose level, which the patient has to adhere to for many years. It is important to reduce the dose as gradually as you have been increasing it. Observe any reactions in this period. The maintenance dose is very individual. Usually it is half of the therapeutic dose. In some cases the patient's maintenance dose is the same as the therapeutic.

A lot of patients ask: Why do we have to have the maintenance dose? In other words why do we have to carry on taking the probiotic? The reason is this: we have been designed by Nature to have these bacteria every day with every mouthful of food or drink. We have changed our environment, water and food to such a degree that we are depriving our bodies of these vital bacteria. For people who have good, healthy resident gut flora it may not present a big problem. However, for patients with GAP Syndrome it is a big problem. For GAPS people it is particularly vital to consume probiotic bacteria every day of their lives, because they do not possess their own. Their gut has been populated by pathogens instead of beneficial bacteria, and these pathogens are extremely difficult to drive out because they occupy different niches in the gut. To get into any of those niches the beneficial bacteria have to fight quite a battle. In fact, probably the only time in our lives we have to populate our gut with beneficial bacteria is at birth, when the gut is sterile. Unfortunately most supplemental probiotics do not settle or colonise on the gut wall. They do their work in the lumen of the gut and then come out of the system. We have not yet found a way to replace the pathogens on the gut wall with beneficial bacteria. So, patients with GAP syndrome need to carry on taking probiotic indefinitely. To maintain the probiotic you do not have to carry on taking commercial preparations. You can supplement your diet with fermented foods in the form of homemade yoghurt, kefir, sauerkraut and other homemade fermented foods.

One of the concerns about probiotic bacteria is that many of them do not survive the stomach acid. Patients with GAP Syndrome usually have low stomach acidity, so this is not a big problem for them. But to make sure that your probiotic survives the stomach acid the general rule is to take it with food or after food, when most stomach acid is bound to food particles. Some manufacturers put an enteric coating on their probiotic capsules to protect them from stomach acid. I do not support this practice for two reasons. First, the stomach needs probiotic bacteria just as much as any other part of your digestive system. In a stomach with low acidity all sorts of pathogens grow on the stomach walls. We need probiotics to deal with these pathogens. Second, patients with digestive abnormalities are often not able to break down the enteric coating on capsules. These capsules go in and out almost unchanged without doing any good.

Perhaps not all bacterial species in your probiotic will survive the stomach acid. But, an important point to make here is that even dead the probiotic bacteria will do a lot of good in your gut. Their cell walls contain substances to stimulate immune response and they will also absorb toxins, removing them from the body. A lot of food manufacturers have picked up on this fact and are planning to start adding dead probiotic bacteria into various foods.

In conclusion, probiotic supplementation is absolutely vital for treating any of the GAPS conditions. Even in those cases where the patient does not present with severe digestive problems, I find that with the use of diet and probiotics a considerable improvement can be achieved.

2. Fats: the Good and the Bad

A human brain is about 60% fat (dry weight). Every membrane of every cell and every organelle inside of cells are made of fats. Many hormones, neurotransmitters and other active substances in the body are made of fats. Fats are extremely important in our diet. The question is what fats?

There has been a great deal of conflicting information and misinformation about fats. In our modern society fats have been pronounced evil and an industry has sprung up to produce an abundance of low fat and no fat products. Animal fats, including those in meats, butter and eggs, have been blamed for all sorts of ills, so industry again has been quick to provide us with synthetic substitutes, butter replacements and spreads. People heard that vegetable oils are better for you, so a variety of different vegetable oils have become the cooking oils instead of traditionally used lard, goose fat and pork dripping. What the public does not know is how all these processed oils and fats are made, what exactly they contain and what effect they have on human health.

Processed fats

Vegetable oils, cooking oils, margarines, butter replacements, spreadable butter, hydrogenated oils, shortenings and many other artificial fats are processed; they are alien to human physiology and must not be consumed by anybody, let along GAPS patients. You can find processed fats and oils in most processed foods: breads and pastries, pre-prepared meals, crisps, snacks, chocolates, ice cream, biscuits, cakes, takeaway meals, condiments, mayonnaise, etc. The basis of most processed fats is vegetable oils, extracted from seeds and plant matter (corn, soy, sunflower seeds, rapeseed, etc.). They are cheap to produce and are very profitable for the food industry. In their natural state these oils have very unstable unsaturated fatty acids, which are easily damaged by heat, oxygen, pressure and light. In the process of extraction very high temperatures, pressure and various chemicals are employed, which change the chemical structure of fragile fatty acids in the natural seeds and plants creating a plethora of unnatural harmful fatty acids. These oils are then sold as cooking oils in large bottles in all the supermarkets. Due to decades of relentless advertising and propaganda these oils have replaced the natural animal fats which people have used in cooking for millennia.

To make vegetable oils solid and to increase their shelf life they are hydrogenated. Hydrogenation is a process of adding hydrogen molecules to the chemical structure of oils under high pressure at a high temperature (120–210°C or 248–410°F) in the presence of nickel, aluminium and sometimes other toxic metals. Remnants of these metals stay in the hydrogenated oils. Nickel and aluminium are both toxic metals, adding to the general toxic load which the body has to work hard to get rid of. Toxic metals have been linked to many degenerative conditions, including learning disabilities, Alzheimer's disease and dementia.

Processing changes the chemical structure of the natural oils producing a whole host of very harmful fats. Many of these changed fats have not been studied very well yet and we don't know what havoc they can wreck in the body. But a group called trans fats have received a great deal of attention. These are unsaturated fatty acids, beneficial for us in a natural state, whose chemical structure has been changed through processing. Trans fatty acids are very similar in their structure to their natural counterparts, but they are somewhat "back to front". Because of their similarity they occupy the place of essential fats in the body while being unable to do their jobs. Because of that they make cells disabled in a way. All organs and tissues in the body get affected. For example, trans fats have great immune-suppressing ability, playing a detrimental role in many different functions of the immune system. They have been implicated in diabetes, atherosclerosis, cancer, neurological and psychiatric conditions. They interfere with pregnancy, normal production of hormones, ability of insulin to respond to glucose and ability of enzymes and other active substances to do their jobs and have damaging effects on liver and kidneys. A breastfeeding mother would have trans fats in her milk fairly quickly after ingesting a helping of a "healthy" butter replacement. A baby's brain has a high percentage of unsaturated fatty acids. Trans fats would replace them and interfere with the brain development. Trans fats are so harmful that there is simply no safe limit for them established. And yet a packet of crisps will provide you with about 6 grams, a snack packet of processed cheese or cheese biscuits (mainly advertised to children) will provide 8 grams of trans fats, a tablespoon of a common margarine will give you 4–6 grams, a portion of French fries, cooked in vegetable oil, will serve you with 8–9 grams of trans fats. It is estimated that an average intake of trans fatty acids in the Western diet can be as high as 50 grams a day. This is a few times more than our consumption of other unnatural substances in foods. Given their ability to impair bodily functions on the most basic biochemical levels, there is no doubt that the role of trans fats in our modern epidemics of degenerative disease is greatly underestimated.

I would like to repeat that no processed fats are allowed on GAPS diet: all common cooking and vegetable oils, hydrogenated oils, margarines, spreads, vegetarian fats and shortenings, butter replacements and spreadable butter. This means that all processed foods are out, as processed fats are one of the main ingredients of processed foods.

What fats are good for GAPS patients? First things first!

The most important fats for GAPS patients, which should be consumed daily and which should constitute the bulk of all fat consumption, are animal fats: fats in fresh meats, fats rendered from meats, dairy fats (butter, cream and ghee) and fats in egg yolks. Animal fats contain largely saturated and monounsaturated fatty acids.

I almost hear you asking a number of very common questions: What about the "deadly" saturated fats? Don't they cause heart disease? Aren't animal fats all saturated? This is the result of the relentless efforts made by the food industry to fight their competition. What is their competition? The natural fats, of course. There is not much profit to be made from the natural fats, while processed oils and fats bring very good profits. So, it is in the food industry's interest to convince everybody that natural fats are harmful for health, while their processed fats, hydrogenated and cooking oils are good for us. We have been subjected to this propaganda for almost a century now; no wonder that many of us have succumbed to it.

The saturated fats in particular were singled out by the food industry. How did that happen? Dr Mary Enig, an international expert in
lipid biochemistry, explained: "In the late 1950s, an American
researcher, Ancel Keys, announced that the heart disease epidemic was
being caused by the hydrogenated vegetable fats; previously this same
person had introduced the idea that saturated fat was the culprit. The
edible oil industry quickly responded to this perceived threat to their
products by mounting a public relations campaign to promote the
belief that it was only the saturated fatty acid component in the hydrogenated oils that was causing the problem... From that time on, the
edible fats and oils industry promoted the twin idea that saturates
(namely animal and dairy fats) were troublesome, and polyunsaturates
(mainly corn oil and later soybean oil) were health-giving."

The wealthy food giants spend billions on employing an army of
"scientists" to provide them with "scientific proof" of their claims. In
the meantime the real science was, and is, providing us with the truth.
However, it is the food giants who have the money to advertise their
"science" in all the popular media. Real science is too poor to spend
money on that. As a result, the population hears only what the
commercial powers want them to hear.

So, what is the truth? What does the real science tell us?

1. Processed fats, hydrogenated fats and cooking vegetable oils cause
    atherosclerosis, heart disease and cancer. This is a fact, proven
    overwhelmingly by real, honest science.
2. Animal fats have nothing to do with heart disease, atherosclerosis
    and cancer. Our human physiology needs these fats; they are
    important for us to eat on a daily basis.
3. Saturated fats are heart protective: they lower the Lp(a) in the blood
    (Lp(a) is a very harmful substance which initiates atherosclerosis in
    blood vessels), reduce calcium deposition in the arteries and are the
    preferred source of energy for the heart muscle. Saturated fats
    enhance our immune system, protect us from infections and are
    essential for the body to be able to utilise the unsaturated omega-3
    and omega-6 fatty acids. One of the most saturated fats that Nature
    has provided is coconut oil. It has been shown to be wonderfully
    healthy and therapeutic in most degenerative conditions.

4. Animal fats contain a variety of different fatty acids, not just satu-
    rated ones (M.G. Enig, 2000). Pork fat is 45% monounsaturated,
    11% polyunsaturated and 44% saturated. Lamb fat is 38%
    monounsaturated, 2% polyunsaturated and 58% saturated. Beef
    fat is 47% monounsaturated, 4% polyunsaturated and 49% satu-
    rated. Butter is 30% monounsaturated, 4% polyunsaturated and
    52% saturated. This is the natural composition of animal fats and
    our bodies use every bit, including the saturated part. If you want
    to understand how important every bit of the animal fat is for us,
    let us have a look at the composition of human breast milk. The
    fat portion of the breast milk is 48% saturated, 33% monounsatu-
    rated and 16% polyunsaturated. Our babies thrive beautifully on
    this composition of fats, and the largest part of it is saturated.
5. We need all of the natural fats in natural foods, and saturated and
    monounsaturated fats need to be the largest part of our fat intake.
6. The simplistic idea that eating fat makes you fat is completely
    wrong. Consuming processed carbohydrates causes obesity.
    Dietary fats go into the structure of your body: your brain, bones,
    muscles, immune system, etc. – every cell in the body is made out
    of fats to a large degree.

These are the facts which honest science has provided. Unfortunately,
as already mentioned, most of us do not hear about the discoveries of
honest science. Spreading any information in this world costs money.
So, the population at large mostly gets information that serves somebody with a fat wallet. In order to get the real, true information on any
subject, we have to search for it, rather than relying on the "news" and
"scientific breakthroughs" unleashed on us by the popular media.

I would like to draw your attention to the fat composition of human
breast milk again: it is 48% saturated, 33% monounsaturated and 16%
polyunsaturated. Mother Nature does not do anything without good
reason! Human breast milk is the best and the only suitable food for a
human baby! Human physiology does not change as babies grow, so
our requirements for a particular fat composition in food stay about
the same throughout our lives: 48% saturated, 33% monounsaturated
and 16% polyunsaturated. This is what we need, this is how we were
designed by Mother Nature! The only dietary foods that provide us

with this composition of fats are animal products: meats, eggs and dairy; and these are the foods that should provide us with the bulk of all fats we consume.

Fats which plants contain have a very different fatty acid composition, they are largely polyunsaturated. Polyunsaturated fatty acids are very fragile, they are easily damaged by heat, light and oxygen. That is why Mother Nature has locked them up and protected them very well in the complex cellular structure of seeds and nuts. When we eat seeds and nuts in their whole natural state we get those fatty acids in their natural state, unchanged and beneficial to health. When we extract oils from seeds and nuts in our big factories, we damage fragile polyunsaturated fatty acids and make them harmful to health. But the most important point is this: when we consume whole natural seeds and nuts, we get their polyunsaturated oils *in small amounts*, amounts which are compatible with our human physiology: we do not need a lot of polyunsaturated fats, the bulk of our fat consumption should be saturated and monounsaturated fatty acids. When we consume vegetable and cooking oils, we consume their polyunsaturated fatty acids in excess, far too much for healthy human physiology. It is excessive omega-6 polyunsaturated fatty acids from vegetable and cooking oils that are to a large degree causing an epidemic of inflammatory degenerative conditions in our modern world, from heart disease and various autoimmune problems to cancer.

What about cholesterol?

When we talk about animal fats, a question about cholesterol invariably comes up, because everybody has heard about cholesterol "clogging up your arteries" and "causing heart disease". This idea came from **the diet-heart hypothesis**, first proposed in 1953. Since then this hypothesis has been proven to be completely wrong by hundreds of scientific studies. George Mann, eminent American physician and scientist, called the diet-heart hypothesis "the greatest scientific deception of this century, perhaps of any century". Why? Because while the science was working on proving the hypothesis wrong, the medical, political and scientific establishments have fully committed to it. To admit that they were wrong would do too much damage to their reputation, so they are not in a hurry to do that. In the meantime their closed ranks give complete freedom to the commercial companies to exploit the diet-heart hypothesis to their advantage. Their relentless propaganda through the popular media insures long life for the faulty diet-heart hypothesis. Please, read about it in detail in my book *Put your heart in your mouth. What really causes heart disease and how to prevent and even reverse it.*

Thanks to the promoters of the diet-heart hypothesis, everybody "knows" that cholesterol is "evil" and has to be fought at every turn. If you believe the popular media you would think that there is simply no level of cholesterol low enough.

The truth is that we humans cannot live without cholesterol. Let us see why?

Every cell of every organ in our bodies has cholesterol as a part of its structure. Cholesterol is an integral and very important part of our cell membranes; the membranes that make the cell wall and the walls of all organelles inside the cells. And we are not talking about a few molecules of cholesterol here and there. In many cells, almost half of the cell wall is made from cholesterol. Different kinds of cells in the body need different amounts of cholesterol, depending on their function and purpose. The human brain is particularly rich in cholesterol: around 25% of all body cholesterol is taken by the brain. Every cell and every structure in the brain and the rest of our nervous system needs cholesterol, not only to build itself but also to accomplish its many functions. The developing brain and eyes of the foetus and a newborn infant require large amounts of cholesterol. If the foetus doesn't get enough cholesterol during development the child may be born with a congenital abnormality called a cyclopean eye (Strauss 1998). Human breast milk provides a lot of cholesterol. Not only that, mother's milk provides a specific enzyme to allow the baby's digestive tract to absorb almost 100% of that cholesterol, because the developing brain and eyes of an infant require large amounts of it. Children deprived of enough cholesterol in infancy end up with poor eyesight and brain function. Manufacturers of infant formulas are aware of this fact, but following the anti-cholesterol dogma, they produce formulas with virtually no cholesterol in them.

One of the most abundant materials in the brain and the rest of our nervous system is a fatty substance called myelin. Myelin coats every nerve cell and every nerve fibre like an insulating cover around electric wires. Apart from insulation, it provides nourishment and protection for every tiny structure in our brain and the rest of the nervous system. People who start losing their myelin develop a condition called multiple sclerosis. Well, 20% of myelin is cholesterol. If you start interfering with the supply of cholesterol in the body, you put the very structure of the brain and the rest of the nervous system under threat. The synthesis of myelin in the brain is tightly connected with the synthesis of cholesterol. GAPS people often test positive for the same antibodies against myelin, as people with multiple sclerosis. Due to these antibodies both groups of patients have ongoing damage to their myelin in the brain and the rest of the nervous system. In order to rebuild myelin their bodies require a lot of cholesterol. In my clinical experience, foods with high cholesterol and high animal fat content are an essential medicine for people with GAPS and multiple sclerosis.

One of the most wonderful abilities we humans are blessed with is an ability to remember things – our human memory. How do we form memories? By our brain cells establishing connections with each other, called synapses. The more healthy synapses a person's brain can make, the more mentally able and intelligent that person is. Scientists have discovered that synapse formation is almost entirely dependant on cholesterol, which is produced by the brain cells in a form of apolipoprotein E. Without the presence of this factor we cannot form synapses, and hence we would not be able to learn or remember anything. Memory loss is one of the side effects of cholesterol-lowering drugs. In my clinic I see growing numbers of people with memory loss who have been taking "cholesterol pills". Dr Duane Graveline, MD, former NASA scientist and astronaut, suffered such memory loss while taking his "cholesterol pill". He managed to save his memory by stopping the pill and eating lots of cholesterol-rich foods. Since then he has described his experience in his book *Lipitor – Thief of Memory, Statin Drugs and the Misguided War on Cholesterol.* Dietary cholesterol in fresh eggs and other cholesterol-rich foods has been shown in scientific trials to improve memory in the elderly. In my clinical experience, any person with memory loss or learning problems needs to have plenty of these foods every single day in order to recover.

Let us see which foods are rich in cholesterol.

1. Caviar is the richest source; it provides 588mg of cholesterol per
    100g. Obviously, this is not a common food for the majority of us,
    so let us have a look at the next item on the list.
2. Cod liver oil follows closely with 570mg of cholesterol per 100g.
    There is no doubt that the cholesterol element of cod liver oil
    plays an important role in all the well-known health benefits of
    this time-honoured health food.
3. Fresh egg yolk takes third place, with 424mg of cholesterol per
    100g. I would like to repeat – fresh egg yolk, not chemically muti-
    lated egg powders (they contain chemically mutilated cholesterol)!
4. Butter provides a good 218mg of cholesterol per 100g. We are talk-
    ing about natural butter, not butter substitutes.
5. Coldwater fish and shellfish, such as salmon, sardines, mackerel
    and shrimps, provide good amounts of cholesterol, ranging from
    173mg to 81mg per 100g. The proponents of low-cholesterol diets
    tell you to replace meats with fish. Obviously, they are not aware
    of the fact that fish is almost twice as rich in cholesterol as meats.
6. Lard provides 94mg of cholesterol per 100g. Other animal fats
    follow.

These foods give the body a hand in supplying cholesterol so it does
not have to work as hard to produce its own. What a lot of people
don't realise is that most cholesterol in the body does not come from
food! The healthy human body produces cholesterol as it is needed.
Cholesterol is such an essential part of our human physiology that the
body has very efficient mechanisms to keep blood cholesterol at a
certain level. When we eat more cholesterol, the body produces less;
when we eat less cholesterol, the body produces more. However,
cholesterol-lowering drugs are a completely different matter! They
interfere with the body's ability to produce cholesterol, and hence they
do reduce the amount of cholesterol available for the body to use. If we
do not take cholesterol-lowering drugs, most of us don't have to worry
about cholesterol. However, GAPS patients are different: due to toxicity and nutritional deficiencies their bodies are unable to produce
enough cholesterol. Research shows that people, who are unable to

produce enough cholesterol are prone to emotional instability and behavioural problems. Low blood cholesterol has been routinely recorded in criminals who have committed murder and other violent crimes, people with aggressive and violent personalities, people prone to suicide and people with aggressive social behaviour and low self-control. The late Oxford professor David Horrobin has stated: "reducing cholesterol in the population on a large scale could lead to a general shift to more violent patterns of behaviour. Most of this increased violence would not result in death but in more aggression at work and in the family, more child abuse, more wife-beating and generally more unhappiness." People whose bodies are unable to produce enough cholesterol do need to have plenty of foods rich in cholesterol in order to provide their organs with this essential-to-life substance.

What else do our bodies need cholesterol for?

After the brain the organs hungriest for cholesterol are our endocrine glands: adrenals and sex glands. They produce steroid hormones. Steroid hormones in the body are made from cholesterol: testosterone, progesterone, pregnenolone, androsterone, estrone, estradiol, corticosterone, aldosterone and others. These hormones accomplish a myriad of functions in the body, from regulation of our metabolism, energy production, mineral assimilation, brain, muscle and bone formation to behaviour, emotions and reproduction. Our stressful modern lives consume a lot of these hormones, leading to a condition called "adrenal exhaustion". This condition is diagnosed a lot by naturopaths and other health practitioners and it is common amongst GAPS patients. There are some herbal preparations on the market for adrenal exhaustion. However, the most important therapeutic measure is to provide your adrenal glands with plenty of dietary cholesterol.

Cholesterol is essential for our immune system to function properly. Animal experiments and human studies have demonstrated that immune cells rely on cholesterol in fighting infections and repairing themselves after the fight. It has been recorded that people with high levels of cholesterol are protected from infections: they are four times less likely to contract AIDS, they rarely get common colds, and they recover from infections more quickly than people with "normal" or low blood cholesterol. On the other side of the spectrum, people with low blood cholesterol are prone to various infections, suffer from them longer and are more likely to die from an infection. A diet rich in cholesterol has been demonstrated to improve these people's ability to recover from infections. So, any person suffering from an acute or chronic infection needs to eat high-cholesterol foods to recover. Cod liver oil, the richest source of cholesterol (after caviar), has long been prized as the best remedy for the immune system. Those familiar with old medical literature will tell you that until the discovery of antibiotics a common cure for tuberculosis was a daily mixture of raw egg yolks and fresh cream (rich in cholesterol).

In conclusion: cholesterol is one of the most essential substances in the body. We cannot live without it, let alone function well. GAPS patients are in particular need of cholesterol; that is why the GAPS diet provides plenty of it.

Essential fatty acids

Many fatty acids our bodies can make. But there is a group of fatty acids which our bodies cannot make. These are essential fatty acids. Essential means – we can not live without them.

Essential fats contain fatty acids, which our human bodies cannot make, so we have to get them from food. These are omega-3 and omega-6 fatty acids. Every cell in the body depends on them for proper function and survival. These oils take part in a myriad of functions in the body on the most basic level. Our bodies, the brain in particular, are, to a degree, made of them. Hundreds of clinical studies using omega-3 and omega-6 oils, have shown them to be effective in treating every health condition under the sun, including autism, ADHD, dyslexia, dyspraxia, diabetes, depression, obsessive-compulsive disorder, schizophrenia, infections, cancer and so on. Due to food processing most of us don't get enough essential fats in our diets, particularly omega-3. Because of impaired digestion, there is no doubt that GAPS people are deficient in essential fatty acids and should have them added to their diet. So, let us have a look at this subject in detail.

There are two parent essential fatty acids, from which all others are made:

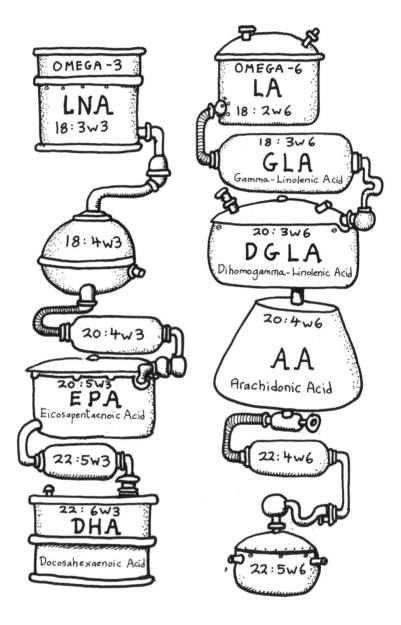

Fig 5   Conversion of parent omega fatty acids (LNA and LA) into various derivatives in the body

omega-3: Alpha-Linolenic Acid or **LNA** for short and
omega-6: Linoleic Acid or **LA** for short.

The richest sources of LNA (omega-3) are flaxseed oil (linseed oil), hemp oil and some exotic oils from kukui (candlenut) and chia. In smaller amounts this fatty acid is present in walnuts, soybeans, pumpkin seeds, rapeseed, rice bran, dark green leafy vegetables, egg yolk, animal fats (particularly from wild animals), animal milk and of course in human breast milk.

The richest sources of LA (omega-6) are evening primrose oil, safflower, sunflower, walnut, hemp oil and pretty much all seeds and nuts. In smaller amounts it is found in egg yolks, milk and human breast milk.

LNA and LA are called "the parent fatty acids". From these two fatty acids the healthy human body can make other fats to be used in pretty much every function in every cell (Fig 5).

Omega – 3 fats

From LNA (Alpha-Linolenic Acid) two very important omega-3 fatty acids are formed: **EPA** (Eicosapentaenoic Acid) and **DHA** (Docosahexaenoic Acid). EPA and DHA are absolutely vital for normal brain and eye development. They are found in abundance in brain cells, nerve synapses, visual receptors, adrenal and sex glands. However, to make them from LNA the body needs a good supply of some nutrients: vitamins C, B3 and B6, magnesium, zinc and some enzymes. GAPS patients are almost routinely deficient in these nutrients, so it is not difficult to predict that their bodies will not be able to convert parent omega-3 (LNA) from flax oil for example, into EPA and DHA, so much needed by their brains. Some researchers in the field believe that this inability to convert the parent omega-3 LNA to brain-building omega-3 EPA and DHA in GAPS children and adults plays a big part in their problems (Fig 6). So, just supplementing LNA as a flax seed or any other plant oil is not enough for these patients. They need EPA and DHA ready made. The best sources of these two oils are cold-water fish: salmon, sardines, mackerel, trout and eel. The oil from these fish can be found as supplements. Seawater and freshwater algae and

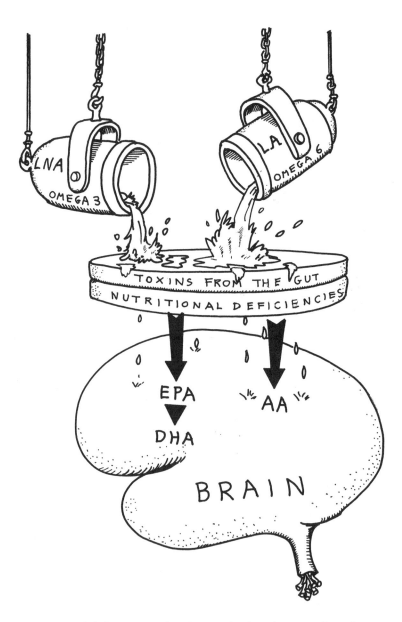

Fɪɢ 6 Nutritional deficiences and various toxins impair conversion of parent omega fats into derivatives vital for the body (EPA, DHA, AA and others)

phytoplankton are very rich in these oils as well. That is where the coldwater fish get their supply of omega-3 fats. Supplementing algae would have been a good way of getting these fats. However, the unpleasant taste of algae is a big problem, particularly with children. Smaller amounts of EPA and DHA are found in seal fat, whale blubber, pike, carp, herring and haddock. Cod liver oil is a good source of DHA and EPA and one of the oldest ways of supplementing these essential fats. But apart from that it is a good source of natural vitamins A and D and cholesterol. Despite concerns about water pollution and quality control in different brands of cod liver oil, again and again it has been shown to be most beneficial for GAPS children and adults. What about just eating fish? Eating fresh fish at least once a week is the best way of getting EPA and DHA for healthy individuals. However, for GAPS children and adults that may not be enough, due to their inability to digest foods properly. Until they recover, they do need supplementing with EPA and DHA in the form of cod liver oil and other fish oils.

Most fish oils, including cod liver oil, contain roughly equal amounts of EPA and DHA. However, there is an opinion that GAPS children and adults need more EPA than DHA. A British psychiatrist, Dr Basant Puri, has described a patient with severe drug resistant depression who recovered completely after supplementation with EPA-rich fish oil. But the most astonishing result was seen on this patient's MRI scans of the brain. Before treatment with EPA this patient showed a typical-for-depression reduction in the thickness of the grey matter in the brain. After nine months of EPA his grey matter was restored to normal thickness. David Horrobin, the late professor of Oxford University and an expert on fat metabolism, described a similar example with a schizophrenic patient where, apart form dramatic clinical improvement, restoration of the brain tissue was seen on MRI scans. There are supplements on the market now with a higher ratio of EPA to DHA and some patients report good effects from these oils. In a healthy body DHA can be made from EPA, but again it is questionable whether the GAPS body can covert EPA into DHA. DHA is considered to be essential for building the brain structure, whereas EPA is considered more important for the functioning of the brain. Both need supplementing in order to help GAPS patients.

Omega – 6 fats

LA (Linoleic Acid) is a parent fatty acid for **GLA** (Gamma-Linolenic Acid), **DGLA** (Dihomogamma-Linolenic Acid) and **AA** (Arachidonic Acid). These fatty acids are essential for the structure and function of the brain, the immune system, hormone metabolism, inflammation, blood clotting and many other functions in the body. Many seeds and nuts contain these oils. Just as with omega-3 oils, to convert LA into GLA, DGLA and AA the body needs magnesium, zinc, vitamins B3, B6 and C. So, this conversion will also be a problem for GAPS patients, which means that derivatives have to be supplemented as well as LA. GLA and DGLA are found in evening primrose oil (9%), borage oil (24%), blackcurrant seed oil (18%), hemp oil (2%) and some other oils. Omega-6 oils can be very efficiently supplied through regular consumption of nuts (walnuts, hazelnuts, pecans, pine nuts, Brazil nuts, etc.) and seeds (sunflower, sesame and pumpkin). Hemp oil, evening primrose oil, unrefined sunflower oil, borage oil and safflower oil are concentrated sources of omega-6 fatty acids available on the market.

One omega-6 fatty acid deserves particular attention as far as the GAPS conditions are concerned – **Arachidonic Acid (AA)**. It is by far the most abundant fatty acid in the brain: it makes up about 12% of all brain fat. Research shows that patients with autism, schizophrenia, bipolar disorder and depression have low levels of AA in their bodies. What is happening in these patients is that AA leaks out of the cell membranes, where it is naturally located. This loss of AA is thought to be largely responsible for the shrinkage of the brain matter seen on the MRI scans in severe patients. Deficiency in AA means that any function, no matter how small or large, cannot be accomplished efficiently between the brain cells, immune cells and other cells in the body. Why are GAPS patients losing AA from their cell membranes? The reason is not yet clear. However, a lot of research points in the direction of an enzyme, called Phospholipase A2 or PLA2, whose function is to release AA from the cell membranes. In GAPS patients this enzyme is overactive, leaching AA from brain cells and leaving them deficient in this vital fatty acid. There are a number of things which can cause PLA2 overactivity. Bio-toxins coming from bacteria, viruses, fungi and parasites in the gut are usually the major cause. Chronic inflammation in the body activates PLA2 and we know that GAPS patients have chronic inflammation in their digestive systems. Exposure to heavy metals, pesticides and other chemicals is known to cause PLA2 overactivity. High levels of insulin, caused by the consumption of processed carbohydrates and sugars, is also a strong stimulant for PLA2 activity. Cutting out grains, starch and sugar will help to preserve a lot of AA and other essential fats in the brain of a GAPS patient. Aspartame, heparin, snake and bee venom, brain injury and lack of oxygen can induce PLA2 overactivity. Due to this enzyme GAPS patients actively lose AA and other essential fatty acids from their brains and other tissues in the body. That is why it is vital to supplement them in large amounts. We have talked about LA, LNA, EPA, DHA, GLA and their dietary sources. Where do we get AA from? Here is the surprise: AA comes from meat, eggs and dairy products. You cannot find it anywhere else! The GAPS diet is rich in these foods and provides large amounts of AA, so vital for GAPS patients to have. At the same time the GAPS diet cuts out the foods which cause the loss of AA and other fatty acids from cell membranes – processed carbohydrates and sugar.

We need both omega-3 and omega-6 oils. However, due to wide consumption of vegetable oils, which are quite rich in omega-6, people generally get more omega-6 than omega-3 oils in their diets, which predisposes them to various inflammatory diseases. Clinical experience shows that for people with health problems it is important to have more omega-3 oils than omega-6 in their diet. The ideal ratio is disputed as it is probably very individual, but generally it is accepted that 2:1 of omega-3:omega-6 is the correct ratio in oil blends. For GAPS people it is vital to have not only parent essential oils (LNA and LA) but their derivatives as well (EPA, DHA and GLA). That is why it is important to supply not only seed and nut oils, but fish oils as well.

There are good blends of seed/nut oils available on the market, where flax oil is the main source of parent omega-3 LNA and evening primrose oil is the main source of omega-6 LA and GLA. Look for the brands with more omega-3 fatty acids than omega-6. Look for high quality blended oils which have not been refined, deodorised or adulterated in any way. Heat, light and oxygen destroy seed/nut oils very quickly, so they have to be cold extracted, supplied in dark glass bottles and refrigerated at all times. Never use them for cooking. They can be mixed with cold or warm food to give to the GAPS child or adult as supplements.

Apart from seed/nut oil blends make sure that you supplement EPA and DHA through good quality cod liver oil and fish oil. These oils are also highly perishable and should be refrigerated and protected from light and oxygen.

To summarise: GAPS children and adults should have a group of essential oils supplemented.

1. **A good seed/nut oil blend** in the ratio of 2:1 of omega-3:omega-6 fatty acids. It will supply the parent omega-3 and omega-6 fatty acids. Make sure that the oil is high quality, in dark glass and refrigerated. Depending on the age of the child start with a very small amount (a few drops added to the cold/warm food) and slowly build the dose up to 1–3 tablespoons a day. For children under the age of 18 months 1–2 tea spoons are usually enough. For GAPS adults start with a teaspoon a day and slowly increase to 4–5 tablespoons a day. I recommend introducing these oils gradually to avoid any reactions, which are possible in individuals with severe fatty acids deficiency.

2. **Cod liver oil**, which will supply EPA, DHA, vitamin A and vitamin D. Please, read the next chapter for more information on cod liver oil.

3. **Fish oil with a higher ratio of EPA to DHA**, as more EPA seems to be beneficial for GAPS patients. Start with a small amount added to your child's food (not hot) and slowly build the dose to 1–3 teaspoons a day (up to 1 teaspoon for children under the age of 24 months). An adult should start with a small amount and build the dose up to 3–4 teaspoons a day. Fish oil does not provide vitamins A and D, only EPA and DHA. That is why we need to supplement cod liver oil as well as the fish oil.

There are some oils which patients ask about the most, as they contain both omega-3 and omega-6 fats in considerable amounts. These are hemp oil and flax seed oil.

Hemp oil is a fairly recent oil on the market. It contains both omega-3 and omega-6 fatty acids in the ratio of 1:3. It is too heavy on omega-6 fatty acids to be supplemented on its own to GAPS children and adults.

Flax seed oil is too heavy on omega-3 LNA; it contains four times as much omega-3 as omega-6 fatty acids, and also should not be supplemented on its own.

Olive oil is a time-proven health-giving food, used by Mediterranean countries for centuries. The long list of benefits include lowered risk of heart diseases, healing and anti-inflammatory effects, stimulation of bile flow, activation of liver enzymes, antioxidant activity, stimulation of pancreatic enzymes, anti-cancer effects, anti-bacterial and anti-viral activity, membrane development, cell formation and cell differentiation. Virgin cold-pressed olive oil has been shown to improve brain cell maturation and function. And yet it doesn't have much in the way of essential fatty acids, which shows us that we need much more than just omega-3 and omega-6 oils. It contains some LA (omega-6) in a range from 3.5% to 20% and LNA (omega-3) from 0.1% to 0.6%. It is an excellent source of oleic acid (omega-9) – a monounsaturated fatty acid, which has an ability to strengthen the Th1 arm of the immune system. But the most important elements in olive oil are its minor components: beta carotene, vitamin E, chlorophyll, squalene, phytosterols, triterpenic substances, polyphenols and many others. Many health-giving properties of olive oil are probably due to these minor components. However, heat, deodorization, refining, degumming and other processing destroys and removes these vital substances. That is why it is very important to buy unrefined extra virgin cold-pressed olive oil. "Virgin" means that the oil has been extracted from whole, undamaged olives without refining. If it does not say "virgin" on the bottle then it is refined. There is no international standard for cold pressing of oils, so different manufacturers mean different things when they say that their oil is "cold-pressed". However, there is a distinct difference in taste between cold-pressed virgin olive oil and just virgin olive oil, so I recommend buying cold-pressed as well as virgin and using it on ready served meals and salads. It is not a good idea to cook with it, as the heat will destroy the minor components and change unsaturated fatty acids into harmful trans fatty acids. Cooking should be done with stable fats: ghee (clarified butter), butter, coconut oil, goose and duck fat, pork dripping, lamb fat and lard, because they do not alter their chemical structure when heated, and are beneficial to health.

Coconut oil is a rich source of saturated fats. That is why coconut and products made out of it (coconut oil and butter, coconut milk, coconut cream, etc.) have been out of favour in the last decades. Based on ill-founded research and commercial interests, coconut and other tropical fats have been blamed for raising blood cholesterol and risk of atherosclerosis, which made them unpopular. And yet tropical fats have been used by indigenous people for thousands of years. These people generally are known for very low incidence of atherosclerosis and heart disease.

About 50% of fatty acids in coconut is lauric acid. Resent research shows that in the body lauric acid gets converted into a highly potent anti-viral, anti-bacterial and anti-fungal substance, called monolaurin. Such pathogens as *candida albicans*, *helicobacter pylori*, HIV virus, measles virus, herpes virus, cytomegalovirus, Epstein-Barr virus, influenza and many others are susceptible to monolaurin. Lauric acid is also one of the natural ingredients of human breast milk, protecting the baby from infections.

Other fatty acids found in coconut are caprylic and myristic acids, which also have pronounced anti-viral, anti-bacterial and anti-fungal properties. For example, caprylic acid has been in use as an anti-fungal, anti-candida supplement for decades in the form of capsules and tablets.

It is a good idea for GAPS patients to have coconut on a regular basis. Coconut can provide a natural source of anti-fungal, anti-bacterial and anti-viral substances for these patients as well as many other nutritional factors. The question is – in what form?

People in the tropics use coconut in its natural state. The nut and juice inside are very rich in saturated fats, fibre, vitamins, minerals, vitamin E, tocotrienols, carotene and many other micro-nutrients. Fresh virgin coconut oil, full of flavour, contains most of these useful substances and is used extensively in tropical countries for cooking. Due to the fact that coconut oil contains saturated fats, it is good to use for cooking as it is stable when heated. Unfortunately, coconut oil available in Western countries is often very different from its natural virgin tropical counterpart. It has been hydrogenated to make it harder and to increase its shelf life. The hydrogenation process requires the use of aluminium and nickel, traces of which stay in the hydrogenated coconut oil. At the same time, the process of hydrogenation destroys vitamins, including vitamin E, carotene, tocotrienols and many other useful nutrients. And, as if that is not enough, many brands of coconut oil and coconut butter in the West go through a refining process which uses heat and solvent chemicals. Not surprisingly, studies of this sort of coconut oil show that it is unhealthy.

As usual, the best thing is to follow Nature and have coconut in its natural form. You can get fresh coconuts in most supermarkets. Please, look in the recipe section for different ways of serving it. Many companies now produce good quality virgin coconut oil, coconut milk and cream. Dried coconut and coconut flour can also be used for GAPS patients. Make sure that these products are pure, without any additives.

In conclusion

We should consume **natural** fats in their **natural** state. It is processed foods, which contain masses of unnatural adulterated fats, that should be blamed for our modern health problems: the crisps and chips, margarines and butter replacements, breads and pastries, biscuits and cakes, sweets and chocolates, our TV dinners and other pre-prepared lazy meals, takeaway meals, our cooking oils and spreads, our salad dressings and mayonnaise, our snacks and condiments, etc, etc. Eat fats in the form that Nature provided us with, and you will not go wrong.

The most important fats to consume for GAPS patients are animal fats: pork, goose, lamb, beef, duck, chicken, ghee, butter, etc. These fats have the most physiological profile of fatty acids for the human body and are the most natural fats for us to eat. They should constitute the bulk of all the fats your patient consumes. Apart from eating meats with good fat covering, render these fats at home (see the recipe section) and use them for all your cooking, baking and frying in generous amounts.

I would like to emphasise that GAPS children and adults need plenty of natural fats. Let them eat the fat on the meats, the skin on the poultry and the skin on oily fish, pour plenty of cold-pressed virgin olive oil on their served meals and use good quality coconut oil in your baking and cooking. Supplement their diet with good quality cod liver oil and fish oil on a daily basis. Supplement their diet with small amounts of good quality blends of cold-pressed nut/seed oils with 2:1 ratio of omega-3:omega-6 fatty acids (LNA, LA, GLA). As well as olive oil, you can use these oils as a dressing on salads and ready served meals. Contrary to popular beliefs, fat is a preferred source of energy in the human body. Remember, the brain and the rest of the nervous system, as well as our immunity, are largely made of fats.

There are some added benefits in supplying your GAPS patient with good amounts of natural unprocessed fats. The more natural fats the GAPS person has with his/her meals the less he/she will crave sweet and processed carbohydrates, which will make it easier to remove these harmful foods from the diet. And as you remove processed foods from the diet, you will automatically remove the bulk of harmful processed fats and trans fats as well.

A good supply of natural dietary fats has another benefit, important for GAPS patients. It stimulates bile production. Secreting bile is the natural way for the liver to rid itself of toxins. GAPS children and adults are very toxic people. The bulk of detoxification in the body happens in the liver. Allowing the liver to drain itself on a regular basis will help the patient to detoxify quicker.

We live in a world of fat phobia, created by commercial interests and funded by them research. Fats constitute a large part of our bodily structure and functions. That is why every health problem can be linked to abnormalities in fat consumption: lots of unnatural fats and deficiencies in natural fats. Stick to the natural fats and make sure that your GAPS patient gets plenty of them. You will see the results for yourself!

3. Cod Liver Oil

Cod liver oil has been around for a very long time. For centuries northern populations of Russia, Scandinavia, Iceland, Scotland, Greenland and Canada have fermented fish livers and guts, and consumed the oil rendered by the fermentation process. In the Roman Empire a product called *garam* was produced by fermenting fish livers and fish guts and used as food and medicine. From the 18th century European doctors started to use cod liver oil as medicine, a practice which continued well into the 20th century. Many people of older generations remember how their parents gave them a spoon of this oil every day to keep them strong and healthy. Oil collected from fermenting shark livers is still used as medicine in Tahiti and other islands in the southern hemisphere.

Amongst its health-giving properties cod liver oil provides omega-3 essential fatty acids (DHA and EPA), cholesterol, vitamin A and vitamin D. We have discussed the omega-3 fatty acids and cholesterol in the previous chapter. Let us have a look at vitamins A and D.

Vitamin A

Vitamin A is a fat soluble vitamin, which means that it comes as part of dietary fats. It exists in many biochemical forms. The parent vitamin A is called retinol. Common dietary sources are organ meats such as liver and kidneys, dairy products, eggs and oily fish. The richest sources are liver oils from marine fish, such as cod, halibut and shark and from marine mammals. The most accessible liver oil available to us is cod liver oil.

Cod liver oil contains vitamin A in its natural preformed biochemical shape. Due to digestive problems GAPS children and adults usually cannot absorb or use other forms of vitamin A, commonly found in supplements: retinyl palmitate, retinyl acetate and others. A natural form of vitamin A found in animal foods, oily fish and cod liver oil is the best form for these patients.

But why do GAPS patients need supplementation with vitamin A?

Vitamin A deficiency is a big problem in the less developed world.

Approximately 350,000 preschool children become blind each year because of vitamin A deficiency and the majority do not survive (WHO 1996). But in Western countries deficiency in this vitamin is considered to be rare, because of wide consumption of dairy, eggs and meats. Also the body has a good ability to store enough vitamin A, mainly in the liver, to last for at least three months. On top of that, theoretically vitamin A can be manufactured in the body from a large group of plant-based substances, called carotenoids. There are approximately 600 different carotenoids in nature (in green, leafy and brightly coloured vegetables and fruit), 50 of which can be converted to vitamin A. Based on all this knowledge the Western population generally is not advised to supplement vitamin A by the authorities.

Many nutritional gurus tell people that they can get all their vitamin A from converting carotenoids from fruit and vegetables. This may apply to some healthy people with very healthy digestive systems and metabolism, but for the majority of the Western population this conversion is very problematic. In people with digestive problems, such as GAPS children and adults, it is virtually impossible to obtain vitamin A from fruit and vegetables. The absorption rate of carotenoids can be less than 5%, which makes them largely useless as a source of vitamin A. Also in order to convert carotenoids into vitamin A the body needs magnesium, zinc, many amino-acids and other vital nutrients, which in a person with poor digestion are always in short supply. Various toxins have an ability to block the conversion of carotenoids into vitamin A, and GAPS patients are very toxic people. To absorb retinol (the preformed vitamin A) from dairy, liver, eggs and other foods a good supply of bile and pancreatic enzymes is needed. Many GAPS patients have whitish pale stools indicating that their bile production and fat digestion are very poor. In clinical practice, people who cannot digest fats always present with vitamin A deficiency.

Digestive system problems and vitamin A deficiency are in a "chicken and egg" relationship. As we have already discovered, poor digestion causes vitamin A deficiency. But vitamin A deficiency can cause digestive problems. In fact, gut disease is one of the symptoms of vitamin A deficiency, because the gut lining is one of the most active sites of cell production, growth and differentiation. Neither of these processes can happen properly without a good supply of vitamin A.

Leaky gut and malabsorption are the typical results of vitamin A deficiency.

According to WHO (1996) in Western countries lactating women and infants are two groups at high risk of being deficient in vitamin A. Lactating mothers need to have much more of this vitamin in their diet, than the rest of us. Due to all the modern factors many women in our society may have poor reserves of vitamin A. So many infants do not get a good supply of this vitamin in the first months of life, which makes their digestive systems prone to developing problems later on. As always, the health of the baby starts from the health of the mother.

It isn't just the digestive system that suffers from an inadequate supply of vitamin A. Its functions in the body are multiple, involving pretty much every aspect of health. It is essential in immune response, brain development, vision, cell differentiation, embryogenesis, reproduction, growth and many other functions.

One of the functions of vitamin A is its role in immunity. In fact, the earliest name for vitamin A was "anti-infective vitamin". In vitamin A deficiency both specific and non-specific immunity are impaired: the humoral response to bacterial, parasitic and viral infections, cell-mediated immunity, mucosal immunity, natural killer cell activity and phagocytosis. Supplementation of vitamin A in children shows proliferation of normal B and T cells and better response to antigens. Acute deficiency of vitamin A with night blindness and xerophthalmia in the West is indeed rare. But vitamin A inadequacy in the absence of clinical acute deficiency is not rare at all. More than 200 million children around the world suffer from vitamin A inadequacy (WHO 1996). These children do not have any visual problems, typical for deficiency. Instead they are very prone to infections, because their immune system does not function properly. Infections, particularly with a high fever, destroy a lot of vitamin A in the body. In clinical practice patients with febrile conditions require supplementation with this vitamin. GAPS children go through numerous ear and chest infections with fever in the first years of life, which reduce their vitamin A reserves in the body (if they had any reserves) and predispose them to further infections.

Obviously the best way to establish whether your child has a vitamin A deficiency is to test for it. But simply by analysing the clinical picture and health history, I would say that most GAPS children and adults need supplementation with a **natural** form of vitamin A, the best source of which is cod liver oil. As always, Nature knows best. Clinical experience and some studies show that synthetic forms of supplemental vitamin A (retinyl palmitate, retinyl acetate, etretinate, accutane and others) do not work for these patients.

Many people are concerned about overdosing on vitamin A. Indeed, in excess, this vitamin can be toxic. However, to reach toxic levels you have to have more than 10 times the recommended daily allowance for a period of weeks to years. For an adult that is 20 teaspoons of cod liver oil every day for weeks or years. For a small child it is 10 teaspoons a day. I cannot imagine anybody taking that amount of cod liver oil once, let alone on a regular basis. To cause an acute toxicity an adult has to have 100 times more than the recommended dose and a child 20 times more, which translates into 20 teaspoons of cod liver oil for a child of 3 years of age. So, taking a teaspoon of cod liver oil per day is not going to cause an overdose of vitamin A. It is synthetic forms of this vitamin, which are often added to processed foods, that can cause an overdose.

Vitamin D

Cholesterol is the major building block of vitamin D: vitamin D is made from cholesterol in our skin when it is exposed to sunlight. Our recent misguided fear of the sun and avoidance of cholesterol-rich foods have created an epidemic of vitamin D deficiency in the Western world.

Sunlight is by far the most important source of this vital vitamin for us, as the typical diet can only be considered as a trivial source of vitamin D (Fraser 1983). So, sunbathing is not only good for us, it is essential! The skin cancer, blamed on sunshine, is not caused by the sun. It is beyond the scope of this book to go into this subject in detail, but it is a fact that skin cancer (just like any other cancer) is caused by our modern processed foods and our modern toxic lifestyles. Trans fats from vegetable oils and margarine and other toxins stored in the skin are a particular culprit. In addition, some of the sunscreens that people use contain chemicals which have been proven to cause skin cancer. Just as with cholesterol, the misguided idea/hypothesis of one person (about sunlight causing skin cancer) has been picked up by commercial powers and made "the common knowledge". We, humans, have spent our lives outdoors in the sunlight for millions of years before we started hiding from the sun. All the time we are exposed to sunlight, even in cold weather, we produce vitamin D. In those times of the year when there isn't much sunlight vitamin D production drops. So, these are the times when we have to pay particular attention to our diet, making sure we consume plenty of foods with a good amount of this vitamin: cod liver oil, eggs, butter and liver.

I would like to draw your attention to the richest natural source of vitamin D – cod liver oil: it contains around 210 micrograms/100g, which puts it way above all other foods. The next richest source is egg yolk, and that only provides 4.94 micrograms/100g, almost 40 times less than cod liver oil (pay attention, please – it is per 100g of egg yolks, not per egg yolk). After egg yolks, butter provides only 0.76 micrograms/100g and calf liver 0.2-1.1 micrograms/100g. The recommended daily allowance in the UK for vitamin D is 10 micrograms per day. In order to receive that amount one would have to consume 200g of egg yolks per day or more than a kilogram of butter. On top of that this allowance is minimal, set only to avoid developing rickets or osteomalacia. To have optimal health, the majority of people need more vitamin D per day than the recommended allowance. GAPS patients, due to poor digestive function and toxicity in the body, require much larger amounts of vitamin D than the recommended allowances. Spending time outdoors in sunlight and sunbathing are the best ways of getting vitamin D. In winter, when there is very little sunlight, supplementing cod liver oil is the best way to get good amounts of vitamin D, as cod liver oil is by far the best food source of this vital vitamin. That is why when we look at the traditional diets of people around the world, the further from the equator we move, the more people prized and consumed fish livers and polar animal livers, particularly in the winter.

What does it mean for our bodies to be deficient in vitamin D?

A long list of suffering:

- Diabetes, as vitamin D is essential for blood sugar control
- Heart disease

- Mental illness
- Auto-immune illness, such as rheumatoid arthritis, lupus, inflammatory bowel disease, multiple sclerosis and other
- Obesity
- Osteoarthritis
- Rickets and osteomalacia
- Muscle weakness and poor neuro-muscular co-ordination
- High blood pressure
- Cancer
- Chronic pain
- Poor immunity and susceptibility to infections
- Hyperparathyroidism, which manifests itself as osteoporosis, kidney stones, depression, aches and pains, chronic fatigue, muscle weakness and digestive abnormalities

Unfortunately, apart from sunlight and cholesterol-rich foods there is no other appropriate way to get vitamin D. Of course, there are supplements, but most of them contain vitamin D2, which is made by irradiating mushrooms and other plants. This vitamin is not the same as the natural vitamin D. It does not work as effectively and it is easy to get a toxic level of it. In fact, almost all cases of vitamin D toxicity ever recorded were cases where this synthetic vitamin D2 had been used. It is impossible to get toxicity from natural vitamin D obtained from sunlight or cholesterol-rich foods, because the body knows how to deal with an excess of those things.

Vitamins A and D are partners!

Vitamin D has been designed to work as a team with vitamin A. They do not work properly without each other and a deficiency in one creates an excess in the other (to the point of making it toxic). In the last decades many Western processed foods have been fortified with synthetic vitamin A (without any idea of supplying vitamin D). Because of the widespread deficiency in vitamin D, this synthetic vitamin A becomes toxic in the body, causing various health problems. This is just another example of how much risk we put ourselves at when we consume processed foods!

Recent testing revealed that a large part of the Western population has "too much" vitamin A stored in their bodies thanks to fortification of processed foods. When both A and D vitamins are present in the body in the right amounts, they do not allow each other to get out of control. If the person has stored too much vitamin A, it means that this person is deficient in vitamin D. And indeed that is the case for the majority of the Western population – vitamin D deficiency is rampant. As a result of these findings cod liver oil has come under attack, as it provides more vitamin A than D. As often happens in nutritional science, the immediate "knee-jerk" reaction was that we must not consume cod liver oil! As the authorities still tell the population to stay away from the sun and avoid cholesterol-rich foods, in order to obtain vitamin D they have left themselves no alternatives but to recommend synthetic supplements.

Vitamin A and vitamin D are partners – they have been designed to work together. Who designed it that way? Mother Nature! That is why natural foods rich in one are usually rich in the other. By taking cod liver oil we can obtain both vitamins at the same time.

How much cod liver oil should we supplement?

Before talking about doses we have to think about quality. Unfortunately, today mass-produced cod liver oil is very different from the oil our grandparents used to consume. Today the industrial process of oil extraction involves heat, pressure, solvents, alkali refining, bleaching, deodorization, etc. Apart from small traditional cultures around the world and one pioneering manufacturer in the USA, nobody uses traditional fermentation for producing cod liver oil. The industrial production destroys most of the vitamins A and D in the oil, so their synthetic counterparts are then added to the oil in different amounts. Some manufacturers add natural vitamins A and D into the oil, but this practice is becoming more and more rare, as synthetic counterparts are less expensive. It is important to find good quality cod liver oil to use as a supplement for your GAPS patient, and the best oil is produced using traditional fermentation methods. If it is not possible to find fermented cod liver oil, try to find a brand of oil with natural vitamins A and D added. I do not recommend consuming synthetic vitamins.

It is difficult to assess exact amounts of vitamins A and D in natural fermented cod liver oil, as these vitamins exist in many different forms in nature. Testing methods are being improved all the time, but we cannot fully rely on them at present. The cod liver oil in your local pharmacy or supermarket has exact amounts of A and D listed on the label because the manufacturer knows how much they added into the oil after it has been refined and deodorised. The trouble is that these vitamins are likely to be synthetic, which makes it difficult to predict how much good they are going to do in the body. Add to that the fact that we are all different. Every one of us, humans, has a unique metabolism and a unique set of circumstances, which would dictate unique requirements for various nutrients. On top of that our nutritional needs change all the time: from day to night, from winter to summer, from being stressed and overworked to being relaxed, etc. So, working out individual doses of any nutrient, including cod liver oil is more of an art than a precise science.

The only manufacturer of fermented cod liver oil in the Western world suggests the following daily doses for their product: 2–2.5 ml (about 1/2 a teaspoon) for adults, double that dose for pregnant and lactating women, and half that dose for children. In my clinical experience, it is safe to double these doses for a few weeks at the beginning of the programme, as GAPS patients are in particular need of all the nutrients the fermented cod liver oil will provide. For babies and very small children it works to rub cod liver oil into their skin (the nappy area is usually the best), as the skin only absorbs what the body needs. If ordinary cod liver oil is used (with natural vitamins added), then it is generally recommended to look for oil with a ratio of vitamin A to vitamin D around 10 to 1. As all manufacturers add different doses of vitamins to their oil, it is a good idea to consult the manufacturer about dosages. The typical recommended daily doses are: one teaspoon for adults, half that dose for children and a third of a teaspoon for babies and very small children. Lactating mothers and pregnant women can have 1.5–2 teaspoons per day.

These amounts of cod liver oil on a regular basis over time would gently help to correct A and D deficiency. And let us not get too focused on the exact ratios of these vitamins in the oil, as cod liver oil is not the only source of these vitamins for a GAPS patient. The GAPS diet is going to be the main source of vitamin A and a good source of vitamin D. Sunlight exposure is going to provide the remaining vitamin D for your patient, so make sure to spend a good amount of time outdoors every day. Keep in mind that we supplement cod liver oil only to remove the tip of the deficiency iceberg; diet and lifestyle are the most important changes to make.

4. Digestive Enzymes

1. Hypochlorhydria

People with abnormal gut flora, almost without exception, have low stomach acid production. Toxins produced by overgrowth of *Candida* species, *Clostridia* and other pathogens have a strong ability to reduce secretion of stomach acid.

What does it mean and why is it important?

The stomach is the place where protein digestion begins. Hydrochloric acid produced by the stomach walls activates **pepsin**, a protein-digesting enzyme, which starts breaking down the very complex structure of dietary proteins into peptides and amino acids. To do its work properly pepsin needs the pH of the stomach to be 3 or below. In hypochlorhydria not enough acid is produced, so the pH in the stomach is not low enough for pepsin to do its job properly.

The most studied proteins in connection with GAPS conditions, particularly autism and schizophrenia, are gluten and casein. In these patients the digestive system converts them into opiate-like substances, called casomorphin and gliadomorphin, which are thought to find their way to the patient's brain and block a lot of normal brain activity and development. The digestion of casein and gluten, just as digestion of all other proteins, starts in the stomach. In a child or an adult with low stomach acidity this digestive process goes wrong from the beginning, which sets up the scene for the formation of casomorphin and gliadomorphin. Dr W. Shaw, in the revised edition of his book *Biological Treatments for Autism and PDD*, gives an interesting example of a child, who had a very severe withdrawal reaction when casein and gluten were taken out of his diet, with violent behaviour and refusal to eat or drink. Indeed withdrawal of opiates in drug addiction can be extremely dramatic. But in this child the withdrawal symptoms were temporarily relieved by regular administration of Alka-Seltzer Gold. Now why would the simple bicarbonate Alka-Seltzer Gold have such an effect? Maybe the answer is that by neutralising whatever little stomach acid the child had, Alka-Seltzer Gold interfered with the digestion of other dietary proteins with production of other opiate-like peptides, which gave this child a temporary "morphine fix", reducing the withdrawal symptoms?

As a result of low stomach acid production the whole process of protein digestion in the body goes wrong from the very beginning. The maldigested protein then passes through into the small intestine. The intestinal wall and pancreatic enzymes, which accomplish further steps in the protein digestion, expect the protein to arrive from the stomach in a particular form in order to do their job properly. It is like a conveyer belt or an assembly line in a factory. If the first person does a poor job, then no matter how well the rest of the people in the line may work, the end product is likely to be of a poor quality. However, what happens in the body is even worse. The problem is that in the body "the rest of the line" cannot work properly either, because it is regulated by the "first person". This first person is the stomach acid. Stomach acidity is the major regulator of pancreatic and liver ability to respond to arriving food. In a normal situation food coming from the stomach into the duodenum has to have a pH of 2 or below to stimulate production of two very important players in the whole digestive process. These players are two hormones, produced by the walls of the duodenum, which get absorbed into the blood and carried to the pancreas, liver, stomach and many other organs in the body. These hormones are **secretin** and **cholecystokinin**. The first hormone, secretin, gives the stomach a command to stop producing its juices, stimulates the liver to produce bile and lets the intestinal lining know that food is coming, so it makes enough mucus to protect itself. But the most important thing that it does is to stimulate the pancreas to produce alkalising bicarbonate solution to neutralise the acid in the food which has just arrived from the stomach, because normally the duodenum and the rest of the small intestine have a far more alkaline pH. This alkaline pH is essential for pancreatic enzymes to do their job of digesting proteins, fats and carbohydrates. By stimulating production of bicarbonate, secretin prepares the food for the digestive enzymes coming from the pancreas.

To produce these digestive enzymes the pancreas needs the command of the second hormone – cholecystokinin. If cholecystokinin is not made by the walls of the duodenum because of too little acid coming from the stomach with the food, then the pancreas will be sitting there idly and not producing its digestive enzymes to deal with that food. In addition, cholecystokinin tells the stomach to stop its activity, makes the gallbladder empty its bile into the duodenum, ready to digest fats, and opens the gates for pancreatic juices to flow and start digesting arriving food. (Fig 7)

These two hormones are so important in normal food digestion that without them this digestion simply cannot happen. Unfortunately, in a person with low stomach acidity that is exactly what happens. The food comes from the stomach not acid enough to trigger the production of secretin and cholecystokinin. So, the pancreas does not produce its juices and bile is not secreted to work on the fats. Maldigestion and malabsorption follow. Partially digested proteins, like casomorphin and gliadomorphin and many others get produced and absorbed through the damaged leaky intestinal wall, acting as opiates in the brain. Other maldigested proteins cause allergies and autoimmune reactions, draining an already compromised immune system even further. A lot of essential vitamins, amino acids and minerals do not get absorbed, causing nutritional deficiencies. Maldigested carbohydrates get consumed by abnormal flora, which converts them into alcohol, acetaldehyde and a whole host of other toxins. Fats do not get digested, which makes the person deficient in extremely important fat soluble vitamins A, D, E and K, essential fatty acids, and gives the person pale floating stool or diarrhoea. Undigested food simply rots in the digestive tract, poisoning the whole body.

Secretin has received a lot of publicity in autistic circles since some cases of great improvements were seen after injecting autistic children with secretin. Soon homeopathic forms of this hormone became available. Cholecystokinin is available as a supplement in the USA and some parents who tried it with their children apparently reported on effect similar to secretin. Unfortunately, the majority of autistic children show very little or no response to this treatment, because secretin is only one factor in a very complex digestive process. Normalising stomach acid production is a far more important intervention in order to put the whole digestive process right from the beginning.

Apart from literally ruining the whole digestive process, lack of acid in the stomach has other serious implications.

Stomach acid is the first barrier for huge numbers of microbes that

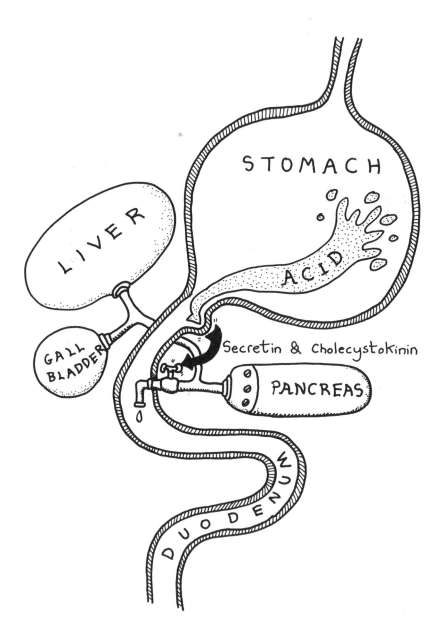

FIG 7   Regulation of digestive process by the stomach acid

arrive with every bit of food or drink we put into our mouths. If the stomach is not acid enough, these microbes have a good chance of getting into the intestines, which they would colonise and then cause trouble. They even start growing in the stomach itself ! Normally the stomach is the least-populated area of the digestive system due to its extremely acid environment. However, in a person with hypochlorhydria all sorts of pathogenic and opportunistic bacteria and fungi can grow on the stomach wall, such as *Helicobacter pylori*, *Campylobacter pylori*, *Enterobacteria*, *Candida*, *Salmonella*, *E. coli* and *Streptococci*. The most research in this area has been done in stomach cancer patients, the majority of which show low levels of stomach acid production. Microbes which populate low acid stomach play a very important role in causing stomach cancer, ulcers and gastritis.

Of course, most of these microbes love to eat carbohydrates, particularly the processed kind. The digestion of carbohydrates starts in the mouth with the action of saliva. When the food reaches the stomach normally stomach acid stops this digestion. So, carbohydrates have to wait until they arrive at the duodenum to be digested. But in the stomach with low acidity, overgrowing microbes start fermenting dietary carbohydrates, often with the production of various toxins and gas, which can make it very uncomfortable for the GAPS child or adult and make them refuse food. Accumulating gases cause excessive belching and burping. Apart from that some pathogens grow around the sphincter muscle at the top of the stomach. This round muscle normally separates the stomach from oesophagus and does not allow food to go back up. Pathogens, growing in that area, and the toxins they produce, partially paralyse the sphincter muscle which causes reflux: regurgitation of food back up into the oesophagus. Even with low stomach acid production there is some acid in the regurgitated food, which burns the walls of the oesophagus, giving the person typical symptoms of "acid indigestion". Antacids are usually prescribed for acid indigestion and reflux, which may alleviate the immediate symptoms, but in the long run make the whole situation worse as they reduce stomach acid production even further.

So, what do we do?

I believe that GAPS patients need supplementation with stomach acid. The most physiological preparation available on the market is

Betaine HCl with added Pepsin. One capsule usually provides 200–300 mg of Betaine HCl and 100mg of Pepsin. It should be taken at the beginning of each meal. The capsules usually contain an adult dose. However, I find that children as young as eight can take this dose without any trouble. To determine the right dose for your child start with a small pinch of the powder added to the first spoonfuls of the meal. In two to three days increase to two pinches and so on. For children from 18 months to 24 months one pinch is usually enough. For two to three-year-olds two to three pinches. For four to six-year-olds half a capsule is enough. For six and older from half to a full capsule. Children older than 10 and adults may need two capsules at the beginning of each meal. A lot of parents report great improvement in their child's stool in just a few days from starting Betaine HCl with Pepsin. Make sure that you do not give probiotic to your child together with Betaine HCl as the acid is likely to destroy the probiotic bacteria. Give the probiotic first thing in the morning, between food or after food when the stomach acid is at its lowest.

Apart from supplementing stomach acid there are natural things we can do to stimulate the body to produce its own stomach acid. Cabbage juice is one of the strongest stimulants. Having a few spoonfuls of cabbage juice or a small cabbage salad before the meal will help to digest that meal. Sauerkraut and its juice are even stronger. A small helping of sauerkraut or a few tablespoons of its juice will prepare the stomach for the arriving food. Having a cup of homemade meat stock with your meal will also help to increase stomach acidity. With children the easiest thing to do is to give them a cup of homemade meat stock with a few spoonfuls of sauerkraut juice or cabbage juice mixed in it.

2. Pancreatic Enzymes

These are the enzymes that people are talking about when they say "digestive enzymes". They usually include a mixture of proteases, peptidases, lipases, amylase, lactase and cellulase, which normally would break down your food in the small intestine. In a healthy digestive tract most of these enzymes are produced by the pancreas. If we can restore normal stomach acidity then this stage in digestion should go without any problem, because the stomach acid would trigger the pancreas to produce its own enzymes. That is why I consider restoring the stomach acid level far more important than supplementing pancreatic enzymes.

There has been a polemic in autistic circles about supplementing some peptidases and proteases to replace the diet (meaning the GFCF diet, of course). The idea was that these enzymes would break down gluten and casein, so that there would be no need to struggle with implementing the diet. Not surprisingly this approach did not work for the majority of people, because enzymes can never replace a diet. The diet which we describe in this book is designed to heal the gut and to re-establish normal gut flora. No enzyme can do that!

Generally in my clinical experience I see a lot of improvement from supplementing stomach acid. However, I do not see much happening from supplementing pancreatic enzymes. If the patient feels that they really help then there is no reason why he or she should not take them, providing the tablet does not contain fillers or binders, which may interfere with the healing processes in the gut. In my experience the majority of patients do very well with just supplementing stomach acid, because it will trigger production of their own pancreatic enzymes through secretin and cholecystokinin, as well as triggering bile secretion and many other important players in the digestive process, making it far more natural.

Digestive enzymes do not need to be taken permanently. As the gut starts healing the person can slowly withdraw the stomach acid supplementation and/or pancreatic enzymes, taking them only with heavy meals or if something not allowed on the diet has been eaten.

5. Vitamin and Mineral Supplementation

A vitamin is a substance that makes you ill
if you don't eat it.
Albert von Szent-Gyorgi (1893–1986)
Hungarian-born US biochemist

GAPS patients have many nutritional deficiencies, so it is a natural desire to get rid of them. The question is: how?

Is it a matter of simply testing how much magnesium, for example, a person is missing and then supplementing that amount? Or is it a matter of taking a supplement "specifically designed" for autism or ADHD or schizophrenia, using the "one size fits all" approach? Maybe we should just give megadoses of all the nutrients which the person is deficient in, hoping that the body will sort it all out?

Many health practitioners turn to testing for nutritional deficiencies. For every nutrient there are optimal tests, which are considered to give the most accurate information about that particular nutrient, and there are less optimal tests, which may be quite misleading. Trying to use the most optimal test for every nutrient is impractical and can be very expensive. So, usually one or two tests are performed for all the nutrients at once, which does not represent the true picture. So, trying to work out a nutritional supplementation protocol based on these tests is shaky from the start.

On top of that, many supplements on the market have a very low absorption rate, some only about 9%, so the amount the patient's body would actually get can be way below what it says on the bottle. But, of course, the majority of manufacturers would not tell you on the bottle how low the absorption rate of their supplement is, even if they knew. So, choosing a supplement can be quite difficult.

Absorption of supplements is a complicated process which, apart from the quality of the supplement, also depends on the state of the patient's digestive system. Two different people may absorb different amounts of nutrients from the same supplement. GAPS digestive system is generally not in good shape and may not absorb any of those nutrients particularly well.

To complicate the whole matter even further, many nutrients compete for absorption sites in the gut. So, if we supplement too much calcium, for example, it may impair absorption of other nutrients: magnesium, zinc, copper, iron, some amino acids and others, creating deficiencies in those nutrients.

Indeed this is a very confusing area of nutrition. The truth is nobody knows how to prescribe vitamins and minerals because we do not have enough research or knowledge on this subject. Every nutritionist or medical practitioner has his/her own collection of favourite supplements and that is what they usually use on most of their patients. Just as with mainstream psychiatry, where drugs are used mostly on a trial-and-error basis, the same method is used in prescribing vitamin and mineral supplements.

Taking vitamin and mineral supplements has become very common not only because many of us take "health-pills", but because a lot of foods are fortified with vitamins and minerals to compensate for the loss of those nutrients in the food processing, not to mention the fact that many foods are grown using intensive farming techniques, which makes them nutrient poor from the start. Unfortunately, a lot of these supplemented nutrients are synthetic. The body has been designed to use natural forms of these nutrients and often does not recognise the synthetic forms and does not know what to do with them. There is a growing suspicion that a lot of cases of kidney stones, for example, are caused by supplementing synthetic forms of vitamin C, which would represent most vitamin C supplements available in the shops.

There is a highly publicised opinion that in our modern world we cannot be healthy without taking nutritional supplements, because our diet cannot provide us with optimal amounts of nutrients. Indeed, if you live on cereal and toast for breakfast, sandwiches for lunch and a standard dinner you will not provide your body with optimal amounts of nutrition and you will have to take supplements. The diet which is described in this book will provide you with concentrated amounts of nutrition in a natural form, which the body recognises and knows what to do with. Juicing will add more concentrated amounts of vitamins, minerals and other useful substances. A good probiotic on average increases absorption rate of nutrients from food by 50% or more. On top of that probiotic bacteria are supposed to be the main source of vitamins B, K, biotin and many other substances in the body. Indeed, that is the first group of nutritional deficiencies which usually disappear when the patient starts taking therapeutic doses of a strong probiotic. The diet and probiotic will start healing the digestive system, so the patient will start absorbing the nutrients from the food properly.

Another important point we have to consider when it comes to our GAPS patients is that their digestive system is inflamed and damaged. A lot of synthetic supplements, fillers and binders in tablets and capsules will aggravate and irritate already sensitive GAPS gut lining and interfere with the healing process. I have seen many patients who put a lot of effort into implementing the diet, but did not achieve the best results until they removed most of their supplements.

That is why I normally do not recommend any vitamin or mineral supplementation at the beginning of the programme. I recommend putting most effort into implementing the diet first and starting the healing process in the gut. Once the digestive system starts working properly in many patients their nutritional deficiencies disappear without any supplementation! They disappear the natural way through the body sorting it out for itself.

Of course, all patients are different and some of them require targeted supplementation. But that is a matter for a qualified practitioner to decide. Here are some important points to keep in mind.

- Choose supplements without any ingredients which may aggravate the gut condition. Supplements in a liquid form are better than in powder, tablet or capsule. Substances which are not allowed on the diet should also be out.
- Choose supplements with a high absorption rate, for example, vitamin and mineral supplements with added fulvic acid. Fulvic acid (not to be confused with folic acid) is produced by bacteria in soil. It can ensure a very high absorption rate for a supplement the natural way. It also has good chelating properties for heavy metals. Soil bacteria in your probiotic will provide your gut with this acid.
- Keep supplements to an absolute minimum!

Detoxification for People with GAP Syndrome

Never go to a doctor whose office plants have died.
Erma Bombeck

We live in a polluted world. Every day we breathe in car fumes and industrial wastes. We eat foods containing pesticides, herbicides and other agricultural chemicals. We drink milk and eat meat from animals which are routinely given antibiotics, steroids and other drugs. We eat a countless number of chemicals in processed foods. We use personal care products full of chemicals shown to be carcinogenic and generally toxic for humans. Our modern energy-conserving homes and offices have become toxic places. Modern building materials, insulation, paints, domestic cleaning chemicals and fire retardants all outgas toxic substances which we breathe day in and day out. For example, chemical analysis on outgassing of common carpets and carpet adhesives in modern homes found considerable amounts of toxic substances such as formaldehyde, toluene, xylene, benzene, methacrylate, tetrachloroethylene, methyl naphthalene, phthalates and styrene. All these chemicals are known toxins for a human and we breathe them in large quantities all the time we are at home. Hospitals and shopping centres have even higher amounts of toxic substances in the air, which is why many people feel so tired and drained after a shopping trip or a long visit to a hospital. And as if all that is not enough, we routinely take prescription drugs, drink alcohol and smoke tobacco.

So, how do we survive? How do we manage to live our lives, go to work, have children, without just dropping dead after our first breath of traffic-jam air in the morning?

We survive thanks to a very important system in our bodies. A system which until recently we did not know much about – a DETOXIFICATION SYSTEM.

This system is like a cleaner in the body. It constantly cleans out all the toxins produced as a result of normal body metabolism, as well as toxins arriving from the outside. Its headquarters are in the liver and it has departments in every cell of the body. The sophistication and complexity of this system is staggering to even the most knowledge-able biochemists and there is a lot we still don't know about how it works so efficiently. But what we do know is that this system, in order to function well, has to have a constant supply of certain nutrients: zinc, magnesium, selenium, molybdenum and other minerals and trace elements, hundreds of enzymes, many amino acids and essential fats – all the substances which our GAPS children and adults are defi-cient in. Due to these deficiencies the detoxification system cannot function at an optimum level in a GAPS person. At the same time this system is overloaded with work, because GAPS patients are very toxic people. Imagine a worker, who is being starved of food and drink, and at the same time is being given more and more work to do. How is he going to cope? He is going to put most of this work into a backlog, hoping for easier times when he will be able to attend to it. That is exactly what the detoxification system does in a GAPS patient – it stores various toxic substances in different tissues in the body in order to deal with them later. That is why when these patients are tested for heavy metals, petrochemicals and other toxins they always test posi-tive. Unfortunately, a lot of these chemicals have an affinity for fats and therefore get stored in body fats. A human brain and the rest of the nervous system have a very high proportion of fats in their tissues and become storage sites for these toxins. A brain clogged with toxic-ity cannot develop or function well. We see this very clearly in GAPS patients.

So, what do we do? How do we lift this toxic load off the bodies of our GAPS children and adults to allow them to develop and function properly?

The first and most obvious thing to do is to remove the main source of toxicity, which means cleaning up and healing the gut.

However, removing the major source of toxicity is not enough. What do we do with all the toxins stored over the years in these patient's bodies? What do we do with all the heavy metals, which GAPS children and adults test positive for?

In recent years a new treatment has emerged – **chelation of heavy metals** with chelating drugs, mainly DMSA (Dimercapto Succinic Acid) and Alfa-Lipoic Acid. This group of drugs was initially used in the army for treating acute exposure to heavy metals and other toxic substances. It is a hot topic at the moment within the circles of parent groups of autistic children. There are a number of practitioners, mainly in the USA, who will administer these drugs to autistic children and who claim benefits for this treatment. We hear stories from parents who feel that chelation has helped their child. However, there are a number of issues here, which a lot of people, including me, do not feel comfortable about. Chelating drugs are drugs. Like any drug they come with side effects and complications. These are not benign substances. I have grave concerns about the idea of using these drugs without direct local medical supervision, let alone without regular blood monitoring. Let's have a look at some known problems.

1. DMSA and other chelating drugs cause dose-related bone marrow suppression, which manifests as neutropenia and thrombocytopenia, which can affect blood clotting and blood immune response to infections and other toxins. Patients who are on a chelation programme have to have their blood composition monitored on a regular basis. In some children and adults this reaction is serious enough to discontinue chelation.

2. Chelating drugs cause an explosion of pathological fungal and bacterial growth in the gut, probably due to the immune system suppression. That is why doctors who practise chelation advise their patients to deal with their gut dysbiosis first before trying to chelate. Anybody who has any experience with treating gut dysbiosis knows how difficult it is to deal with it. GAPS patients have gut dysbiosis as their most basic and primary pathology and with all the experience in treating it we still cannot say whether you can completely get rid of it.

3. In addition to taking out heavy metals chelating drugs bind essential minerals and also take them out of the body. They chelate zinc, for example, which is why zinc has to be supplemented in very high doses prior to and during chelation. However, doctors who have experience with supplementing zinc know that it has a very complex absorption mechanism, which requires normal stomach acidity. GAPS patients do not have normal stomach acidity, which

impairs absorption of supplemented zinc. On top of that we know that GAPS patients are already quite severely deficient in this essential mineral. Apart from zinc, chelating drugs also chelate other essential minerals which these patients are already deficient in, like magnesium, molybdenum and others. That is why chelation protocols include very heavy supplementation with a large number of different nutrients.

4. Patients on chelating drugs show high amounts of enzymes called transaminases in their blood, which is an indication of liver damage, specifically damage to hepatocytes (liver cells).

5. Chelating drugs are contraindicated in people with any renal problems because they have a damaging effect on kidneys. Kidney function, as well as liver function, has to be regularly monitored during chelation.

6. During chelation a long list of side effects are reported by the parents of autistic children: regression in autistic symptoms, anorexia, fatigue, irritability, nausea, sleep disturbances, diarrhoea, flatulence, macular-papular skin rash. In some cases doctors have observed such serious complications as Stevens–Johnson Syndrome (severe toxic reaction with high fever, diarrhoea, polyarthritis, erosive skin rash, myalgia, pneumonitis – usually treated with steroid medication), hemolysis (red blood cell destruction), serious neutropenia (low count of blood cells, called neutrophils, which are involved in immune response) and thrombocytopenia (low count of thrombocytes, which are blood cells mainly responsible for blood clotting).

7. A number of autistic children are reported to improve while taking chelation drugs, but they regress back to their previous state as soon as chelation stops. One explanation for this phenomenon may be that these children re-accumulate heavy metals from the environment as soon as the chelation stops, because their own detox system is unable to deal with these metals.

There is no hard or soft data available yet to prove that chelation really works, only anecdotal evidence. There are a few studies on the way, which are trying to assess any improvements from chelation, but the success rate is still unknown. If GAPS patients do improve after chelation, we do not know yet to what extent they improve to justify putting them through all the risks and side effects of this treatment, not to mention the expense.

So, what do we do about all these heavy metals and other toxins lurking in our patients' bodies? We can't just forget about them. Well, there is a time-proven way of detoxifying, taking out of the body not just the heavy metals but a lot of other poisons as well without any side effects or harmful complications. And a very tasty way too. Children in particular love it! This way is **JUICING**. Thousands of people all over the world freed themselves from the most deadly diseases with juicing. Dozens of books have been published on this subject full of testimonies and hundreds of wonderful recipes. Some very big names in natural medicine have strongly advocated juicing and used it actively in the treatment of their patients – people like Dr Gerson and Dr Norman Walker for example. Hundreds of scientific studies have been published on the health benefits of fresh raw fruit and vegetables. Juices provide all the goodness from these fruit and vegetables in a concentrated form and in large amounts. For example, to make a glass of carrot juice you need a pound of carrots. Nobody can eat a pound of carrots at once, but you can get all the nutrition from them by drinking the juice. On top of that juicing removes the fibre, which impairs absorption of many nutrients in fruit and vegetables and aggravates the condition in the already sensitive digestive system of a GAPS patient. The digestive system has virtually no work to do in digesting juices, they get absorbed in 20–25 minutes, providing the body with a concentrated amount of nutrients. With juicing you can consume large quantities of fresh vegetables and fruit every day in the most digestible and pleasant form. Many GAPS children and adults will not eat fresh vegetables and fruit due to their texture. Drinking juices can solve this problem very efficiently. Some GAPS children will not drink enough liquids either. Juices, being so tasty, can provide a good solution to this problem too. Drinking at least two cups of freshly extracted juice will provide your patient with many essential vitamins, magnesium, selenium, zinc and other minerals, amino acids and lots more nutrients which GAPS people are deficient in. A combination of pineapple, carrot and a little bit of beetroot in the morning will prepare the digestive system for the coming meals, stimulating stomach acid production and pancreatic enzymes production. A mixture of carrot, apple, celery and beetroot has a wonderful liver-cleansing ability. Green juices from leafy vegetables (spinach, lettuce, parsley, dill, carrot and beet tops) with some tomato and lemon are a great source of magnesium and iron and good chelators of heavy metals. Cabbage, apple and celery juice stimulates digestive enzyme production and is a great kidney cleanser. There is an endless number of healthy and tasty variations you can make from whatever fruit and vegetables you have available at home. To make the juice taste nice, particularly for children, generally try to have 50% of less tasty but highly therapeutic ingredients: carrot, small amount of beetroot (no more than 5% of the juice mixture), celery, cabbage, lettuce, greens – spinach, parsley, dill, basil, fresh nettle leaves, beet tops, carrot tops, white and red cabbage – and 50% of some tasty ingredients to disguise the taste of the rest of the ingredients: pineapple, apple, orange, grapefruit, grapes, mango, etc. (for more detail look in the recipe section).

What about fibre? Drinking juices doesn't mean that the patient stops eating fresh fruit and vegetables. Providing there is no diarrhoea the GAPS person should carry on eating fruit and vegetables as usual. Treat the juices like a supplement of concentrated amounts of nutrients in a glass. They should be taken on an empty stomach 20–25 minutes before food and 2–2½ hours after a meal.

But can't we just buy juices in the shops? The answer is a big NO! Juices in the shops have been processed and pasteurised, which destroys all the enzymes and most vitamins and phytonutrients. They are a source of processed sugar, which will feed abnormal bacteria and fungi in the gut. In freshly extracted juice the natural sugars are balanced with enzymes, minerals, and other nutrients, which turn them into energy for the body. When you make your juice at home you know what you put into it, you know that it is fresh without any contamination and oxidation, and you can have great fun by mixing different fruit and vegetables together, making different tasty combinations. There are a large number of books on juicing with wonderful recipes for every health problem and every occasion. To turn your juices into a powerful immune remedy, consider adding black elderberries to it.

Black Elderberry

Black elderberry is a small tree, which grows pretty much everywhere from cold to very warm climates. In spring it bears clusters of tiny whitish flowers, which at the end of the summer turn into small juicy black berries. Medicinal properties of this plant have been appreciated for centuries. Its flowers, berries, leaves and bark were traditionally used for treating colds, pneumonia, flu, sore throat, hay fever, wounds, eye infections and many other ailments. In England the berries are still used for making elderberry wine, in Scandinavia the flowers are used for making elderflower cordial. Black elderberry has strong immune-stimulating properties and it is one of the most powerful anti-viral remedies known to man.

You do not have to be an experienced herbalist to use this plant. Many people have this tree in their gardens as it is quite decorative. At the end of the summer collect clusters of berries, a small bucket would be enough. Make sure that you collect ripe berries – ripe berries are very black and squashy. At home separate the berries from their twigs using a fork. Put the berries into small plastic bags or small containers and freeze them. From the end of summer / beginning of autumn make it your bedtime routine to take 1–2 tablespoons of berries out of the freezer and leave them at room temperature to defrost over night. In the morning juice them together with pineapple, carrot or any other fruit and vegetables you planned to use. If you do it every day or every other day throughout the cold season your family will not have any colds. A small amount of 1–2 tablespoons of berries is enough for a family of four. If you are juicing just for one person, then one teaspoon is enough. Apart from juicing you can add elderberries into your cakes.

You can also collect flowers in spring and freeze them. During the winter they make a very pleasant aromatic tea or you can just crush them, while frozen, with your hand and add them to your salads. The flowers also have strong immune-stimulating properties. Use them as a tea to remedy colds, flu and fever. The same tea can be used topically on wounds and grazes, sunburn, frostbites and sore eyes. It is also a traditional remedy for hay fever.

I can just hear somebody saying "I am a very busy person and do not have time to collect berries and flowers!" But even the busiest person has got weekends. Isn't it a pleasure to spend a day with your family out in the country, when you can collect elderberries? When you come home in the evening and slump in front of your TV, you can separate the berries from their twigs with a fork and put them into small freezer bags, while watching your favourite programme. When the programme is finished, you can put the bags into your freezer. Not that much of an effort for having a winter supply of a wonderful immune-stimulating remedy. And it will cost you absolutely nothing!

The general toxic load

An important part of the treatment is reduction in the **general toxic load** on the patient's detoxification system as much as possible. What is a general toxic load? Anything toxic we eat, breathe, touch or put on our skin absorbs very quickly and puts another workload on our detox-ification system. In a GAPS person his or her gut is the major source of the toxicity overloading the detox system with too much work. It is not sensible to add more to that workload by exposing the patient to toxic and carcinogenic substances from the environment. What substances are we talking about?

The patient's house should be kept as chemical free as possible by using minimal amounts of domestic cleaning chemicals, paints, carpet pesticides and other toxic substances. All widely available domestic chemicals are toxic. Bathroom detergents, floor cleaners, polishes, etc. all stay in the air and on the surfaces, contributing to the general toxic load on the patient's detox system. Toxic domestic chemicals can be replaced with safer bio-degradable alternatives from various conscien-tious companies. However, generally try to use as little as possible. A lot of cleaning around the house can be done with just water and a bit of vinegar or lemon juice, bicarbonate of soda and olive oil. You can clean your wood floors with strong tea. You can polish your furniture with a mixture of 1 cup of olive oil and ? cup of white vinegar. You can pour white wine on red wine spills on your carpet to remove the stain.

It is wise **not** to redecorate the house or install new carpets or furni-ture while the patient is trying to detoxify. Paints, many building materials, new carpets and new furniture outgas a plethora of extremely toxic chemicals, which we absorb through our lungs, skin and mucous membranes. New carpet can outgas considerable amounts of highly carcinogenic formaldehyde for a few years. New furniture is full of fire retardants, which are great contributors of antimony (a toxic metal) in our systems. Fresh household paints outgas dozens of extremely toxic chemicals into the air of the house for at least six months. Just recently I had a phone call from a parent of an autistic child who, apart from severe autism, had epilepsy. After implementing the GAPS Nutritional Protocol the seizures disappeared completely and the child was doing very well. Then, unfortunately, the parents decided to paint the walls in the house. The day the painter started work the child had a major epileptic fit. Epilepsy in a majority of cases, particularly in children, is caused by toxicity. Obviously, this child's detoxification system was not ready to take an onslaught of the extremely toxic chemicals which we can breathe in from paints.

Very important contributors to the general toxic overload in the body are *cosmetics, toiletries, perfumes and other personal care products.* The personal care products industry is generally not regulated. More than a thousand carcinogenic and toxic chemicals are widely used in the formulation of shampoos, soaps, toothpaste, cosmetics, perfumes, creams, etc. The old opinion that our skin is a barrier and does not let toxins in has proven to be completely wrong. Human skin absorbs most things from the environment very efficiently, in some cases even better than our digestive system. Toxins, which go into the body through the digestive system, have to pass through the liver, where most of them get broken down and rendered benign. That is why the pharmaceutical industry has recently started producing more and more drugs which are applied to the skin as patches, because the skin absorbs them better than the digestive system and they get straight into the bloodstream without passing the test of the liver. The wide use of personal care products is a major contributor to our cancer epidemic. Children, women and men are unknowingly exposing themselves to huge amounts of carcinogenic substances, which they apply to their skin. A good example is breast cancer. Cells removed from a cancerous breast in many cases are full of aluminium – a toxic metal. Where does all this aluminium come from? Probably from not far away – from deodorants, which are absorbed through the skin in the woman's armpits. Recent research into toxic metals showed that when a pregnant animal is exposed to these metals they accumulate in large amounts in the foetus. That is why it is particularly important for a pregnant or breastfeeding mother to be careful about the personal products and cosmetics she puts on her skin, face and hair. In this book we cannot go into the details of all the toxins present in our toiletries and cosmetics. But let us list some of the most common ones.

- Talc or talcum powder can cause ovarian cancer. Do not use it, particularly on babies!
- Sodium Lauryl (Laureth) Sulfate (SLS) – a highly toxic detergent that is present in most shampoos, soaps and toothpaste.
- Fluoride – a terrible poison for every system in the body. Widespread in toothpaste and other dental care products, it is also added to some water supplies and given to babies as drops. If you are not familiar with its toxicity I would strongly advise you to learn more about it and avoid it like the plague.
- Titanium dioxide – carcinogenic.
- Triethanolamine (TEA) and Diethanolamine (DEA) form carcinogenic nitrosamines.
- Lanolin, itself a non-toxic natural substance, is often contaminated with DDT and other carcinogenic pesticides.
- Dioxanes are inhaled and absorbed through skin – highly carcinogenic.
- Saccharin – carcinogenic.
- Formaldehyde – a toxic and carcinogenic substance.
- Propylene glycol – carcinogenic.
- Lead, aluminium and other toxic metals are present in many personal care products, particularly in deodorants and make-up.

In patients with GAP syndrome the use of personal care products should be reduced to an absolute minimum. The body does not need washing with soaps, shower gels or bubble baths. They not only contribute to the general toxic overload, but also wash off important oils, which protect the skin from infections and drying out. Washing with water and a sponge should be quite enough.

A child does not need any personal care products apart from natural toothpaste. There are number of companies which produce safe personal care products without the harmful substances listed above.

To assist elimination of toxins through the skin, give your patient a bath every night before bed. Instead of bath soaps, add a cup of cider vinegar, bicarbonate of soda or seaweed powder to the bath; they will help to normalise the pH of the skin and encourage appropriate skin flora, as well as assisting the detoxification process. On alternate days add a cup of Epsom salt to the bath, which will also assist in the detoxification process. Air your house regularly and let your patient spend as much time as possible in the fresh air.

Swimming pools are very toxic places. People generally believe that going to the swimming pool is a healthy exercise. This cannot be further from the truth. Apart from a few rare pools sterilised with ozone, the rest of them use chlorine-based chemicals for sterilising the water. Chlorine is a poison, which affects every system in the body, particularly the immune system and liver. It absorbs quite well through the skin. In addition a thick layer of chlorine gas floats above the swimming pool water, which children and adults inhale while swimming. Inhaled chlorine absorbs extremely well through the lungs into the bloodstream. GAPS patients are already very toxic. Swimming in a chlorinated pool would add to that toxicity.

GAPS people should swim in the natural waters of lakes, rivers and the sea instead of the toxic chemical soup of swimming pools. Natural waters are full of life, biological energy from plants and different creatures, minerals, enzymes and many other beneficial substances. Swimming in natural living waters has been prized as a therapy for many health problems for centuries. Obviously, you have to make sure that the water you swim in is as far as possible from any source of industrial pollution.

Washing powders and liquids all stay in the fabric of our clothes, bedding and towels and also contribute to the toxic overload. Try to look for safer ecologically friendly alternatives.

Houseplants are our great friends when it comes to keeping our houses toxin free. They consume the toxic gases and replace them with oxygen and other beneficial substances. Fill your house with geraniums, ivies, spider plants, Aloe vera, ficuses and many other varieties of houseplants. The more the merrier, particularly in your bedrooms!

Keep your houseplants healthy, don't let them become mouldy, as some GAPS people may react to moulds.

Detoxification and reducing exposure to environmental toxins has to be an important part of the treatment of GAP Syndrome. Normalising gut flora, appropriate nourishing diet, clean water, juicing and avoiding exposure to toxins are the natural measures which work very well and without any side effects!

A healthy body is clean inside!

Happy cleaning!

Part Three: DIFFERENT ISSUES
1. Ear Infections and Glue Ear

Ear infections and glue ear are the most common reasons why GAPS children are prescribed so many antibiotics in their first years of life. But if we look at ear infections and glue ear on their own, we will see another epidemic. Ear infections account for more than a third of all visits to GPs. Around two-thirds of all children in the Western world have ear infections at some time every year, with one-third having more than four ear infections a year.

Why do we have this epidemic? Why do so many children finish up with ear grommets after endless courses of antibiotics for acute ear infections?

To understand this phenomenon we have to look at the structure of the ear. (Fig 8)

Ear infections happen in the middle ear, which is quite a small closed space – its volume is about 1 cubic cm. Its main function is to pass the sound from your eardrum to the inner ear, which it does very efficiently with a system of three interconnected tiny bones, called hammer, anvil and stirrup. Your middle ear is filled with air and is separated from the outer ear canal by the eardrum. However, it is connected to the outside world with a tube called the auditory or Eustachian tube. This tube is the most important player in ear infections and glue ear, so I would like to concentrate on it in detail.

The Eustachian tube stretches from the front wall of the middle ear to the nasopharynx (back of your nose and throat), where it opens quite near the back of your nose. The major function of this tube is to equalise the pressure in the middle ear with the atmospheric pressure. The opening of the Eustachian tube in the pharynx is guarded by a lump of lymphoid tissue, called the Tube Tonsil. These tube tonsils are a part of the immune system. Their function is to prevent infectious agents in the nose and throat from getting into the Eustachian tubes and your middle ear. There is one situation when we feel the presence of tube tonsils very well. I am sure that everybody recalls that blocked ears feeling when flying on aeroplanes. What happens is that the tube

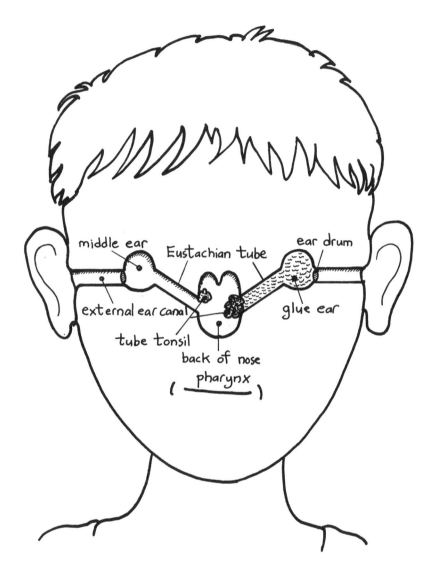

FIG 8 Interconnecting structure of the middle ear and pharynx

tonsils can get inflamed and swollen due to infection in your nose or throat or simply due to the plane's air conditioning. When the tube tonsils get swollen, they block the entrance into the Eustachian tubes. As a result the pressure inside your middle ear cannot be equalised with the changing atmospheric pressure when the plane is taking off or landing, which gives you that muffled hearing and pain in the affected ear. Swallowing, yawning, chewing, and holding the nose and mouth shut while gently trying to force air out of the lungs stretches the opening of the Eustachian tube and allows the air into the middle ear. But if the tube tonsils are swollen too much these measures usually don't work.

The Eustachian tube is the most obvious way for any infection to get into the middle ear. However, it is not so simple.

The mucous membranes of the Eustachian tubes are covered by ciliated epithelium and contain a lot of mucous glands and lymphatic follicles.

Ciliated epithelium is a layer of cells with tiny hairs on them. These hairs normally point away from the middle ear in the direction of the nasopharynx, providing an effective barrier for any food debris or air trying to get into the middle ear from the nose and the mouth. The numerous mucus-producing cells in the mucosa of Eustachian tubes are constantly cleaning the tubes up with their mucous secretions, which are moving along the direction of the tiny hairs of the ciliated epithelium down into the back of your nose. To get into the middle ear an infection would have to struggle against this flow of mucus. But if any infectious agents do manage to get into the Eustachian tube, the lymphatic follicles in its walls, which are part of the immune system, will launch their attack and finish the invader off. And, of course, before the infection even gets into the Eustachian tube it has to pass the first barrier – the tube tonsil, which is a concentration of immune cells specially designed to stop any invader. This combination of factors provides a pretty formidable defence for the middle ear! In healthy children it works very well indeed. Why don't these defences work in so many children? How does the infection get through all these barriers? Why do we have an epidemic of ear infections and glue ear?

Here we come to a very important point. The mouth, nose, throat,

Eustachian tubes and middle ear of a newborn baby are sterile. Fairly soon after birth, mouth, nose and throat get populated by a varied mixture of microbes, coming from the environment, mum, dad and anybody else who is in contact with the child. Just as it happens with the gut, due to various factors which we have discussed, many children develop abnormal flora in that area. This will do two things. First, the epithelium of the Eustachian tubes will start producing too much mucus in order to protect and clean itself. Second, the tube tonsils will be in a chronic state of inflammation, blocking the entrance into the tubes and not allowing the mucus to drain out. Fairly quickly the middle ear fills up with mucus. This situation is called glue ear. Mucus will not allow appropriate passage of sound through the middle, ear impairing the child's hearing and hence development. A lot of children with glue ear do not become autistic, for example, but their general learning abilities suffer. Speech delay is very common amongst these children. The mucus which fills their middle ear would provide a good growing environment for any infection which may come along from the back of the nose through the Eustachian tube. When that happens the child gets the typical symptoms of ear infection – pain and fever, when antibiotics are usually prescribed. Antibiotics clear away the infectious agent, but do not remove the glue ear. In fact, in the long run, they make the situation worse by altering the bacterial flora in the nose and throat even further. So, with the middle ear still filled with mucus, a good medium for growing bacteria, predictably the ear infection happens again and fairly soon. Having suffered numerous ear infections, many children finish up with little pipes, called grommets, put through their eardrum in order to provide another channel for draining the mucus from the middle ear. This operation is a symptomatic measure, but it usually resolves the problem of glue ear and stops the chain of constant ear infections. So, the epithelium of the middle ear and Eustachian tube will still be producing a lot of mucus and the natural channel for draining this mucus will still be blocked, but the mucus will now drain through an artificial pipe – grommet – into the outside.

As we said, grommets are a symptomatic measure, a crutch in a way, which does not remove the real problem. The real problem is the abnormal flora that has developed in the child's nose and throat.

Practice shows that when that flora is normalised, the glue ear and ear infections disappear. Two things have to be done to normalise bacterial flora in that area.

First, the diet should not provide food for abnormal bacteria. As we discussed in other chapters these foods are sugars, milk and processed carbohydrates. It is amazing how quickly glue ear resolves, when these foods are taken out of the diet.

Second, a strong therapeutic probiotic should be added to the child's regimen. The beneficial bacteria in the probiotic help to clear out pathogenic flora and re-establish normal healthy flora in the mouth, nose and throat, which will keep the child clear from ear infections. To do that, apart from adding a probiotic to the food, I routinely suggest to parents of children whom I see in my clinic that they open a capsule of probiotic and put the powder on the child's tongue last thing before bed, after the child has cleaned teeth and is not going to eat or drink any more. This way the probiotic bacteria will have a chance to work on the flora of the mouth and throat all night. As the back of the nose and the back of the mouth both open to the same place, the probiotic bacteria have a good chance to reach the back of the nose, where the tube tonsils are, and deal with any pathogenic flora in that area. On top of that, the stimulation of immune responses, which the probiotics produce, will also help to clear out any infection. As a result, the inflammation will subside and the tube tonsils will resume their normal size and not block the Eustachian tubes any more, allowing mucus to drain from the middle ear. This will resolve glue ear and the constant chain of ear infections.

Another common contributing factor to ear infections is food allergies, particularly allergy to milk. In the previous chapters we have discussed what role gut flora plays in development of food allergies. With the use of diet and probiotic we can improve the state of the gut flora and the immune system in the child's body. Clinical experience shows that a lot of food allergies disappear as the gut heals. In the meantime it is a good idea to remove foods which the child may be allergic to, particularly cow's milk.

However, it takes time to change the child's diet and to establish normal bacterial flora in the throat. What do we do as an immediate response to an ear infection?

Unfortunately, a very common thing that happens is a prescription of antibiotics. It is the routine response of the medical profession pretty much everywhere in the Western world. We have discussed in detail what antibiotics do to the bodily flora (in the gut, on the skin, on all mucous membranes, including the nose, throat and ears). Though the course of antibiotics will clear that particular ear infection, it will also lay the ground for the next one to come. Apart from destroying the beneficial bacteria, antibiotics are usually given to small children in a syrup, which provides concentrated amounts of sugars and starches to encourage growth of pathogenic microbes in the throat, many of which are resistant to the antibiotic in that syrup. As a result these pathogens start growing, even while the antibiotic is being administered. Many children whom I see have another ear infection pretty much as soon as the course of antibiotic finishes. Unfortunately, in these cases, children are put on a permanent antibiotic for many months, which results in very deep damage to the child's bodily flora and immune system.

There have been comparison studies done, where one group of children with an ear infection was treated with antibiotics and another group received no treatment. The result of these studies was the same – there is no difference in the outcome of an ear infection between giving an antibiotic treatment and doing nothing at all.

So, if you leave a child with an ear infection without any treatment, he or she will recover just as well. However, there is no need to leave the child without any help. People treated ear infections very effectively for centuries with simple home remedies. Here are some recommendations.

1. If you can help it keep your child indoors until the ear infection resolves itself. Keep your child warm all the time. Put a knitted woollen hat on your child, and a warm jumper while inside. Let your child wear a warm hat at all times – during the day and at night.

2. Give your child plenty of hot drinks. Just hot water with a slice of lemon and a spoon of honey is sufficient. Sit your child on your lap and give him or her this drink from a teaspoon, taking great care not to burn the child but letting him/her have the drink as

hot as possible. Put some probiotic powder on his/her tongue after finishing the drink. If it is difficult to get your child to take the powder, mix it in a teaspoon of warm water and give him this teaspoon straight after finishing the drink. Remember that probiotic contains live bacteria, which will be killed by hot water, so mix it with warm or cool water.

Instead of just water with lemon and honey, you can make some herbal teas: camomile, calendula, marjoram, eucalyptus and thyme all have anti-inflammatory and antiseptic properties. Make sure that you get the pure herb itself without any additives. Put a teaspoon of the herb into your teapot, pour boiling water over it, cover and let it brew for 5 minutes. Pour this tea through a sieve into a teacup, add some honey and give it to your child spoon by spoon. After finishing the tea, follow with the spoonful of probiotic powder on the tongue.

3. Take 1–2 tablespoons of cold-pressed olive oil and mix in a crushed clove of garlic. Leave it for 30 minutes, strain through a sieve or cheese-cloth. Put a few drops of this oil into your child's ear every hour, particularly before going to bed. Keep this oil at room temperature and warm it up slightly before putting it in your child's ear. To warm this oil up, stand the cup with the oil in a dish of warm water (not hot though, as it will reduce the oil's effectiveness). Do not microwave this oil, as all the enzymes and other active substances in it will be destroyed. Every day make a fresh mixture. The fresher it is the more effective it will be. There are some commercial preparations available as Natural Ear Drops, containing olive oil with some garlic oil, lavender oil, calendula and other natural herbs. Another time-proven oil is mullein, which you can get in most pharmacies.

4. The old onion remedy. Take a large white onion, chop it up finely and wrap it in a piece of cotton cloth. Put it into a microwave or conventional oven and warm it up to fairly hot but tolerable to the touch. Put it on your child's ear and securely cover with a warm hat (a soft woollen knitted hat is best). You can put a piece of cling film between the onion wrap and the hat, so the onion juice does not soak the hat. Keep it on your child's ear until it starts cooling down. Warm it up again and repeat the application. This procedure is very

relaxing for the child and is very good to do at bedtime. It is a bit messy and makes your child smell of onion, but works amazingly well. After this procedure keep the warm hat on your child and let him/her go to sleep on the side of the affected ear to keep it warm.

If your child runs a fever below 38°C (100°F), you do not need to reduce it. The fever is the body's way of fighting the infection. However, a temperature above 38°C (100°F) should be reduced as it can be harmful. Unfortunately, all anti-inflammatory preparations for children are made with syrup, full of sugars and starches, which should be avoided. I recommend that parents use aspirin for children, which is very effective in reducing pain and inflammation. Get soluble aspirin in small 75mg tablets. Dissolve half a tablet in warm water and give to your child as a drink with some honey. You can dissolve it in his/her cup of hot herbal tea. Aspirin should never be given on an empty stomach as it may irritate the stomach lining. Let your child eat something first before giving him/her aspirin.

Aspirin is a very safe medicine and had been given to children for decades until a very rare and obscure condition was described, called Reye's syndrome. A whole host of drugs, pesticides and other chemicals can cause this condition. This association with Reye's syndrome has led to the withdrawal of aspirin from routine use in children in USA and UK, though it is still used for many childhood rheumatic conditions. So, aspirin got replaced by paracetamol for use as a painkiller and anti-inflammatory in children. Yet paracetamol is a far more dangerous drug than aspirin will ever be. Because paracetamol is extremely bitter it has to be mixed with very concentrated sugary substances to disguise its taste. We know that children with GAP Syndrome should avoid sugars. Aspirin has a very mild taste and is very easy to give to children. It is one of the safest and oldest medicines used for all inflammatory conditions. Apart from reducing inflammation and pain it will improve blood circulation in the body. As a result, quite often an administration of aspirin relieves an ear infection very well on its own, possibly by allowing the mucus to drain from the middle ear.

A caution: if your child has any rare genetic condition, liver impairment or kidney impairment, always consult your doctor before using any medication, including aspirin.

All these measures should be applied as early as possible. If after 2–3 days the pain and fever are not getting any better you may have to resort to antibiotics. However, in the majority of cases these natural treatments work very well and the child recovers without any help from your doctor. In the meantime it is a good idea to start the long-term intervention (diet and probiotics) as soon as possible, to prevent any future ear infections.

2. Top Ten Influences which Boost Immunity

1. Fresh animal fats (from meats and dairy) and cholesterol-rich foods (particularly raw egg yolk).

2. Cold-pressed oils: olive oil, fish oils, nut and seed oils.

3. Onions and garlic.

4. Freshly pressed vegetable and fruit juices.

5. Regular consumption of greens: parsley, dill, coriander, spring onion and garlic, etc.

6. Probiotic supplementation and fermented foods.

7. Contact with animals: horses, dogs, etc. Having a pet in the family can do a lot for children's immune status.

8. Swimming in unpolluted natural waters: lakes, rivers and sea.

9. Physical activity *in the fresh air.*

10. Exposure to sunlight and sensible sunbathing.

3. Top Ten Influences which Damage Immunity

1. Sugar and everything containing it: sweets, soft drinks, confectionery, ice cream, etc.

2. Processed carbohydrates: cakes, biscuits, crisps, snacks, breakfast cereals, white bread and pasta.

3. Chemically altered and artificial fats: margarines, butter replacements, cooking and vegetable oils, processed foods prepared with these fats.

4. Lack of high quality protein in the diet from meats and fish, eggs, dairy products, nuts and seeds.

5. Exposure to man-made chemicals: cleaning and washing chemicals, personal care products, paints, fire retardants, petrochemicals, pesticides, etc.

6. Exposure to man-made radiation: electronic screens (TV, computers, play stations, etc.), mobile phones, high-power electricity lines, nuclear stations and nuclear wastes.

7. Drugs: antibiotics, steroids, antidepressants, painkillers, anticancer medication, anti-viral drugs, etc.

8. Lack of fresh air and physical activity.

9. Lack of exposure to sunlight.

10. Lack of exposure to common microbes in the environment. Living in a too sterilised environment is strongly associated with compromised immunity. The immune system needs constant stimulation from the microbes in the environment.

4. Constipation

Many of the GAPS children and adults whom I see in my clinic are constipated. Sometimes the constipation is very severe when the person cannot pass the stool for 5, 7, 10 or more days.

This is one of the common scenarios. A little boy J. would not have a stool for a week or so and then he would pass an enormous stool, screaming with pain. His mother described his stool-passing as similar to going through childbirth. The stool initially would be hard and large, followed by masses of loose or watery faeces. His anus would crack and bleed and as soon as these cracks began healing, the next stool would arrive after seven days tearing his anus again. The boy was obviously fearful of passing his stool and would hold on for as long as possible. This situation is terrible enough, but it is actually not as bad as the next common scenario.

A little girl B. has quite a good appetite and would eat and eat all day. But she would not pass any stool for 10 or more days. Then she would have a very small mushy stool, coming out in thin strips. This sort of stool is an over-spill, squeezed through masses of compacted faeces, which will stay in her bowel for months or longer, poisoning this child. And indeed her learning disability was far more severe than that of the boy J., who managed to empty his bowel, though only once a week.

Constipation is always a sign of deficient gut flora in children and in adults. The beneficial bacteria, that normally populate the bowel play a crucial role in proper stool formation and elimination. The most numerous species of friendly bacteria in a healthy bowel are *Bifidobacteria* and physiological strains of *E.coli*. These microbes produce a whole host of enzymes and other active substances, whose action is essential in proper stool formation. They stimulate the wall of the bowel to produce mucus for lubricating the stool and for passing it out as soon as it is ready. A healthy person should have 1–2 stools a day.

GAPS children and adults do not have normal gut flora and that is why they often have constipation or diarrhoea. Populating their bowel with beneficial bacteria is the most important thing to do in treating

constipation. In many cases the constipation gets resolved by changing the diet and giving the patient a therapeutic probiotic by mouth.
However, in more stubborn cases we have to take other action. Here we
have to talk about enemas.

A lot of people in the West find the subject of enemas repulsive. And
yet this safe and very effective procedure is probably as old as humans.
There is a whole chapter in *Manual of Discipline,* which was recorded
two thousand years ago in the *Dead Sea Scrolls,* describing in detail how
to perform an enema and how beneficial it is for health. Another third-
century manuscript, found in the archives of the Vatican, called *The
Essene Gospel of Peace,* gives a full procedure for performing an enema
and strongly advises doing it as the "holy baptizing by the angel of
water". Famous Arabian physician, Ibn Sina Avicenna in his timeless
work *Canon Medicinae* in the 11th century advocated regular enemas to
clear the body and soul. Regular enemas are an integral part of many
natural treatment programmes for such serious health afflictions as
cancer, psychiatric problems and autoimmunity. The enema kit is a
common tool found in family bathrooms in many Eastern countries,
performed without any medical assistance or prescription on children
and adults alike.

What are the benefits of enema?

- It is the most effective and quick relief of constipation.
- It is the most effective way to clear out faecal compaction from the
  bowel, greatly reducing the amount of toxins coming from this
  putrefaction into the person's body.
- It is the best way to introduce probiotic bacteria directly into the
  bowel.
- It is completely safe, providing that it is performed correctly.

The enema procedure

You can get an enema kit from various health shops and health
companies.

Boil 2 litres of filtered or bottled water and cool it down to around
40°C (80°F).

Prepare the enema. To do that assemble the enema kit and hang the enema bucket about a metre above the place where your patient is going to lie down. Fill the enema bucket with clean water, open the tap at the end of the enema pipe and let all the water flush out through the pipe. Close the tap and fill the enema bucket with your warm boiled water. Let some of it flush through the pipe to wash out any impurities. Close the enema tap.

In order to introduce probiotic bacteria directly into the bowel dissolve a probiotic in the remaining warm boiled water in the enema bucket. Use a therapeutic strength probiotic with predominantly *Bifidobacteria* species in it and make sure that the enema contains at least 4–5 billion viable bacterial cells. Obviously you cannot use probiotics in a tablet form, as it will have fillers and binders and other additives. Probiotics in a powder or a capsule form may have a medium of maltodextrin or FOS, which are acceptable to use in enemas but not ideal as they may cause excessive gas production for a day or two. Pure probiotics without any additives are the best to use for enemas. If you cannot find a suitable probiotic just use clean boiled water or a pure weak camomile tea (make sure that there are no other ingredients but camomile herb). A few tablespoons of homemade yoghurt added to the enema water can be very soothing for an inflamed or irritated rectum.

With a child make sure that you have an adult helper, who will either perform the enema or distract the child. You need to make this procedure as comfortable for the child as possible. Make a nice soft place for him/her to lie down underneath the enema bucket and not far from the toilet or have a potty ready. Have some favourite toys, books or a video handy to occupy him/her. Lie your child on the right side with bent knees close to his/her chest. Apply olive oil or Aloe vera gel as a lubricant on the nozzle of the enema and on the anal area of your child. It is a good idea to warm up the nozzle before doing the enema by placing it in warm water. Insert the nozzle into the anus of your child 1–2 cm deep and open the tap of the enema. Because you positioned the enema bucket at least a metre higher than the child the water will flow by gravity through the enema pipe into the rectum. Initially 100ml of water may be enough, later on you may use more water (up to one litre). The more water you can comfortably get in, the better cleaning will take place. Close the enema tap and take the nozzle out. Let your child lie on the right side for as long as he/she feels comfortable. The longer your child keeps the water inside, the better the cleaning. Your child will let you know when he/she is ready to go on the toilet or a potty. Let your child sit on the toilet for at least 10–15 minutes to empty his/her bowel completely. Occupy him/her with toys, books, videos or anything that works to keep the whole experience pleasant. It is particularly important to make the first enema pleasant, so your child will accept it next time without any apprehension.

If you feel uncomfortable about performing the enema yourself for the first time, employ a nurse or a trained colonic therapist to do it for you. Never give your child an enema with salt or anything else apart from clean boiled water, water with probiotic, homemade yoghurt or pure weak camomile tea.

With an adult the whole procedure can be much simpler. The amount of water in the enema for an adult should be 1–2 litres.

After performing the enema you need to clean the enema kit by flushing it through with water. After that sterilise it by pouring 20–30 ml of 3%–6% hydrogen peroxide through it and hang it to dry with the enema tap open. You can get hydrogen peroxide in any pharmacy without prescription. If you cannot find it, use any sterilising solution, suitable for baby bottles or other children's plastic equipment. You will need to wash and sterilise the nozzle separately.

A patient with persistent constipation should have a daily enema every night before bed, followed by a warm bath with one of the following: $^1/_2$–1 cup of Epsom salt, seaweed powder, cider vinegar, bicarbonate of soda or sea salt. After the bath rub some Udo's oil, hemp oil, cold-pressed sunflower oil, castor oil or cold pressed virgin olive oil on the skin of the abdominal area. These oils absorb quite well through skin and will help to relieve constipation in the long run. The whole procedure should be repeated every bedtime until the patient starts producing a regular stool on his/her own.

Of course, the diet which we have discussed is very important in reestablishing normal gut flora and normalising all functions of your patient's digestive system, including elimination.

I do not support the use of any laxatives, drug or herbal, particularly in children. They are designed to work on fairly healthy digestive systems. For a person with abnormal gut flora they usually are inappropriate. A combination of the diet and supplementation which we have discussed would relieve constipation in most cases. In those cases when it is not enough the enemas would do the job very effectively.

In conclusion I would like to say that GAPS patients, whether a child or an adult, should never be left constipated! Constipation is extremely harmful for the whole body. It lays the ground for all sorts of digestive disorders, including bowel cancer, and it produces a huge amount of various toxins, which poison the whole body. Diet and probiotics as a long-term treatment and an enema as an immediate remedy would effectively put constipation in the past for your patient.

5. Genetics

The word genetics is mentioned a lot in connection with the GAPS conditions. Now and then we see articles in various journals reporting that some part of some gene has been found, which may have something to do with autism, or schizophrenia, or ADHD/ADD, or dyslexia, or dyspraxia or depression. We are assured that scientists are working on it and that the genetic cause of these conditions will be found! Not that it will help the patients or their families, but it will put our minds at rest in that our children were meant to be disabled and there was nothing we could do about it!

In our modern world genetics is a popular concept. Almost every health problem is commonly blamed on genetics. We pollute the water we drink, the food we eat, the air we breathe with industrial and nuclear wastes and when we get ill we blame it all on genetics. We deplete our soils of minerals and other nutrients and replace them with pesticides, organophosphates, weedkillers and lots of other chemicals, we grow our crops on these soils, we eat these crops, we get ill and blame it all on genetics. We damage our children's immune systems with vaccinations and antibiotics and blame it all on genetics. We regularly consume processed foods with virtually no nourishment for the body that are full of chemicals and detrimental to health, and when we get ill we blame it all on genetics. We regularly intoxicate ourselves with alcohol, tobacco and drugs and when we get ill we blame it all on genetics.

If we look at all the epidemics of degenerative disease we have in our modern times which are blamed on genetics, it is easy to come to the conclusion that we all must have very poor genetics indeed! In fact I don't know how human kind survived for millennia with such poor genetics! According to the scientific establishment genetics are pretty much to blame for every misery we suffer. We have epidemics of cancer, heart disease, diabetes, psychological and psychiatric maladies, learning disabilities, autoimmune disorders, obesity, etc. etc., the list is very long. These are all conditions which doctors very rarely encountered 100 years ago. Have our genetics changed so quickly to cause these epidemics?

Well, for the last few decades genetic research or molecular biology has received the most research money in the Western world. A lot of laboratories which used to do basic science have been converted into genetic research. Billions have been poured into this area in every Western country. So, if every other scientist works in genetics then that is what they know and that is what they are going to think about when it comes to identifying the course of any disease. As the old English proverb states: "If the only tool you have is a hammer, then everything looks like a nail." Obesity? Don't worry about your eating habits. Just wait, we will find a gene to blame for it!... Cancer? Do not torment yourself with questions about your lifestyle, we will pinpoint a gene which caused it!... Learning disabilities? Oh, definitely must be genetic!

Before the discovery of *Helicobacter pylori* the medical professionals talked a lot about genetics causing stomach ulcers, gastritis and stomach cancer. When the *H. pylori* was discovered and it was proven to cause stomach ulcers, gastritis and stomach cancer, nobody talked about genetics anymore in connection with these disorders, because the real cause had been found. This example shows just how easy it is for us to blame things on genetics in order to fill a gap in our knowledge.

Genetics are a very convenient scapegoat. It is something we are born with, there is nothing we can do about it at the moment. So, wouldn't it be wonderful not to worry about our food, environment or our lifestyles? Wouldn't it be so convenient to just put all the responsibility for our state of health on our genetics?

Fortunately, life is not that simple!

Of course there are clearly identified genetic conditions, like phenylketonuria, haemophilia and many others, where specific faulty genes have been discovered. However, these conditions are relatively rare, their incidence is fairly stable and they are not the main concern in the modern world. The real problem in our modern world are the epidemics mentioned before of cancer, heart disease, autoimmune and psychiatric conditions, learning disabilities, diabetes, obesity and many other modern maladies, where the numbers of sufferers are growing at a rapid pace. Despite huge amounts of money spent on genetic research, none of these conditions has had any clear genetic causes allocated to them. A number of different genes are thought to have something to do with them, and the more research is done the clearer it becomes how unclear it all is. GAPS conditions are not an exception. A number of research studies have been published here and there, where scientists suspect different genes, but there is no conclusive evidence for any specific gene or combination of genes which we can blame for these disorders.

As with other modern epidemics, there is a conclusion that there may be a genetic predisposition to the disorder rather than a genetic cause. This predisposition can be made of tens or even hundreds of various genes, nobody knows yet how many and in what combinations. But what we do know is that before any predisposition materialises into a disease it has to have certain environmental conditions – in other words things that happen to us after we are conceived. Diet is a major part of this environmental conditioning.

Let us have a look at studies on identical twins. Identical twins are two people who have the same genetics and consequently they should have the same predisposition to the same diseases. However, there are many studies showing that when identical twins are separated at an early age and live in different environments with different diets and lifestyles, they do not develop the same health problems at all. Even in schizophrenia, which is commonly perceived as a "genetic" disease, in 50–60% of identical twins, only one twin develops schizophrenia.

Studies on ethnic emigration also confirm the fact that in the majority of cases environment, specifically diet, is more important than genetics. For example, Chinese people who live in China are generally shorter than the Western population. However, Chinese people who were born and grew up in Western countries are generally as tall as Westerners. Western diet is obviously a more important factor here than genetics.

To make the matter even more interesting, there is a large body of research showing that maternal diet during pregnancy and the diet of a baby have a major impact on the genetics of that baby. Apparently, there are many genes in a child which never become active. For a gene to become operational it has to have certain conditions to express itself. Depending on the diet of the mother during pregnancy and the diet of the infant after birth different genes will get expressed. This process does not stop at the infant stage. Throughout our whole lives our diet has a profound influence on gene expression, in other words what we eat changes our genetics. So, which is the chicken and which is the egg – genetics or the environmental factors?

Environment: our diet, lifestyle, pollution, stress, infections, etc. has a profound effect on what happens to the child's health after conception. The environment will shape a lot of the genetics of the child. Genetics is a very complicated area and despite all our investment in molecular biology we are still very far away from a full understanding of the role genetics may play in our health. What the science has learned so far we can't put into practical use, in other words there is nothing we can do with our genetics directly. But, there is a lot we can do with our environment! By changing the environment (diet, lifestyle, etc.) we can make sure that whatever genetic predisposition the child may have, this predisposition will not develop into a disease, and at the same time we can alter gene expression with the correct diet which will indirectly improve our genetics.

Another aspect of GAPS conditions, where genetics are usually mentioned, is a family history. In almost every family with an autistic child, for example, there is a history of autoimmune disease and digestive problems. Routinely it is assumed that if a mother or a grandmother had asthma, arthritis, lupus or any other autoimmune disease, then the immune imbalances in the child must be genetic. There are two factors here that are usually overlooked.

The first one is the gut flora. The gut flora with its unique composition is passed mainly from the mother to the child. Let's look at a very common scenario. If a maternal grandmother of an autistic child had an abnormal gut flora, which in her case resulted in arthritis, she passed this flora to her daughter. Quite commonly for her generation she opted not to breastfeed her daughter, because it was not fashionable at the time. This deepened the damage to the gut flora of the daughter, who developed asthma and eczema and/or a digestive disorder as a result. In her generation most girls were put on a contraceptive pill from late teens for quite a few years before they had children. The pill altered her gut flora even further. Then she had a child, to whom she passed her deeply abnormal gut flora. This child develops autism. In the previous chapters we have looked in detail at how abnormal gut flora cause autoimmune disorders. Whether genetics may play a role in passing these immune abnormalities to the next generation the science has yet to demonstrate. But, rather than assuming that it is genetics, let's not lose sight of a proven and significant factor, passed through generations, the gut flora.

Another familial factor, which is often overlooked, is learned behaviour. What is a learned behaviour? These are all the things that children learn from their parents: what to eat, how to cook, what foods to choose from, personal values and priorities. These learned behaviours can vary quite dramatically from family to family. This is something being passed through generations without any genetic involvement. But it is as important as genetics if not more so, because it will alter the gut flora, the pH, the metabolism and the biochemistry of the body. And if the grandmother, daughter and granddaughter follow the same family behaviour then they will predispose themselves to similar health problems. For example, imagine a family where rich sugary deserts were always a tradition together with a lot of bread, pies, biscuits and cakes. This diet will alter the gut flora and promote an overgrowth of pathogenic microbes in the gut, which always has an unbalancing effect on the immune system. At the same time this is a very house-proud family, so there is a lot of cleaning and polishing with domestic chemicals, air fresheners, deodorants, personal care products and perfumes – all highly allergenic and toxic substances and another onslaught on already compromised immune systems. We did not even come close to genetics here, but already you can see how the family can make you immune-compromised simply through learned behaviours.

In conclusion: it is possible that there are some non-specific genetic predispositions to autism, schizophrenia and other GAPS conditions, which quite likely overlap with a predisposition for autoimmune and digestive disorders and some weakness in the blood-brain barrier. It is very likely that this predisposition is very widespread and that modern environmental factors make it materialise into disease much more often than 100 years ago, when the environment was different. A century ago people may have had this predisposition just as much, but it did not show itself because the environment for it was not right – the diet was more natural, there was less pollution, less stress, no vaccinations, no antibiotics, contraceptive pills or other drugs, no nuclear contamination just to mention a few factors. One hundred years ago the majority of doctors did not see autism in their practice at all, for example. Today we have a growing epidemic of autism. Genetics just don't work this way. This epidemic can only be due to environmental factors: modern diet, lifestyles, vaccinations, drugs and pollution.

Rather than dwelling on genetics, which we can do nothing about, I see this conclusion as positive, because there is a lot we *can do* to change the environment to help our children. And those who have done so know that it works!

6. A Few Words about Education

I have probably learned more in the first five
years of my life than during the rest of it.
Leo Tolstoy

Education of GAPS children is a huge subject. It is beyond the scope of this book to cover it in detail. However, it is important to make one point clear. I have seen many parents in my clinic who have put a lot of effort into the physical side of their child's disorder but did not do much in terms of organising their child's education. These children usually do not do as well as the children who had both issues addressed at the same time.

From the moment children are born, what do they do most of the time?

They learn!

Every moment, they are awake, they learn from the environment and from the people around them how to communicate, how to behave appropriately, how to play with toys appropriately, how to play with their peers and, later on, as they go to school, they learn how to acquire academic skills. This is one of the most important abilities we human beings are born with – to be able to learn in order to survive and to fit in the world.

A normal child learns from the moment it is born. Have you ever observed babies and toddlers? They are like little sponges, listening to everything, watching everybody around them, absorbing every little bit of information from their environment and learning, learning, learning. Their brain cells develop very vital connections and circuits, which will serve these children for the rest of their lives.

GAPS children miss a lot of this learning. Due to their toxicity their brains are not able to process information properly, so these children are not sponges in those very important first formative years. They have normal ears, eyes, taste buds and sensors in their skin. But all the information these organs receive is then passed to the brain to be processed. A brain clogged with toxicity cannot process this sensory input appropriately, so GAPS children may not hear, see, taste or feel the same way a normal child would do.

Highly functioning autistic individuals, who lecture about their disorder, tell us that they cannot hear certain frequencies, that certain sounds hurt their ears, that they may not hear parts of words said to them or hear them in a distorted way. They say that they cannot see certain parts of the light spectrum and some parts of written words, they get lost or disoriented in fractionated light, for example the shadow of a tree or flickering electric lights and some parts of the light spectrum hurt them. They describe touch from certain fabrics and people's hands as unpleasant, like the "pins and needles" feeling we can get after sitting uncomfortably. A lot of these autistic individuals say that many foods taste bland and that the texture of the food can be offensive. All the sensory input from eyes, ears, skin and mouth turns into a jumble in their heads, disorienting, sometimes pleasant, sometimes unpleasant and sometimes frightening. That is why these children develop all sorts of behaviours which look bizarre to us, but would probably make perfect sense if we took into account what happens to the sensory input in their brains. Their brain cells do not develop normal connections and circuits. Instead they develop abnormal brain cell connections and circuits. Some of these circuits show themselves as self-stimulatory behaviour or self-destructive behaviour.

Depending on the severity of the GAPS condition this abnormality in processing sensory input may range from an absence of speech development in an autistic child, for example, to very slight abnormalities in semantics and pragmatics of the language, commonly seen in ADHD/ADD and dyslexia. Many dyslexic children may not show any obvious problems with processing sensory input until they need to learn reading and writing. However, looking back parents of these children would describe other sensory issues, like unusual fears of certain sounds and objects, strange taste preferences and fussiness with food, unexplained tantrums and unusual play routines. Children with ADHD/ADD, apart from their behavioural problems, almost without exception have deficits in pragmatics of the language, which may not be obvious to parents, but can be identified on testing. These are the finer points of the language development concerning conversational skills, answering/responding, greeting, informing, naming, labelling, negotiating, reasoning, etc. This language deficiency leads to problems in social skills and learning.

In the case of severe GAPS conditions like autism the longer this situation goes on, the more normal learning these children miss and the more they fall behind their normal peers. Normal children never stop learning, so for an autistic child to have any chance of catching up with them he or she has to learn at double speed. The earlier this intensive learning starts the more chance there is for an autistic child to catch up, simply because he or she misses less. The older the child, the more he or she has missed and the more he/she has got to catch up on. Apart from learning all the normal things, the teaching has to undo all the abnormal patterns and behaviours the child has developed. Again, the older the child, the more difficult it becomes to break abnormal brain cell circuits and build normal ones. So there is a definite sense of urgency for parents of newly diagnosed children in starting appropriate education as soon as possible.

The question is – what education?

Let us start from autism, as these children are at the most severe end of the GAP Syndrome.

Helping an autistic child

I will not attempt to describe here all the existing methods of educating autistic children. There are many of them and you can find many sources of information on this subject. Some methods aim to create an artificial environment to suit the child's needs. Other methods try to change the child so that he or she can fit in the normal world and lead as normal a life as possible. At the end of the day the method chosen comes down to the parents and their abilities and determination.

However, no matter what method is chosen, any educationalist with experience in teaching autistic children would agree that to be able to achieve the most, an autistic child needs **one-to-one teaching**. This teaching has to be **intensive** and very **structured**. It cannot be just any teaching. It has to be **conducted by specially trained people**. Every skill has to be broken down into the tiniest possible steps, manageable for an autistic mind, and taught step-by-step, making sure that all the previous steps are solidly learned and used by the child. A normal child learns every minute he or she is awake, so the teaching has to go on for **as many hours a day as possible**, every day. And we must not forget the sense of urgency if your child stands any chance of catching up with the same age typically developing children. Those children are not standing still in their development, so the goal post is constantly moving. There is not a moment to waste. I personally know only one method which can achieve all that.

This method is Behaviour Modification or Applied Behaviour Analysis (ABA). Based on behaviour modification principles a very effective teaching programme for autistic children was developed by Norwegian psychologist Dr O. Ivar Lovaas and his colleagues at the University of California in Los Angeles (UCLA). Dr Lovaas started his groundbreaking work in the 1960s and the programme is still evolving. It is the only programme for autistic children in existence which has solid published scientific basis behind it. The initial study on the efficacy of this programme was done by Lovaas and his team. It produced an astonishing result: 47% of children completing this programme achieved normal intellectual and educational functioning, with normal range IQ scores and successful performance at mainstream schools. Another 42% were mildly retarded and went to special classes for the language delayed, and only 10% were profoundly retarded and assigned to classes for autistic children. In contrast, only 2% of the control group children achieved normal educational and intellectual functioning; 45% were mildly retarded with language delay and 53% severely retarded and placed in special schools for autistic and retarded children. The treatment group received 40 hours of intensive one-to-one behaviour modification teaching a week, while the control group received 10 hours one-to-one teaching a week. The children started the treatment before the age of four and the programme lasted for at least two years. The results of this study were published in the *Journal of Consulting and Clinical Psychology* in 1987. Since then this study has been replicated in many other universities, mainly in the US, with similar results. All these studies concentrated on children under the age of five. Based on that, for many years there was a general understanding that ABA could only be done with small children. However, in 2002 Dr Svein Eikeseth and his colleagues published the results of their study, which demonstrated that older autistic children, aged from four to seven, could make large gains with intensive behavioural treatment. In parallel with that articles published mainly in the *Journal of Applied Behaviour Analysis* show that the ABA programme works not only for children but for adolescents and adults with autism.

So, although developed initially for small children with autism, the ABA programme can be effective with all autistic individuals – children and adults. However, one point still remains – the earlier you start this programme the better results you can expect.

As one of the parents, who was doing the ABA programme with her autistic boy, put it: "It is amazing how powerful this method of teaching is! With this programme you probably can teach a hippopotamus to speak and behave properly!" Whether you can teach a hippopotamus or not I don't know, but in combination with appropriate nutritional management the ABA programme has shown an ability to achieve the best outcomes for autistic children.

An example: From *Entering the world of autism: a mother's story* by Carolyn Lewis. You can read the full story in the books: *Treating Autism. Parent Stories of Hope and Success* (2003) and *Recovering Autistic Children* (2006, revised edition), edited by Stephan M. Edelson and Bernard Rimland.

Apart from nutritional intervention Brian had the ABA programme running at the same time.

"Brian's ABA program began August 1, 2001. I'll never forget that weekend because he cried and had tantrums for much of the three-day workshop. I was drained by the end of the third day. The only thing that kept me from breaking down was the hope that this program would pull our son out of the world of autism. His first task was to sit quietly on a chair for approximately five seconds. As he didn't want to do this, all of his crying and tantrums were in protest. Actually, this was a lot to ask of him, but it was the key to getting him into a teachable setting."

"Now Brian looks forward to each session of therapy, and he even hand-leads the therapist to the therapy room."

"Fifty percent of his time in therapy is play, and he gets much reward from success and the interaction with his therapists. Some have criticised ABA because they believe it 'kills the spirit'. I believed in the beginning, and still believe now, that without ABA we may never have known Brian's spirit.

Brian's daily schedule is full, and I am much more homebound than before ABA started. We schedule six hours of therapy a day seven days a week in our home. We plan two three-hour shifts of therapy each day. We allow time for naps, meals, and playtime between sessions. It is not always perfectly regimented, and I use the times when therapists can't make it to spend time in new adventures with Brian and Rachael." (Rachael is Brian's sister)

"Brian now (March 2003) behaves much like a typical three-year-old. His eye contact and his facial expressions are normal. He plays with other children and toys appropriately. There are a few social quirks that need to be worked out, but I believe the pre-school environment and playing with typical children more often will address those issues."

"He has come so far in the short period of intervention that many of us who see him and work with him cannot help but comment on how many ways he has improved. Brian is a loving, affectionate, playful little boy who prefers to interact with others instead of watching TV. Brian has acquired many skills including pretend play, and he is a practical joker. He is speaking in sentences and will request what he wants with the appropriate words. He points to and comments on things. He has mastered many programs in his ABA therapy. He likes animals and can make many animal sounds. Brian especially loves trains, cars, and aeroplanes. He also enjoys frequent trips to the pet store, and he plays with the neighbour's Boston terrier. Brian is no longer a stranger in our house, and he gives love back to us in so many ways. Brian is a miracle beyond belief to those of us who knew where he used to be."

Helping children with other GAPS conditions

Behaviour modification is a cornerstone of helping hyperactive children as well. Parents and teachers alike have to be trained in this valuable technique in order to provide consistent and structured help to an ADHD/ADD child. To learn in detail about how best to educate and handle a hyperactive child I highly recommend two books by Sandra Rief *The ADD/ADHD Checklist* and *How to Reach and Teach ADD/ADHD Children*. Parent and teacher training, language therapy, work on social skills and many other aspects have to be addressed in order to help a hyperactive child.

As a result of abnormalities in processing sensory input GAPS children often do not develop normal social skills. So, making friends and sustaining relationships becomes a problem. If these problems are not addressed, then through the years the child's self-esteem suffers. Feeling rejected for years may create withdrawal or vindictive and anti-social behaviours. Working on speech and language pragmatics with a qualified therapist is partly important in addressing this problem. However, in parallel, there is a lot the parents can do to help their GAPS child in developing good social skills. I highly recommend a book and a manual by Myrna B. Shure *Raising a Thinking Child.*

Children with GAP Syndrome are eligible to receive a lot of professional help: speech and language therapy, occupational therapy, psychotherapy, special teaching, etc. However, the most important people in children's lives are their parents. So, it is the parents that have to be the main therapists for GAPS children. Behaviour modification is the most practical and sensible way of bringing up a GAPS child. I believe that parents of all GAPS children need to be trained in this valuable method. It allows mom and dad to deal with their child's behaviours in a positive, constructive and effective way, which brings a lot of normality into their family life. We are not trained to be parents. Most of us have no idea how to bring up a child before our first bundle of joy arrives into our lives. Lucky are those of us who are blessed with a healthy, happy and compliant child. Unfortunately, GAP Syndrome parents are blessed with just the opposite. To bring up a child like that you cannot just rely on parental instincts. You need to be specially trained! Behaviour modification works on the common sense premise: *the way the parent responds to what the child does will shape that child's behaviour.* Untrained parents unintentionally reinforce their children's bad behaviours by the way they respond to these behaviours. At the same time these parents unintentionally ignore good behaviour, which does not encourage the child to repeat that good behaviour. As a result the child finishes up with a whole bunch of unpleasant and irritating habits, which then receive negative attention from the parents. The child-parent relationship deteriorates to non-compliance, reprimands and punishments. Both sides suffer and family life becomes a struggle. Being trained in behaviour modification makes you an effective parent. Effective parents have happy children and build happy families.

In conclusion: children with GAP Syndrome have to receive very targeted education from trained people, including trained parents. In those cases where children receive this kind of education the outcome is much, much better than in cases where children's education is left to chance.

Part Four: HAVING A NEW BABY IN THE GAPS FAMILY

To understand what a GAPS family is, please read the chapter *The Families*. Parents who have a child with autism, ADHD, dyslexia, dyspraxia or any other GAPS condition are quite rightly concerned when planning for a new baby. Nobody wants to produce another child with physical and mental problems. In order to give yourself the best chance to produce a beautiful healthy baby it is important to start thinking about it before conception. If you are already expecting a baby, it is best to start making changes straight away.

1. Pre-conception and Pregnancy

The most important change to make before conceiving is in both the parents' diet. The nutritional status of prospective parents is one of the most important factors in producing healthy offspring. Once the pregnancy begins, the mother must continue with her healthy diet. The father does not have to, but if he does, he will be in a much better state (physical and mental) to support his wife though the pregnancy and childbirth.

If there are no serious digestive problems, allergies, chronic fatigue, lethargy or any other typical GAPS symptoms in the partners, then I recommend following the full GAPS diet for 4–5 months prior to conception.

If there is pronounced GAP Syndrome in any of the parents, particularly in the mother, follow the whole GAPS Nutritional Protocol until you are much healthier and feel that you are ready to conceive and go through pregnancy.

If you are already pregnant go straight into the Full GAPS Diet. However, read carefully the section on the Introduction Diet and follow the recommendations for introducing fermented foods, as they need to be introduced gradually (if you have never had them before).

The diet is explained in the relevant chapters. Here I will add a few important points.

- Religiously avoid all processed foods (all packets and tins), soft drinks, sugar and food additives. Avoid eating out! Eating out will make it impossible for you to avoid harmful processed fats and oils, chemical additives, poor quality proteins and carbohydrates and many other dangers for your future baby. Make fresh food at home from fresh ingredients. For those who are not used to eating at home, this may feel like a major change. But if you stop and think: pregnancy only lasts for nine months; think of it as an investment in your baby's health and future life. I am sure you will agree that your baby deserves it!

- Remember that about 85% of everything you eat on a daily basis should be savoury: made out of fresh meats, fish, eggs, good quality dairy, vegetables and natural fats. Sweet things: baking (with nut flour and dried fruit), honey and fruit should be limited to snacks between meals.

- Consume homemade meat/bone stock on a daily basis as soups, stews or hot drinks. Meat/bone broth will provide your baby and you with countless benefits: strong digestive and immune systems, strong bones and muscles, and good stamina. Consume gelatinous meats around bones and joints after making the stock with them. Drinking warm meat stock (with some live yoghurt, kefir or sour cream added) will help with morning sickness during pregnancy.

- Please pay particular attention to the fats you consume, as they are the main agents that balance our reproductive hormones. Consume *only* natural animal fats (butter, cream, fats on meats and animal fats you rendered yourself), cold-pressed good quality olive oil or coconut oil; consume more fats than usual as your baby will need these fats very much. The majority of fats you consume should be animal fats.

- Introduce fermented foods gradually. Fermented foods are *not* optional, particularly in pregnancy! They will ensure proper digestion and absorption of nutrients and provide you and your baby with B vitamins, vitamin K and many other benefits.

- Do your best to find raw organic dairy products from a local farm: the nutritional value of raw milk, butter, yoghurt, cheese and cream can never be compared to their commercial pasteurised processed counterparts. If you cannot find unpasteurised organic milk, do not drink milk at all: instead every single day consume plenty of organic butter and fermented dairy – live natural whole yoghurt, kefir, traditionally produced cheese and sour cream.

- Eat liver and other organ meats regularly. Liver is the richest source of folic acid (not to mention many other nutrients) and will prevent many common problems.

- If your digestion is normal you can have potatoes, sourdough bread and whole grains cooked at home in moderate amounts. Remember that all these carbohydrates must be consumed with good amounts of natural fats to slow down their digestion and improve their nutritional value: let people say about you: "She likes a bit of bread with her butter!"

Apart from good food, you may want to take a good quality probiotic at a maintenance level. However, if you consume plenty of fermented foods on a daily basis, you may not need to take any commercial preparations.

Take good quality cod liver oil at a maintenance level. Don't forget to eat small oily fish (not farmed) on a regular basis, such as fresh sardines, mackerel and herring.

Other relevant issues to consider before and during pregnancy

1. Reduce general toxic load on your body and, as a result, on your baby

Everything toxic a pregnant woman is exposed to gets into her foetus. Nowadays, in our polluted world, many babies are born with a considerable toxic load, which undermines their constitution and makes them vulnerable physically and mentally. Avoiding common pitfalls will allow you to produce a baby with a smaller toxic load and hence a stronger constitution. Please read the chapter *Detoxification for People with GAPS*, particularly the part about reducing the general toxic load. In order to have a successful pregnancy it is essential to keep your body toxin free.

Avoid all man-made chemicals as much as possible: personal care products, make-up, perfume, hair dyes, domestic cleaning chemicals, carpet pesticides, dry cleaning, professional chemicals, household paints, etc. Pregnancy is not a good time to redecorate your house or buy new furniture, as these things will bring a plethora of toxic chemicals into the household toxic for your baby. Avoid going to toxic places such as hairdressers, chlorinated swimming pools, shopping centres and hospitals and anywhere with chemical smells.

Avoid dentists, as most materials they use are toxic. If you absolutely have to have a filling, avoid amalgams. Ask for a white filling and discuss with your dentist less toxic options.

Avoid taking drugs. Avoid medical tests, unless it is something absolutely essential: tests lead to drugs and medical procedures.

Avoid electronic screens, as they emit harmful radiation: don't spend much time working on computers or in front of the TV. Use mobile phones and radio phones only as necessary and for as short period of time as possible, as they also emit radiation, the consequences of which are not well studied yet.

Think very carefully what in your immediate daily environment may negatively affect your baby: radiation, pollution, high voltage masts, poor quality water, industrial factories polluting the area, etc.; take steps to avoid these problems.

2. Enjoy your pregnancy!

Your emotions, thoughts and attitudes during pregnancy have a considerable effect on your baby's development. Positive emotions create positive biochemistry in the body while negative emotions create destructive hormones and other chemicals in the body, which can affect your baby negatively. That is why it is essential for you to be relaxed, content and happy during your whole pregnancy. That is easier said than done, you would say! Here are a few ideas to accomplish that goal.

From the moment of conception your baby must become your priority. Everything else has to take a second place. So, no matter what you are planning to do, your first thought must be – "How will that affect my baby?" Whether this is a job, a holiday, a trip to visit family or friends – everything has to be done (or cancelled) from the point of view of doing the best for your baby. Do not overexert yourself and do not try to do too much, because you are already doing a full-time job carrying your baby; everything else is an extra strain. Consider very carefully whether it is fair to you or your baby to put that extra strain on yourself.

Stress is not the event itself, but the way we react to it. So, try to control your reactions to life situations. Be calm and philosophical. Don't place any demands on yourself or others around you, try to go with the flow and you will find your life more agreeable as a result. A sense of humour can do wonders in stressful situations. Avoid people who make you feel inadequate, guilty or sad. Seek the company of people who make you happy and good.

Good sleep is essential. Make your bed soft and comfortable so you can sleep well, particularly in the later stages of pregnancy. Every afternoon take a nap: this is not optional for a pregnant woman! Plan your day in such a way that you can have your afternoon rest, even if you do not fall asleep.

A daily walk in the fresh air is another essential for a pregnant woman. Walking at a comfortable pace in pleasant natural surroundings is the best exercise.

One more thing to add to your daily checklist: you must laugh every day at least once. So, find things that will make you smile and laugh: a good book, a comedy film, a friend with a good wit, your pet, etc. Think of all the positive hormones and health-promoting active chemicals your body produces when you laugh. Research shows that these hormones and chemicals may bring you a baby with a smiley happy personality.

3. Prepare for birth and breastfeeding

It is essential to prepare your birth canal for the baby, which is something women used to do in traditional societies. In order to prepare the birth canal you need to populate it with beneficial flora. To do that, every day after your bath or shower apply a handful of your home-made yoghurt or kefir all over your genital area, as well as all over your breasts and armpits. Let the kefir or yoghurt dry on you before dressing. If you have an unusual vaginal discharge or thrush (which is very common in pregnancy), once or twice a week insert a capsule of a good quality probiotic into your vagina at bedtime and leave it there to dissolve. Alternatively you can use a piece of cotton wool soaked in kefir or yoghurt as a tampon, inserted into the vagina for a few minutes. As those areas get populated by beneficial flora, they will be protected from anything pathogenic, and when your baby goes through the birth canal it will acquire beneficial flora from you. Populating your breasts and armpits with good bacteria will help to prevent mastitis and supplement your baby with probiotics, so carry on with this procedure after your baby is born.

Mentally prepare to breastfeed your baby for at least a year. Following the GAPS Programme should ensure that you will provide your baby with excellent nourishing milk. However, it does happen sometimes that a woman does not produce enough breast milk or there are problems with its quality. So, before your baby arrives, it is a good idea to establish a network of expectant mothers in your area (perhaps at the maternity classes), who would agree to share their milk, if any of them have a problem with breastfeeding. Wet nursing used to be an established practice for centuries in all cultures, and is the best alternative for your baby if you cannot provide it with your own breast milk. No commercial formula will ever come close to the quality of breast milk for your baby. Look for strong young women, who do not have established health problems and who do not take any medications.

2. New Baby

Your baby has arrived! Congratulations!

The first thing we need to think about is feeding.

Feeding your baby

I cannot emphasise strongly enough, how important it is to breastfeed your baby! Particularly in those first few days, when colostrum is produced.

If you cannot do it yourself, try to find a wet nurse or a breast milk donor: a good place to start looking for one is in your antenatal classes during pregnancy and in your maternity ward before giving birth (if you arrived at the hospital in a planned fashion) or straight after giving birth. In order to ensure a good supply of breast milk for your baby, it is practical to look for 2–4 wet nurses or breast milk donors. Look for healthy women who live not too far away from you. Even in the case of formula feeding, supplementing your baby's diet with some breast milk (even occasional) will do wonders for your baby's development and overall health. No commercial formula will ever get close to the quality of breast milk!

If you have no alternative but to feed your baby formula (even supplemented occasionally with breast milk), add good quality probiotics into every bottle feed right from the start.

Breastfeeding is wonderful! However, in the first few weeks you may have sore nipples, which may bleed and make you wince with pain as your baby latches onto them. Just survive that short time, it will not last, your nipples will heal and breastfeeding will become comfortable, relaxing and a pleasure for you. The majority of women remember breastfeeding their babies as a beautiful experience, which they would not have missed for anything in the world!

Mastitis

Mastitis is an integral part of breastfeeding. Most breastfeeding women get it and often not once. If the mother gets mastitis, the last thing she should do is to stop breastfeeding! Carry on feeding your baby with the inflamed breast as it will bring benefits for both you and the baby.

For you: emptying the breast regularly is an essential treatment for mastitis; you must not allow milk to stagnate in your breast.

For your baby: the infection from your breast is one of the nature's fist ways of maturing your baby's immune system. Babies are born with an immature immune system, which requires education. The environment educates your baby's immune system by exposing it to common pathogens. Mastitis is a safe way to introduce common microbes into your baby's body to train her immune system: the milk from the inflamed breast will supply these microbes in a complex with antibodies and many other immune factors, which will interact with your baby's immune system and teach it the right response.

Mastitis creates a very high temperature in the body: this is essential, though can be hard to cope with! The high temperature allows the body to dissolve blockages in the milk ducts in the breast. Your baby suckling will remove those blockages. A qualified homeopath can help you with both the temperature and the mastitis. Freshly brewed willow tea or plain aspirin will also help you to cope with the high temperature.

Antibiotics are usually prescribed for mastitis. However, there is no consensus amongst medics as to whether antibiotics really help: the important thing is to open up the blocked milk ducts, and your baby can do that for you very effectively. If you have to take antibiotics, carry on breastfeeding. Yes, your baby will be exposed to those antibiotics, but in a mixture with many protective immune factors in your milk. As the mastitis gets resolved your milk will restore normal balance in your baby's digestive system. Make sure to take probiotics and eat plenty of fermented foods while on the antibiotic treatment.

Introducing solids

For a bottle-bed baby introduce solids from the age of 4 months. A breastfed baby can often wait till 6 months of age, unless she is a very hungry baby and you have to introduce solids earlier.

Solids should be introduced gradually, starting from just one very small meal a day. The rest of the meals should be breast milk or, if your baby is formula fed, her usual formula with some probiotic added.

Before introducing any food, particularly at the beginning, do the **Sensitivity Test**. Take a drop of the food in question (if the food is solid, mash and mix with a bit of water) and place it on the inside of your baby's wrist. Do it at bedtime. Let the drop dry on the skin and let your baby go to sleep. In the morning check the spot: if there is an angry red or itchy reaction, avoid that food for a few weeks, and then try again. If there is no reaction, then go ahead and introduce it gradually, starting with a tiny amount. Always test the food in the state you are planning to introduce it: for example, if you are planning to introduce raw egg yolks, test the raw egg yolk and not the whole egg or cooked egg.

First week:

*   Start with homemade meat stock. To make good meat stock,

simmer a piece of meat on the bone (whole or half a chicken) for 2–3 hours without adding salt or anything else to the water. You can make fish stock the same way, using a whole fish or fish fins, bones and heads. Take the bones and meat out and sieve the stock. It can be frozen or it will keep well in the fridge for a week. Start with 1–2 teaspoons of warm meat stock before every breast feed. Make sure to give the breast only as a reward/top up after your infant has had some meat stock from a bottle, a spoon or a beaker. As your baby accepts that amount, gradually increase it. Do not use commercially available soup stock granules or bullion cubes; they are highly processed and are full of detrimental ingredients. Chicken stock is particularly gentle on the stomach. Do not take fat out of the stock; it is important for your baby to have fat with it.

- Give your baby one or two teaspoons of freshly pressed vegetable juice mixed with some warm water between meals. Start with pure carrot juice, then in a week or so try adding a dash of cabbage, celery or lettuce to the carrot. Do the Sensitivity Test first with the juice, before introducing it. Do not give your baby any commercially available vegetable or fruit juices; babies can only have juices freshly pressed by you at home. These juices do not keep: they need to be consumed within half an hour after pressing.

Second week:

- Continue with the previous foods, gradually increasing daily amounts.
- Start adding probiotic foods to the meat stock. They will provide your baby with beneficial bacteria and easy-to-digest nutrients. Begin with ½ a teaspoon of any probiotic food per day and gradually increase the daily amount.

  You have two choices: homemade whey (from dripping homemade yoghurt) or juice from your homemade sauerkraut or fermented vegetables. In the majority of babies both homemade whey and sauerkraut juice are well tolerated. Do the Sensitivity Test on your baby's skin first before introducing whey or the sauerkraut juice. It may be a good idea to start with goat's whey, as it is often better tolerated than cow's. If whey is well tolerated, try to introduce yoghurt without dripping it. Start with ¹/₂ teaspoon per day and gradually increase the daily amount. If yoghurt is well tolerated and you are gradually increasing its daily amount, introduce sour cream, fermented with yoghurt culture.

- Start making vegetable soup or puree from peeled, deseeded and well-cooked vegetables. Cook them in your homemade meat stock without adding salt or anything else. Use non – starch vegetables (no potato, sweet potato, yams or parsnips). Suitable vegetables are carrots, marrows, squashes, leeks, onions, garlic, broccoli, cauliflower and courgettes (peel and deseed marrows, squashes and courgettes). Cook the vegetables well, until very soft, cool them down to warm and puree with a little natural fat, choosing from: a teaspoon of any animal fat (pork, beef, lamb, duck, goose, chicken, etc.), a teaspoon of organic coconut oil, a teaspoon of cold-pressed olive oil, 5 drops of cod liver oil, a teaspoon of ghee (made by you from unsalted organic butter) or a teaspoon of raw organic butter (unsalted!). Give your baby different fats and oils on different days. When the vegetable soup or has puree cooled down to body temperature (test by putting a little on your wrist), add one teaspoon of homemade organic yoghurt. Start with 2–4 teaspoons of this soup or puree a day and gradually increase the amount. Start with quite a liquid puree and gradually increase its thickness.

Third week:

- Carry on with the previous foods.
- Start adding boiled meats (cooked for a long time in water and then pureed) to your baby's vegetable soups and puree. Start with a small bit of organic chicken and gradually increase: make sure to put meat and skin from wings, legs and carcass with a little meat from the breast of the chicken (skin, brown meats and all the fatty bits are the most valuable for your baby). After organic chicken introduce other meats (preferably gelatinous around bones and joints) well cooked in water. The most suitable meats are the ones you used for making the meat stock: well cooked and gelatinous. When making the meat stock cook a piece of liver together with the meats and bones. When cooked blend the liver with some meat stock and

put it through a metal mesh or a sieve. Keep the mixture in the fridge and add it to your baby's meals (about a teaspoon per serving), together with meats.

Don't forget to make fish stock regularly and serve your baby with cooked fish with vegetable puree or soup. When blending the fish it is important to use fish skin as well as the meat, the skin will provide excellent nutrients for your baby. That is why it is essential to de-scale the fish before cooking.

- If your baby is on formula milk, keep replacing it with the soups and vegetable puree with meat or fish. If breastfeeding, carry on topping up with breast milk after every feed.
- Increase the amount of homemade yoghurt and sour cream to 1–2 teaspoons with every meal. Continue adding 1 teaspoon of sauerkraut juice in soups and stews.
- Introduce ripe avocado, starting with a teaspoon added to the vegetable pure. Gradually increase the amount.

Weeks 4 and 5:

- Carry on with the previous foods.
- Start adding raw organic egg yolk to the vegetable puree. Do the Sensitivity Test with raw egg yolk first. Start with ? a teaspoon of raw egg yolk a day. Watch for any reaction. If there is none, gradually increase the amount of raw egg yolk and start adding it to every bowl of soup or vegetable puree.
- If all the previous foods are well tolerated try adding cooked apple as an apple puree: peel and core *ripe* cooking apples and stew them with a bit of water until soft. When cooked add a generous amount of butter, coconut oil or ghee. This apple puree will keep very well in the fridge for at least a week or it can be frozen. Warm it up to body temperature (or at least room temperature) before giving it to your baby. Start with a few teaspoonfuls a day. Watch for any reaction such as loose stool. If there is none, gradually increase the amount. Do not use microwave ovens for warming up or cooking, as microwaves destroy food. Use a conventional stove or oven for warming up; an apple puree you can warm up by standing the dish in some hot water.

Weeks 6 and 7:

- Carry on with the previous foods.
- Increase the amount of homemade yoghurt or sour cream to 3 teaspoons with every meal. You can start adding it to your baby's juice and water in her bottle.
- Gradually increase raw egg yolks to two a day, added to your baby's soup or cups of meat stock. Increase the meat intake, particularly gelatinous meats around joints and bones (well cooked in water).
- Stop the milk formula completely. If breastfed, then carry on.

Weeks 8 and 9:

- Carry on with the previous foods.
- Add pancakes made with nut butter (almond butter or hazelnut butter), courgette or squash (peeled and blended) and eggs, starting with one small pancake a day and gradually increasing the amount. Fry them gently in ghee, coconut oil or any animal fat (which you rendered yourself from fresh meats).
- Increase the amount of freshly pressed juices. Add some yoghurt to the juice. Try to add some fresh apple to the juice mixture.
- Add raw vegetables starting with lettuce and peeled cucumber (blended in a food processor and added to soup or vegetable puree). Start with a tiny amount and gradually increase if well tolerated. After those two vegetables are well tolerated, gradually add other raw vegetables: carrot, celery, soft cabbage, etc., finely blended.

Week 10 and onwards:

- Carry on with the previous foods.
- Try to give your baby a little bit of egg gently scrambled (or an omelette) with a generous amount of raw butter, any animal fat, coconut oil or ghee. Serve it with avocado and raw or cooked vegetables.
- Try some ripe raw apple without the skin. Try some ripe banana (yellow with brown spots on the skin). Fruit should be given to your baby between meals, not with meats.

- Introduce your homemade cottage cheese (made from your home-made yoghurt) starting with a tiny amount and gradually increasing. To make cottage cheese from your yoghurt, stand the pan with the yoghurt in a large bowl with hot water until the yoghurt separates into curds and whey. Line a large bowl with cheese cloth, pour the yoghurt into it, tie the corners of the cheese cloth together and hang it for about 8 hours to drip (overnight works well). You can add this cottage cheese to your baby's meals or give it to her as a dessert with a little cold expressed honey.
- Try to bake bread using recipes in this book. Start with a tiny piece of bread and gradually increase the amount.
- When your baby is on the Full GAPS Diet, you can start adding small amounts of natural salt into the food. This means that you will not have to cook for your baby separately, but can use the meat stock and other GAPS foods you have cooked for your whole family.

You may have to introduce some foods later than in this programme depending on your baby's sensitivities. The best indication is your baby's stool: if she gets loose stool or constipation, take it as an indication that she is not ready for the newly introduced food. Remove it from the diet, wait for a few weeks, then try to introduce it again. Another common reaction is any new skin rash or an eczema flare-up.

When weaning your baby, be confident and relaxed, as babies are like barometers: they sense our anxiety without words and will react accordingly. If your baby has refused a particular food now, try an hour later or tomorrow. Choose times when you are not in a hurry and can be happy and relaxed. From the beginning embrace the wonderful mess of baby feeding: put a plastic sheet on the floor under your baby's chair and don't worry about where the food may fly. Always have two spoons: give one spoon to your baby and let her do with this spoon whatever she wants. Hold the second spoon yourself and use it for feeding. Over time your baby will learn to use her spoon appropriately.

The stage of baby weaning is so short: enjoy it while you can!

Apart from feeding

Apart from good food your baby needs your loving attention, daily walks in the fresh air and good sleep. Nothing else! No vaccinations, no injections, no tests, no unnecessary visits to doctors and no man-made chemicals.

For information on vaccinations please read the relevant chapter. Babies in GAPS families must not be vaccinated until they have developed strong immune systems and good physical and communication skills: this means no vaccines until the child is 3–5 years of age. Even then, if you have to vaccinate, make sure that your child is absolutely healthy and well at the time of the vaccination. Ask to see the ingredients list of the vaccine and demand that they are explained to you. Try to avoid combined vaccines; look for single alternatives.

Avoid all man-made chemicals in your baby's care! No personal care products, even those that are claimed to be natural. Babies do not need to be washed with any soap or shampoo. Clean warm water is all they need. Soaps wash off protective oils from the baby's skin and expose it to drying out and invasion by pathogens. Use coconut oil, olive oil and your homemade yoghurt and kefir on the nappy area or any dry skin.

Make sure that your home is as chemical free as possible: use water and vinegar to clean your house, natural bio-degradable laundry detergents and wash your baby's dishes by hand (rinsing the soap off thoroughly). In the first year of your baby's life try not to redecorate your house or buy new furniture, new kitchen, etc. These things bring a plethora of toxic chemicals into the house, which may affect your baby's development. Avoid taking your baby to toxic places, such as chlorinated swimming pools, shopping centres and hospitals. Do not allow anybody to smoke around your baby or use excessive amounts of perfume.

Use natural bedding for your baby. Wrap your baby's mattress in a plastic sheet: if urine gets into some modern mattresses (particularly an old mattress left from your previous child), it may react with microbes and chemical ingredients in the mattress and release toxic gases (the main cause of cot death!).

On the whole, think what man-made chemicals, radiation or any other environmental dangers your baby may be exposed to and avoid them.

And what about you?

We have talked about what your baby needs. However, we must not forget about your needs! Your beautiful bundle of joy will bring into your life sleepless nights, physical exhaustion, tiring visits from close and distant family, cleaning, washing, cooking and possibly much more. It is important to plan in advance to have help, particularly in the first few months, when you are recovering from labour. For example, delegating shopping and cleaning to a member of the family or a friend can make a huge difference. If you are trying to do too much, while looking after your baby, then neither of you is going to enjoy the experience. A tired parent is rarely an effective parent. Apart from that, stress and tiredness can cause the breast milk to dry up. So, shamelessly take any chance to have a rest, even if you are surrounded by piles of work to do. It is better to prevent tiredness than to deal with it later. Research in this area shows that having several small periods of rest during the day is almost twice as productive, as having one long rest. So, take two or three small naps per day; they will do wonders for you! Make it a rule: when your baby sleeps, you sleep.

While breastfeeding your baby, don't forget to feed yourself very well! If you are to produce good quality breast milk for your baby you must eat a good quality diet yourself. Continue with your Full GAPS Diet with liberal amounts of animal fats, fermented foods and good quality proteins from meat, fish and liver. Just as you did during your pregnancy, continue to avoid any toxin exposure, as everything that gets into your blood will be in your milk.

Good food and frequent, regular small periods of rest will allow you not only to survive your child's babyhood, but to enjoy it. And you should enjoy it, as it is so short!

In conclusion

I am sure that many people will agree that having children is the biggest and the most wonderful thing we will ever do in our lives. Giving life to another human being, then gently guiding and teaching your child to survive in this world and make the best of it is an honour, a thrilling journey and a huge achievement! It is vital to start the whole process right, to lay solid healthy foundations. I hope that this part of the book will help you to do that and become successful, happy and proud parents!

Selected References

To the Parents of Autistic Children – an Open Letter
Introduction

1. The International Autism Research Centre, www.gnd.org .
2. Centre for Disease Control (CDC), April, 2000. "Prevalence of Autism in Brick Township, New Jersey, 1998: Community Report" available on the CDC web-site, http://www.cdc.gov/nceh/prograrams/cddh/dd/report.htm.
3. Testimony on April 25, 2001 before the US House of Representatives Committee on Governmental Reform by James J. Bradstreeet, M.D., director of research for the International Autism Research Centre.
4. 22nd Annual Report to Congress on the Implementation of the Individuals with Disabilities Education Act, Table AA11, "Number and Change in Number of Children Ages, pp. 6–21, Served Under IDEA, Part B."
5. Absolon CM at al. Psychological disturbance in atopic eczema: the extent of the problem in school-aged children. *Br J Dermatology*, Vol 137(2), 1997, pp. 24105.
6. Edelson SM and Rimland B. Treating autism. Parent stories of hope and success. 2003. Published by Autism Research Institute.
7. Rimland B. New hope for safe and effective treatments for autism. *Autism Research Review International* 8:3, 1994.
8. Schauss A. Nutrition and behaviour. *J App Nutr*, Vol 35, 1983, p. 30–5.
9. Shaw W. Biological Treatments for Autism and PDD. 2002. ISBN 0-9661238-0-6
10. Warren RP et al. Immunogenetic studies in autism and related disorders. *Molecular and Chemical Neuropathology*, 1996, 28, pp. 77–81.
11. World Health Organisation. The World Health Report 2001 – Mental Health: New Understanding, New Hope. See www.who.int/whr/2001/

All Diseases Begin in the Gut (Part 1: Chapter 1)

1. Baranovski A, Kondrashina E. Colonic dysbacteriosis and dysbiosis. Saint Petersburg Press, 2002.
2. Baruk H. 1978. Psychoses of digestive origins. In: Hemmings and Hemmings (eds), Biological Basis of Schizophrenia. Lancaster MTP Press. Coleman M, Gillberg C, 1985. The Biology of Autistic Syndromes. Praeger. NY.

3.   Cade R et al. Autism and schizophrenia: intestinal disorders. *Nutritional Neuroscience,* March 2000.
4.   Crook W. The yeast connection. 1986.Vintage Books.
5.   Dohan FC. Is celiac disease a clue to pathogenesis of schizophrenia? *Mental Hygiene,* 1969; 53: 525–529.
6.   Horvath K, Papadimitriou JC, Rabsztyn A et al. Gastrointestinal abnormalities in children with autism. *Journal of Paediatrics,* 1999; 135: 559–563.
7.   Kawashima H et al. Detection and sequencing of measles virus from peripheral mononuclear cells from patients with inflammatory bowel disease. *Dig Dis Sci,* 2000 Apr; 45(4): 723–9.
8.   Maki M, Collin P. Coeliac disease. *Lancet,* 1997; 349: 1755–9. IF: 13.251.
9.   McCandless J. Children with starving brains. A medical treatment guide for autism spectrum disorder. 2003. Bramble books.
10. McGinnis WR. Mercury and autistic gut disease. *Environmental Health Perspectives,* 109(7): A303–304 (2001).
11. Melmed FD, Scheneider CK, Fabes RA et al. Metabolic markers and gastrointestinal symptoms in children with autism and related disorders. *J Paediatr Gastroenterol Nutr,* 2000; 31 (Suppl 2): S31.
12. Reichelt KI et al. Probable aetiology and possible treatment of childhood autism. *Brain Dysfunct,* 4: 308–319, 1991.
13. Seeley, Stephens, Tate. Anatomy and Physiology. 1992. Second edition. Mosby Year Book.
14. The International Autism Research Centre, www.gnd.org.
15. Torrente F et al. Enteropathy with T-cell infiltration and epithelial IgG deposition in autism. *Molecular Psychiatry,* 2002; 7: 375–382.
16. Vorobiev AA, Nesvizski UV. Human microflora and immunity. Review.(Russian).*Sovremennie Problemi Allergologii, Klinicheskoi Immunologii I Immunofarmacologii,* M, 1997, pp. 137–141.
17. Vorobiev AA, Pak SG et al. Dysbacteriosis in children. A textbook for doctors and medical students (Russian), M, "KMK Lt", 1998, ISBN 5-87317-049-5.
18. Wakefield AJ, Anthony A et al. Enterocolitis in children with developmental disorders. AIA Journal, Autumn 2001.
19. Wakefield AJ, Murch SH, Anthony A et al. Ileal-lymphoid-nodular hyperplasia, non-specific colitis and pervasive developmental disorder in children. *Lancet,* 1998; 351: 637–41.
20. Wakefield AJ and Montgomery SM. Autism, viral infection and measles, mumps, rubella vaccination. *Israeli Medical Association Journal,* 1999; 1: 183–187.
21. Walker-Smith JA. Autism, inflammatory bowel disease and MMR vaccine. *Lancet,* 1998; 351: 1356–57.

The Roots of a Tree (Part 1: Chapter 2)
Immune System (Part 1: Chapter 3)

1. Alan Jones V, Shorthouse M, Workman E, Hunter JO. Food intolerance and the irritable bowel. *Lancet*, 1982, 633–634.
2. Anthony H, Birtwistle S, Eaton K, Maberly J. Environmental Medicine in Clinical Practice. BSAENM Publications 1997.
3. Balsari A, Ceccarelli A, Dubini F, Fesce E, Poli G. The faecal microbial population in the irritable bowel syndrome. *Microbiologica,* 1992, 5, 185–194.
4. Baranovski A, Kondrashina E. Colonic dysbacteriosis and dysbiosis. Saint Petersburg Press. 2002.
5. Comi AM at al. Familial clustering of autoimmune disorders and evaluation of medical risk factors in autism. *Jour Child Neurol*, 1999, Jun; 14(6): 338–94.
6. Cummings JH, Macfarlane GT (1997). Role of intestinal bacteria in nutrient metabolism. (Review) (104 refs). *Journal of Parenteral & Enteral Nutrition*. 1997, 21(6): 357–65.
7. Cummings JH, Macfarlane GT (1997). Colonic Microflora: Nutrition and Health. *Nutrition.* 1997; vol.13, No. 5, 476–478.
8. Cummings JH (1984). Colonic absorption: the importance of short chain fatty acids in man. (Review) (95refs). *Scandinavian Journal of Gastroenterology* – Supplement. 93: 89–99, 1984.
9. Cunningham-Rundles S, Ahrn'e S, Bengmark S, Johann-Liang R, Marshall F, Metakis L, Califano C, Dunn AM, Grassey C, Hinds G, Cervia J, (2000). Probiotics and immune response. *American Journal of Gastroenterology*, 95 (1 Suppl): S22-5, 2000 Jan.
10. D'Eufemia P, Celli M, Finocchiaro R et al. 1996. Abnormal intestinal permeability in children with autism. *Acta Pediatr* 1996: 85: 1076–79.
11. Finegold SM, Sutter VL, Mathisen GE (1983). Normal indigenous intestinal flora in "Human intestinal flora in health and disease" (Hentges DJ, ed), pp. 3–31. Academic Press, London, UK.
12. Fuller R. Probiotics in man and animals. *J Appl Bacteriol*, 1989; 66: 365–78.
13. Furlano RI, Anthony A, Day R et al. Colonic CD8 and gamma delta T-cell infiltration with epithelial damage in children with autism. *J Pediatr*, 2001; 138: 366–72.
14. Ferrari P et al. Immune status in infantile autism: correlation between the immune status, autistic symptoms and levels of serotonin. *Encephale,* 14: 339–344, 1988.
15. Guarino A, Canani RB, Spagnuolo MI, Albano F, DiBenedetto L (1997). Oral bacterial therapy reduces the duration of symptoms and of visceral excretions in children with mild diarrhoea. *Journal of Paediatric Gastroenterology and Nutrition,* 25(5): 516–9, 1997 Nov.

16. Gupta S at al. Dysregulated immune system in children with autism. Beneficial effects of intravenous immune globulin in autistic characteristics. *Autism Develop Dis,* 26: 439–452, 1996.

17. Gupta S. Immunological treatments for autism. *J Autism Dev Disord,* 2000 Oct; 30(5): 475–9.

18. Krasnogolovez VN. Colonic dysbacteriosis. – M: Medicina, 1989.

19. McCandless J. Children with starving brains. A medical treatment guide for autism spectrum disorder. 2003. Bramble books.

20. McLaren Howard J. Intestinal dysbiosis. Complementary Therapies. *Med* 1993; 1: 153.

21. Petrovskaja VG, Marko OP. Human microflora in norm and pathology. M: Medicina, 1976.

22. Pimentel M. at al. Study links intestinal bacteria to Irritable Bowel Syndrome. *The American Journal of Gastroenterology,* December, 2000.

23. Plioplys AV at al. Lymphocyte function in autism and Rett syndrome. *Neuropsychobiology* 7: 12–16, 1994.

24. Reichelt KL et al (1994). Increased levels of antibodies to food proteins in Downs syndrome. *Acta Paediat Japon.* 36: 489–492.

25. Roberfroid MB, Bornet F, Bouley C, Cummings JH (1995). Colonic microflora: nutrition and health. Summary and conclusions of an International Life Sciences Institute (ILSI) [Europe] workshop held in Barcelona, Spain. [Review] [33 refs]. *Nutrition Reviews.* 53(5): 127–30, 1995 May.

26. Singh V. Neuro-immunopathogenesis in autism. 2001. New Foundations of Biology. Berczi I & Gorczynski RM (eds) Elsevier Science B.V. pp. 447–458.

27. Singh V at al. Changes in soluble interleukin-2, interleukin-2 rector, T8 antigen, and interleukin-I in the serum of autistic children. *Clin Immunol Immunopath,* 61: 448–455, 1991.

28. Singh V et al. Immunodiagnosis and immunotherapy in autistic children. *Ann NY Acad Sci,* 540: 602–604, 1988.

29. Singh V at al. Antibodies to myelin basic protein in children with autistic behaviour. *Brain Behav Immunity,* 7: 97–103, 1993.

30. Singh V et al. Serological association of measles virus and human herpesvirus-6 with brain autoantibodies in autism. *Clinical Immunology and Immunopathology.* 1998: 89; 105–108.

31. Shaw W. Biological Treatments for Autism and PDD. 2002. ISBN 0-9661238-0-6

32. Stubbs EG at al. Depresed lymphocyte responsiveness in autistic children. *JAutism Child Schizophr,* 7: 49–55, 1977.

33. Sullivan NM, Mills DC, Riemann HP, Arnon SS. Inhibitions of growth of Clostridium botulinum by intestinal microflora isolated from healthy infants. *Microbial Ecology in Health and Disease,* 1988; 1: 179–92.

34. Swedsinski A at al. Mucosal flora in inflammatory bowel disease. 2001. PMID: 11781279 PubMed.

35. Tabolin VA, Belmer SV, Gasilina TV, Muhina UG, Korneva TI. Rational therapy of intestinal dysbacteriosis in children. – M.: Medicina, 1998.

36. The International Autism Research Centre. www.gnd.org

37. Vorobiev AA, Nesvizski UV. (1997). Human microflora and immunity. Review (Russian), *Sovremennie Problemi Allergologii, Klinicheskoi Immunologii Immunofarmacologii*. – M., 1997. c.137–141.

38. Vorobiev AA, Pak SG et al (1998). Dysbacteriosis in children. A textbook for doctors and medical students.(Russian). M: "KMK Lt.", 1998. ISBN 5-87317-049-5.

39. Warren R et al. Immune abnormalities in patients with autism. *J Autism Develop Dis*, 16, 189–197, 1986.

40. Warren PP at al. Reduced natural killer cell activity in autism. *J Am Acad Child Phychol*, 26: 333–335, 1987.

41. Warren R. et al. Immunoglobulin A deficiency in a subset of autistic subjects. *J Autism Develop Dis,* 27: 187–192, 1997.

42. Waizman A et al. Abnormal immune response to brain tissue antigen in the syndrome of autism. *Am J Psychiatry,* 139: 1462–1465, 1982.

43. Wilson K, Moore L, Patel M, Permoad P. Suppression of potential pathogens by a defined colonic microflora. *Microbial Ecology in Health and Disease.* 1988; 1: 237–43.

44. Yasui H, Shida K, Matsuzaki T, Yokokuta T. (1999). Immunomodulatory function of lactic acid bacteria. (Review)(28 refs), Antonie van Leenwenhoek. 76(1–4): 38309, 1999, Jul–Nov.

45. Yonk LJ et al. D4+ per T cell depression in autism. *Immunol Lett* 35: 341–346, 1990.

What Can Damage Gut Flora? (Part 1: Chapter 4)
The Opportunistic Flora (Part 1: Chapter 5)
Gut – Brain Connection (Part 1: Chapter 6)
The Families (Part 1: Chapter 7)

1. Anthony H, Birtwistle S, Eaton K, Maberly J. Environmental Medicine in Clinical Practice. BSAENM Publications, 1997.

2. Baranovski A, Kondrashina E. Colonic dysbacteriosis and dysbiosis. Saint Petersburg Press. 2002.

3. Bjarnason I et al. Intestinal permeability, an overview. (Review). *Gastroenterology*, 1995; 108: 1566–81.

4. Bolte ER, (1998). Autism and Clostridium tetani. *Medical Hypothesis,* 51(2): 133–144.

5. Campbell LL, Postgate SR. Classification of the spore-forming sulphate-reducing bacteria. *Bacteriological Reviews*, 1965, 29, 359–363.

6. Capel ID et al. The effect of prolonged oral contraceptive steroid use on erythrocyte glutathione peroxidase activity. *J Steroid Biochem* 1981; 14: 729–732.

7. Coleman M, Gillberg C. 1985. The Biology of Autistic Syndromes. Praeger. NY.

8. Crook W. The yeast connection. 1986. Vintage Books.

9. De Boissieu D et al. Small-bowel bacterial overgrowth in children with chronic diarrhoea, abdominal pain or both. *J Paediatr* 1996; 128: 203–7.

10. D'Eufemia P, Celli M, Finocchiaro R et al. 1996. Abnormal intestinal permeability in children with autism. *Acta Pediatr* 1996: 85: 1076–79.

11. Dunne C, Murphy L, Flynn S, O'Mahony L, O'Halloran S, Feeney M, Morissey D, Thornton G, Fitzerald G, Daly C, Kiely B, Quigley EM, O'Sullivan GC, Shanahan F, Collins JK. 1999. Probiotics: from myth to reality. Demonstration of functionality in animal models of disease and in human clinical trials. (Review)(79 refs). Antonie van Leenwenhoek. 76(104): 279–92, 1999, Jul–Nov.

12. Eaton KK. Sugars in food intolerance and abnormal gut fermentation. *J Nutr Med* 1992; 3: 295–301.

13. Edelson SB, Cantor DS. Autism: xenobiotic influences. *Toxicol Ind Health,* 1998; 14(4): 553–563.

14. Falliers C. Oral contraceptives and allergy. *Lancet* 1974; part 2: 515.

15. Gardner MLG (1994). Absorption of intact proteins and peptides. In: Physiology of the Gastrointestinal Tract, 3rd edn. Chapter 53, pp 1795–1820. NY: Raven Press.

16. Gibson GR, Roberfroid MB (1999). Colonic Microbiota, Nutrition and Health. Kluwer Academic Publishers, Dodrecht.

17. Gobbi G et al (1992) Coeliac disease, epilepsy and cerebral calcifications. *Lancet* 340: 439–443.

18. Grant E. The contraceptive pill: its relation to allergy and illness. *Nutrition and Health* 1983; 2: 33–40.

19. Howard J. The "autobrewery" syndrome. *J Nutr Med* 1991; 2: 97–8.

20. Jackson PG et al. Intestinal permeability in patients with eczema and food allergy. *Lancet* 1981; I: 1285–6.

21. Karlsson H et al. Retroviral RNA identified in the cerebrospinal fluids and brains of individuals with schizophrenia. *Proc Natl Acad Sci.* Vol 98(8), 2001, pp. 4634–9.

22. Kilshaw PJ and Cant AJ (1984). The passage of maternal dietary protein into human breast milk. *Int Arch Allergy Appl Immunol* 75: 8–15.

23. Kinney HC et al (1982). Degeneration of the central nervous system associated with coeliac disease. *J Neurol Sci* 5: 9–22.

24. Krasnogolovez VN. Colonic dysbacteriosis. – M.: Medicina, 1989.
25. Lewis SJ, Freedman AR (1998). Review article: the use of biothera-peutic agents in the prevention and treatment of gastrointestinal disease. (Review)(144 refs). *Alimentary Pharmacology and Therapeutics.* 12(9): 807–22, 1998 Sep.
26. Lindstrum LH et al (1984) CSF and plasma beta-casomorphin-like opioid peptides in post-partum psychosis. *Amer J Psychiat* 141: 1059–1066.
27. Mackie RM. Intestinal permeability and atopic disease. *Lancet* 1981; I: 155.
28. Maki M, Collin P. Coeliac disease. *Lancet* 1997; 349: 1755–9. IF: 13.251.
29. McCandless J. Children with starving brains. A medical treatment guide for autism spectrum disorder. 2003. Bramble books.
30. McGinnis WR. Mercury and autistic gut disease. Environmental Health perspectives 109(7): A303–304 (2001).
31. Melmed FD, Scheneider CK, Fabes RA et al. Metabolic markers and gastrointestinal symptoms in children with autism and related disor-ders. *J Pediatr Gastroenterol Nutr* 2000; 31 (Suppl 2): S31.
32. Ostfeld E, Rubinstein E, Gazit E and Smetana Z (1977). Effect of systemic antibiotics on the microbial flora of the external ear canal in hospitalised children. *Paediatrics* 60: 364–66.
33. Panksepp J. 1979. A neurochemical theory of autism. *Trends in Neuroscience*, 2: 174–177.
34. Petrovskaja VG, Marko OP. Human microflora in norm and pathol-ogy. – M.:Medicina, 1976.
35. Reichelt KL, Knivsberg AM et al. 1996. Diet and autism: a 4 year follow up. Probable reasons and observations relevant to a dietary and genetic aetiology. Conference proceedings from "Therapeutic intervention in autism", University of Durham. 281–307.
36. Reichelt KL et al (1994). Increased levels of antibodies to food proteins in Down syndrome. *Acta Paediat Japon.* 36: 489–492.
37. Reichelt KL et al. (1994) Nature and consequences of hyperpeptiduria of bovine casomorphin found in autistic syndrome. *Develop Brain Dysfunct*, 7: 71–85.
38. Rimland B. New hope for safe and effective treatments for autism. *Autism Research Review International* 8: 3, 1994.
39. Roberfroid MB, Bornet F, Bouley C, Cummings JH (1995). Colonic microflora: nutrition and health. Summary and conclusions of the International Life Sciences Institute (ILSI) [Europe] workshop held in Barcelona, Spain. [Review] [33 refs]. Nutrition Reviews. 53(5): 127–30, 1995 May.
40. Rogers S. 1990. Tired or toxic? A blueprint for health. Prestige Publishers.

41. Rolfe RD. The role of probiotic cultures in the control of gastrointestinal health. *J Nutr*, 2000 Feb; 130(2S) Suppl: 396S–402S Journal Code: JEV.

42. Samonis G et al. (1994). Prospective evaluation of the impact of broad-spectrum antibiotics on the yeast flora of the human gut. *European Journal of Clinical Microbiology and Infections Diseases*, 13: 665–7.

43. Seeley, Stephens, Tate. Anatomy and Physiology. 1992. Second edition. Mosby Year Book.

44. Shattock P et al. 1990. Role of neuropeptides in autism and their relationship with classical neurotransmitters. *Brain Dysfunction*, 3(5), 328–45.

45. Shattock P, Savery D. 1996. Urinary profiles of people with autism: possible implication and relevance to other research. Conference proceedings from "Therapeutic intervention in autism", University of Durham. 309–25.

46. Shaw W. Biological Treatments for Autism and PDD. 2002. ISBN 0-9661238-0-6

47. Stuart CA et al. (1984). Passage of cow's milk protein in breast milk. *Clin Allergy*, 14: 533–535.

48. Summers AO et al. Mercury released from dental silver fillings provokes an increase in mercury – and antibiotic-resistant bacteria in oral and intestinal floras of primates. *Antimicrobial Agents and Chemotherapy*, 1993: 37(4): 825–34.

49. Survey shows link between antibiotics and developmental delays in children. Townsend Letter for Doctors and Patients. October 1995.

50. Tabolin VA, Belmer SV, Gasilina TV, Muhina UG, Korneva TI. Rational therapy of intestinal dysbacteriosis in children. – M.: Medicina, 1998.

51. The International Autism Research Centre. www.gnd.org

52. Toskes PP. Bacterial overgrowth of the gastrointestinal tract. *Adv Int Med*, 1993; 38: 387–407. 27.

53. Troncone R et al. (1987). Passage of gliadin into human breast milk. *Acta Paed Scand*, 76: 453–456.

54. Voronin AA, Taranenko LA, Sidorenko SV 1999.Treatment of intestinal dysbacteriosis in children with diabetes mellitus (Russian).*Antibiotiki I Khimoterapiia*. 1999, 44(3): 22–4.

55. Vorobiev AA, Nesvizski UV (1997). Human microflora and immunity. Review. (Russian). *Sovremennie Problemi Allergologii, Klinicheskoi Immunologii Immunofarmacologii*. – M., 1997. c.137–141.

56. Vorobiev AA, Pak SG et al. (1998). Dysbacteriosis in children. A textbook for doctors and medical students.(Russian). M.: "KMK Lt.", 1998. ISBN 5-87317-049-5.

57. Waring (2001). Sulphate, sulphation and gut permeability: are cytokines involved? In: The Biology of Autism – Unravelled. Conference proceedings 11th May 2001, Institute of Electrical Engineers, London.

58. Wakefield AJ, Anthony A et al. Enterocolitis in children with developmental disorders. *AIA Journal*, Autumn 2001.

Vaccinations. Does MMR Cause Autism? (Part 1: Chapter 8)

1. Anthony H, Birtwistle S, Eaton K, Maberly J. Environmental Medicine in Clinical Practice. BSAENM Publications 1997.

2. Bernard S et al. Autism: a novel form of mercury poisoning. *Med Hypothesis*, 2001 Apr; 56(4): 462–71.

3. Clarkson T. Methylmercury toxicity to the mature and developing nervous system: possible mechanisms. In: Sakar B, ed. Biological Aspects of metals and metal-related diseases. New York: 1983: 183–197.

4. Classen JB. The diabetes epidemic and the hepatitis B vaccines. *N Z Med J* 1996 Sep 27; 109 (1030): 366.

5. Classen JB, Classen DC. Public should be told that vaccines may have long-term adverse effects. *BMJ* 1999 Jan 16; 318 (7177) 193.

6. Coulter H, Fisher BL (1991). A shot in the dark. Avery Publisher Group, New York.

7. Dankova E et al. Immunologic findings in children with abnormal reactions after vaccination. *Chesk Pediatr* 1993 Jan; 48(1): 9–12.

8. Kawashima H et al. Detection and sequencing of measles virus from peripheral mononuclear cells from patients with inflammatory bowel disease. *Dig Dis Sci*, 2000 Apr; 45(4): 723–9.

9. McCandless J. Children with starving brains. A medical treatment guide for autism spectrum disorder. 2003. Bramble books.

10. McGinnis WR. Mercury and autistic gut disease. *Environmental Health Perspectives*, 109(7): A303–304 (2001).

11. Rimland B. New hope for safe and effective treatments for autism. *Autism Research Review International* 8: 3, 1994.

12. Rogers S. 1990. Tired or toxic? A blueprint for health. Prestige Publishers.

13. Shaw W. Biological Treatments for Autism and PDD. 2002. ISBN 0-9661238-0-6

14. Singh V et al. Serological association of measles virus and human herpesvirus-6 with brain autoantibodies in autism. *Clin Immunol Immunopathol*, 1998 Oct; 89(1): 105–108.

15. The International Autism Research Centre. *www.gnd.org*

16. Wakefield AJ and Montgomery SM. Autism, viral infection and measles, mumps, rubella vaccination. *Israeli Medical Association Journal* 1999; 1: 183–187.
17. Walker-Smith JA. Autism, inflammatory bowel disease and MMR vaccine. *Lancet* 1998; 351: 1356–57.
18. Yazbak FE. Autism – is there a vaccine connection? See *www.autism.net/Yazbak1.htm*

Schizophrenia (Part 1: Chapter 9)

1.   Ashkenazi et al. Immunologic reaction of psychotic patients to fractions of gluten. *Am J Psychiatry*, 1979; 136: 1306–1309.
2.   Baruk H. 1978. Psychoses of digestive origins. In: Hemmings and Hemmings (eds), Biological Basis of Schizophrenia. Lancaster MTP Press.
3.   Bender L. Childhood schizophrenia. *Psychiatric Quarterly*, Vol 27, 1953, pp. 3–81.
4.   Cade R et al. Autism and schizophrenia: intestinal disorders. *Nutritional Neuroscience*. March 2000.
5.   Cade et al. The effect of dialysis and diet on schizophrenia. In: *Psychiatry: A World Perspective*, Vol 3. Elsevier Science Publishers, pp. 494–500, 1990.
6.   Calabrese, Joseph R et al. Fish oils and bipolar disorder. *Archives of General Psychiatry*, Vol. 56, May 1999, pp. 413–14.
7.   Conquer, Jilie A et al. Fatty acid analysis of blood plasma of patients with Alzheimer's disease, other types of dementia, and cognitive impairment. *Lipids*, Vol. 35, December 2000, pp. 1305–12.
8.   Crow T (1994). Aetiology of schizophrenia. *Current Opin Psychiat*, 7: 39–42.
9.   Dohan CF. Cereals and schizophrenia: data and hypothesis. *Acta Psychiat Scand*, 1966; 42: 125–152.
10. Dohan CF et al. Relapsed schizophrenics: more rapid improvement on a milk and cereal free diet. *Brit J Psychiat*, 1969; 115: 595–596.
11. Dohan et al. Is schizophrenia rare if grain is rare? *Biology and Psychiatry*, 1984: 19(3): 385–399.
12. Dohan FC. Is celiac disease a clue to pathogenesis of schizophrenia? *Mental Hygiene*, 1969; 53: 525–529.
13. Dohan FC and Grasberger JC (1973). Relapsed schizophrenics: earlier discharge from the hospital after cereal-free, milk-free diet. *Amer J Psychiat*, 130: 685–686.
14. Feinberg I (1982–83). Schizophrenia: caused by a fault in programmed synaptic elimination during adolescence? *J Psychiat Res*, 17: 319–334.

15. Goldman-Rakic PS et al (1983). The neurobiology of cognitive development. In Handbook of Child Psychology: Biology and Infancy development. P Mussen: edit. NY, Wiley. pp. 281–344.

16. Hibbein, Joseph R. Fish consumption and major depression. *Lancet*, Vol. 351, April 18, 1998, p. 1213.

17. Hoffer A. Megavitamin B3 therapy for schizophrenia. *Canad Psychiatric Ass J*, Vol 16, 1971, pp. 499–504.

18. Horrobin D. The madness of Adam and Eve. Bantam Press. ISBN 0 593 04649 8, 2001.

19. Horrobin DF, Glen AM, Vaddadi K. 1994. The membrane hypothesis of schizophrenia. *Schiz Res* 18, 195–207.

20. Joy, CB et al. Polyunsaturated fatty acid (fish or evening primrose oil) for schizophrenia. *The Cochrane Library*, Issue 4, 2000.

21. Kinney HC et al. Degeneration of the central nervous system associated with coeliac disease. *J Neurol Sci* 5: 9–22, 1982.

22. Laughame, J.D.E. et al. Fatty acids and schizophrenia. *Lipids*, Vol. 31, 1996, pp. S163–S65.

23. Mycroft et al. JIF-like sequences in milk and wheat proteins. NEJM 1982; 307: 895.

24. Reichelt K et al. The effect of gluten-free diet on urinary peptide excretion and clinical state in schizophrenia. *Journal of Orthomolecular Medicine*, 5: 1223–39, 1990.

25. Reichelt K et al. Biologically active peptide-containing fractions in schizophrenia and childhood autism. *Adv Biochem Psychopharmacol* 28: 627–47, 1981.

26. Richardson AJ et al. Red cell and plasma fatty acid changes accompanying symptom remission in a patient with schizophrenia treated with eicosapentaenoic acid. *European Neuropsychopharmacology*, Vol. 10, 2000, pp. 189–93.

27. Schoenthaler SJ et al. The effect of randomised vitamin-mineral supplementation on violent and non-violent antisocial behaviour among incarcerated juveniles. *J Nut Env Med*, Vol 7, 1997, pp. 343–352.

28. Singh & Kay. Wheat gluten as a pathogenic factor in schizophrenia. *Science* 1975: 191: 401–402.

29. Sioudrou et al. Opioid peptides derived from food proteins. The exorphins. *J Biol Chem*. 1979; 254: 2446–2449.

30. Tanskanen, Antti, et al. Fish consumption, depression, and suicidality in a general population. *Archives of General Psychiatry*, Vol. 58, May 2001, pp. 512–13.

31. Torrey EF et al. Endemic psychosis in western Ireland. *Am J Psychiatry* 141: 966–970, 1984.

32. Ward PE et al. Niacin skin flush in schizophrenia: a preliminary report. *Schizophr Res*, Vol 29, 1998, pp. 269–74.

33. Wittenborn JR. Niacin in the long term treatment of schizophrenia. *Arch Gen Psychiatry*, Vol 28, 1973, pp. 308–15.

Epilepsy (Part 1: Chapter 10)

1. American Academy of Neurology. Lower IQ found in children of women who took epilepsy drug. AAN Press Release, *Newswise*, Wed 11-Aor-2007. http://www.newswise.com/articles/view/528880/?dc=dwhn.
2. Anthony H, Birtwistle S, Eaton K, Maberly J. *Environmental Medicine in Clinical Practice*. BSAENM Publications, 1997.
3. Appleton R, Gibbs J. *Epilepsy in childhood and adolescence*. 1995. Martin Dunitz.
4. Barbeau et al. Zinc, taurine and epilepsy. *Arch Neurol*, Vol 30, 1974, pp. 52–8.
5. Berg AT, Shinnar S, Levy SR, Testa FM (November 1999). "Childhood-onset epilepsy with and without preceding febrile seizures". *Neurology* 53 (8): 1742–8.
6. Bok LA, Struys E, Willemsen MA, Been JV, Jakobs C. Pyridoxine-dependent seizures in Dutch patients: diagnosis by elevated urinary alpha-aminoadipic semialdehyde levels. *Arch Dis Child*. 2007 Aug; 92(8): 687–9. Epub 2006 Nov 6.
7. Botez et al. Thiamine and folate treatment of chronic epileptic patients: a controlled study with the Wechsler IQ scale. *Epilepsy-Res*, Vol 16(2), 1993, pp. 157–63.
8. Crayton JW et al. Epilepsy precipitated by food sensitivity: report of a case with double-blind placebo-controlled assessment. *Clinical Electorencephalo*, Vol 12(4), 1981, p. 192–9.
9. Dubé CM, Brewster AL, Richichi C, Zha Q, Baram TZ . "Fever, febrile seizures and epilepsy". *Trends Neurosci,* Oct 2007, 30 (10): 490–6.
10. Dupont CL and Tanaka Y. Blood manganese levels in children with convulsive disorders. *Biochem Med*, Vol 33(2), 1985, pp. 246–55.
11. Egger J, Carter CM, Soothill J et al. Oligoantigenic diet treatment of children with epilepsy and migraine. *J Pediatrics*, 1989; 114:5108.
12. Elger CE and Schmidt D. Modern management of epilepsy: a practical approach. *Epilepsy & Behavior,* 2008, 12(4), 501–539.
13. Freeman JM, Kelly MT and Freeman JB. *The epilepsy diet treatment. An introduction to the ketogenic diet*. 2nd Edition. 1996. Demos Vermande.
14. Freeman JM. The ketogenic diet – 1998. *Epilepsy Today*, Dec 1998.
15. Freeman JM, Kossoff EH, Hartman AM. The ketogenic diet: one decade later. *Pediatrics* . 2007 Mar; 119(3): 535–43.
16. French JA, Pedley TA. Clinical practice. Initial management of epilepsy. *N Engl J Med*. 2008; 359(2): 166–76.

17. Garrow JS, James WPT, Ralph A. *Human nutrition and dietetics*. 2000. 10th edition. Churchill Livingstone.

18. Gasior M, Rogawski MA, Hartman AL. Neuroprotective and disease-modifying effects of the ketogenic diet. *Behav Pharmacol*. 2006; 17(5–6): 431–9.

19. Gibberd FB et al. The influence of folic acid on the frequency of epileptic attacks. *Europ J Clin Pharmacology*, Vol 9(1), 1981, pp. 57–60.

20. Gorges LF et al. Effect of magnesium on epileptic foci. *Epilepsia*, Vol 19(1), 1978, pp. 81–91.

21. Gupta SK et al. Serum magnesium levels in idiopathic epilepsy. *J Assoc Physicians India*, Vol 42(6), 1994, pp. 456–7.

22. Huxtable R et al. The prolonged anticonvulsant action of taurine on genetically determined seizure-susceptibility. *Canadian J Neurol Sci*, Vol 5, 1978, p. 220.

23. Kinsman Sl, Vining EPG et al. Efficacy of the ketogenic diet for intractable seizure disorders: review of 58 cases. *Epilepsia* 1992; 33: 1132–1136.

24. Keyser A, De Brujin SF. Epileptic manifestations and vitamin B1 deficiency. *Eur Neurol*, Vol 31(3), 1991, pp. 121–125.

25. Kossof EH, Dorward JL. The modified Atkins diet. *Epilepsia*. 2008 Nov; 49 Suppl 8: 37–41.

26. Lefevre F, Aronson N. Ketogenic diet for the treatment of refractory epilepsy in children: a systematic review of efficacy. *Pediatrics* 2000; 105: e46.

27. Liu YM. Medium-chain triglycerides (MCT) ketogenic therapy. *Epilepsia*. 2008, Nov 49. Suppl 8: 33–6.

28. MHRA (2008b) Anti-epileptics: risk of suicidal thoughts and behaviour. *Drug Safety Update* 2(1), 2.

29. MHRA (2009) Drug safety advice. Anti-epileptics: adverse effects on the bone. *Drug Safety Update* 2(9), 2.

30. Morrow, J., Russell, A., Guthrie, E. et al. (2006) Malformation risks of antiepileptic drugs in pregnancy: a prospective study from the UK Epilepsy and Pregnancy Register. *Journal of Neurology, Neurosurgery, and Psychiatry* 77(2), 193–198.

31. Nakazawa M. High dose vitamin B6 therapy in infantile spasms – the effect of adverse reactions. *Brain and Development*, Vol 5(2), 1983, p.193.

32. Papavasiliou et al. Seizure disorders and trace metals: manganese tissue levels in treated epileptics. *Neurology*, Vol 29, 1979, p. 1466.

33. Pietz J et al. Treatment of infantile spasms with high-dosage vitamin B6. *Epilepsia*, Vol 34(4), 1993, pp. 757–63.

34. Qin P et al. Risk for schizophrenia and schizophrenia-like psychosis among patients with epilepsy: population based cohort study. *BMJ* 2005; 331: 23.

35. Ramaeckers Vt. Selenium deficiency triggering intractable seizures. *Neuropediatrics*, Vol 25(4), 1994, pp. 217–23.
36. Ranganathan IN, Ramaratnam S. Vitamins for epilepsy. Cochrane Database of Systematic Reviews 2005, Issue 2. Art. No.: CD004304. DOI: 10.1002/14651858.CD004304.pub2.
37. Schachter SC. Seizure disorders. *Med Clin North Am.* March 2009; 93(2).
38. Schlanger S, Shinitzky M and Yam D. Diet enriched with omega-3 fatty acids alleviates convulsion symptoms in epilepsy patients. *Epilepsia*, Vol 43(1), 2002, pp. 103–4.
39. Shoji Y. Serum magnesium and zinc in epileptic children. *Brain and Development*, Vol 5(3), 1983, p. 200.
40. Schwartz RM et al. Ketogenic diets in the treatment of epilepsy: short-term clinical effects. *Dev Med Child Neurol* 1989; 31: 145–151.
41. Sirven J et al. The ketogenic diet for intractable epilepsy in adults: preliminary results. *Epilepsia* 1999; 40: 1721–1726.
42. Smith DB and Obbens E. Antifolate-antiepileptic relationships, in Botez MI and Reynolds EH, eds, *Folic Acid in Neurology, Psychiatry and Internal Medicine*, Raven Press (1979).
43. Sohler A and Pfeiffer C. A direct method for the determination of manganese in whole blood: patients with seizure activity have low blood levels. *J Orthomol Psychiat*, Vol 12, 1983, pp. 215–234.
44. Stafstrom CE. Dietary approaches to epilepsy treatment: old and new options on the menu. *Epilepsy Curr*, 2004; 4(6): 215–222.
45. Tanaka Y. Low manganese level may trigger epilepsy. *JAMA*, Vol 238, 1977, p. 1805.
46. Temkin O. *The falling sickness: a history of epilepsy from the Greeks to the beginnings of modern neurology.* 2nd ed. Baltimore: Johns Hopkins University Press; 1971.
47. Turner Z, Kossoff EH. The ketogenic and Atkins diets: recipes for seizure control. *Pract Gastroenterol.* 2006, Jun: 29(6): 53–64.
48. Vestergaard P, Rejnmark L and Mosekilde M. Fracture risk associated with use of anti-epileptic drugs. *Epilepsia,* 2004, 45(11), 1330–1337.

The Diet – a Discussion (Part 2, Diet: Chapter 1)
The Appropriate Diet for GAP Syndrome (Part 2, Diet: Chapter 2)

1. Anthony H, Birtwistle S, Eaton K, Maberly J. Environmental Medicine in Clinical Practice. BSAENM Publications 1997.
2. Boris M, Mandel F. Food and additives are common causes of the attention deficit hyperactive disorder in children. *Annals of Allergy* 72: 462–68, 1994.

3. Carter CM et al (1993). Effects of a few food diet in attention deficit disorder. *Arch Dis Child* 69: 564–568.
4. Ebringer a et al. The use of a low starch diet in the treatment of patients suffering from ankylosing spondyllitis. *Clin Rheumatol* 1996;15, suppl 1: 62–6.
5. Egger J et al (1985). Controlled oligoantigenic treatment of the hyperkinetic syndrome. *The Lancet.* March 9th: 540–544.
6. Egger J et al. (1992). Controlled trial of hyposensitisation with food-induced hyperkinetic syndrome. *The Lancet* 339: 1150–1153.
7. Garrow JS, James WPT, Ralph A. Human nutrition and dietetics. 2000. 10th edition. Churchill Livingstone.
8. Geary A. The food and mood handbook. 2001. Thorsons.
9. Gottschall E. Breaking the vicious cycle. Intestinal health through diet. 1996. The Kirkton Press.
10. Hole K et al (1988). Attention deficit disorders: a study of peptide-containing urinary complexes. *J Develop Behav Paediatrics.* 9: 205–212.
11. Hurst AF, Knott FA. Intestinal carbohydrate dyspepsia. *Quart J Med* 1930–31; 24: 171–80.
12. Kaplan SJ et al (1989). Dietary replacement in preschool-aged hyperactive boys. *Paediatrics* 83: 7–17.
13. Kilshaw PJ and Cant AJ (1984). The passage of maternal dietary protein into human breast milk. *Int Arch Allergy and Appl Immunol* 75: 8–15.
14. Mirkkunen M (1982). Reactive hypoglycaemia tendency among habitually violent offenders. *Neuropsychopharmacol* 8: 35–40.
15. Rowe KS, Rose KJ. Synthetic food colouring and behaviour: A dose response effect in a double-blind, placebo-controlled, repeated-measures study. *Journal of Paediatrics* 12: 691–698, 1994.
16. Rowe KS. Synthetic food colouring and hyperactivity: A double-blind crossover study. *Aust Paediatr J*, 24: 143–47, 1988.
17. Smith MW, Phillips AD. Abnormal expression of dipeptidyl peptidase IV activity in enterocyte brush-border membranes of children suffering from coeliac disease. *Exp Physiol* 1990 Jul; 75(4); 613–6.
18. The International Autism Research Centre. www.gnd.org
19. Ward NI. Assessment of clinical factors in relation to child hyperactivity. *J Nutr Environ Med*, Vol 7, 1997, p. 333–342.
20. Ward NI. Hyperactivity and a previous history of antibiotic usage. *Nutrition Practitioner*, Vol 3(3), 2001, p.12.
21. Schoenthaler SJ et al. The effect of randomised vitamin-mineral supplementation on violent and non-violent antisocial behaviour among incarcerated juveniles. *J Nut Env Med*, Vol 7, 1997, pp. 343–352.

Failure to Thrive (Part 2: Diet, Chapter 5)
Eating Disorders (Part 2: Diet, Chapter 6)

22. Askenazy E. et al. Whole blood serotonin content, tryptophan concentrations and impulsivity in anorexia nervosa. Biological Psychiatry, Vol 43(3), 1998, pp. 188–195.

23. Bakan R. The role of zinc in anorexia nervosa: etiology and treatment. Med Hypotheses, Vol 5(7), 1979, pp. 731–6.

24. Biederman J. Are girls with ADHD at risk for eating disorders? Results from a controlled, five-year prospective study. Dev Behav Pediatr. 2007 Aug; 28(4): 302–7.

25. Birmingham C. et al. Controlled trial of zinc supplementation in anorexia nervosa. Int J Eat Disord, Vol 15(3), 1994, pp. 251–5.

26. Birmingham CL, Gritzner S. How does zinc supplementation benefit anorexia nervosa? Eat Weight Disord. 2006 Dec; 11(4): e109–11.

27. Braun Dl. Psychiatric comorbidity in patients with eating disorders. Psychological Medicine 1994; 24: 854–67.

28. Bryce-Smith D. and Simpson RI. Case of anorexia nervosa responding to zinc sulphate. Lancet, Vol 2(8398), 1984, p.350.

29. Bulik CM et al. Anorexia nervosa treatment: a systematic review of randomized controlled trials. Int J Eat Disord. 2007 May; 40(4): 310–20.

30. Caralat DJ, Carmago CA. Review of bulimia nervosa in men. American Journal of Psychiatry 1991 Jul; 148(7) 831–834.

31. Casper and Prasad, 1980, later confirmed by L. Humphries et al. Zinc deficiency and eating disorders. J Clin Psychiatry, Vol 50(12), 1989, pp. 456–9.

32. Cortese S. et al. Attention-deficit/hyperactivity disorder (ADHD) and binge eating. Nutr Rev. 2007 Sep; 65(9): 404–11. Nutr Rev. 2008 Jun; 66(6): 357.

33. Cowen PJ and Smith KA. Serotonin, dieting and bulimia nervosa. Advances in Experimental Medicine and Biology, Vol 467, 1999, pp. 101–4.

34. Erdmann R. & Jones M. The amino revolution. The most exciting development in nutrition since the vitamin tablet. 1987, Century.

35. Favaro A. Tryptophan levels, excessive exercise, and nutritional status in anorexia nervosa. Psychosomatic Medicine, Vol 62(4), 2000, pp. 535–8.

36. Halmi KA. The multimodal treatment of eating disorders. World Psychiatry. 2005 Jun; 4(2): 69–73.

37. Hudson et al. The prevalence and correlates of eating disorders in the National Comorbidity Survey Replication. Biological Psychiatry. 2007 Feb 1; 61(3) 348–58.

38. Humphries L. et al. Zinc deficiency and eating disorders. J Clin Psychiatry, Vol 50(12), 1989, pp. 456–9.

39. Holford P. *Optimum nutrition for the mind.* 2003, Piatkus.
40. Jimerson DC, et al., Eating disorders and depression: is there a serotonin connection? *Biol Psychiatry.* 1990 Sep 1; 28(5): 443–54.
41. Kaye WH. Et al. Effects of acute tryptophan depletion on mood in bulimia nervosa. *Biol Psychiatry*, Vol 47(2), 2000, pp. 151–7.
42. Kaye WH, Anorexia, obsessional behaviour and serotonin, *Psycopharmacology Bulletin*, 1997; 33(3) 335–44.
43. Kuhne T, Bubl R, Baumgartner R. Maternal vegan diet causing a serious infantile neurological disorder due to vitamin B12 deficiency. *Europ J Pediatrics*, 1991, 150: 205–208.
44. Lask Bryan. Anorexia Nervosa and Related Eating Disorders in Childhood and Adolescence, Rachel Bryant-Waugh Publisher: Psychology Press; 2 edition (October 12, 2000).
45. Leibowitz, The role of serotonin in eating disorders. *Drugs* 1990; 39 Suppl 3: 33–44.
46. Mikami AY et el. Bulimia nervosa symptoms in the Multimodal Treatment Study of Children with ADHD. *Int J Eat Disord.* 2009 Apr 17.
47. Patrick L. Eating disorders: a review of the literature with emphasis on medical complications and clinical nutrition. *Alternative Medicine review*, 2002 Jun; 7(3) 184–202.
48. Rosenvinge et al. The comorbidity of eating disorders and personality disorders: a metanalytic review of studies between 1983 and 1998. *Eating and Weight Disorders,* 2000 June; 5(2): 52–61.
49. Roberts IF, West RJ, Ogilvie D, Dillon MJ. Malnutrition in infants receiving cult diets: a form of child abuse. *BMJ* 1979; 1: 296–268.
50. Sullivan PF. Mortality in anorexia nervosa. *Biological Psychiatry,* 2007 Feb 1; 61(3) 348–58: 1073–1074.
51. Toivanen and E. Eerola. A vegan diet changes the intestinal flora. *Rheumatology,* August 1, 2002; 41(8): 950–951.

Probiotics (Part 2: Supplementation, Chapter 1)

1. Black FT, Andersen PL, Orskov J, Orskov F, Gaarslev K, Laulund S. Prophylactic efficacy of lactobacilli on traveller's diarrhoea. In: Steffen R. ed. Travel medicine. Conference on international travel medicine 1, Zurich, Switzerland, *Berlin: Springer*, 1989: 333–5.
2. Bowden TA, Mansberger AR, Lykins LE. Pseudomembranous colitis; mechanism for restoring floral homeostasis. *Am Surg* 1981; 47: 178–83.
3. Borriello SP. The application of bacterial antagonism in the prevention and treatment of Clostridium difficile infection of the gut. In: Hardie JM, Borriello SP, Anaerobes Today 1988, London; John Wiley & Sons: 195–202.

4. Brigidi P at al. Effects of probiotic administration upon the composition and enzymatic activity of human faecal microbiota in patients with irritable bowel syndrome or functional diarrhoea. *Research in Microbiol,* 2001 Oct; 152(8): 735–41 Journal Code: R6F.

5. Cunningham-Rundles S, Ahrn'e S, Bengmark S, Johann-Liang R, Marshall F, Metakis L, Califano C, Dunn AM, Grassey C, Hinds G, Cervia J, (2000). Probiotics and immune response. *American Journal of Gastroenterology,* 95(1 Suppl): S22–5, 2000 Jan.

6. Drisko JA at al. Probiotics in health maintenance and disease prevention. *Alternative Medicine Review,* 2003, vol 8, number 2.

7. Dunne C, Murphy L, Flynn S, O'Mahony L, O'Halloran S, Feeney M, Morissey D, Thornton G, Fitzerald G, Daly C, Kiely B, Quigley EM, O'Sullivan GC, Shanahan F, Collins JK 1999. Probiotics: from myth to reality. Demonstration of functionality in animal models of disease and in human clinical trials. (Review)(79 refs), Antonie van Leenwenhoek. 76(104): 279–92, 1999 Jul–Nov.

8. Eiseman B, Silem W, Boscomb WS, Kanov AJ. Faecal enema as an adjunct in the treatment of pseudomembranous enterocolitis. *Surgery* 1958; 44: 854–8.

9. Fuller R. Probiotics in man and animals. *J Appl bacteriol,* 1989; 66: 365–78.

10. Gibson GR, Roberfroid MB (1999). Colonic Microbiota, Nutrition and Health. Kluwer Academic Publishers, Dodrecht.

11. Goldin BR (1998). Health benefits of probiotics. *British Journal of Nutrition,* 80(4): S203–7, 1998 Oct.

12. Guandalini S, Pensabene L, Zilri MA, Dias JA, Casali LG, Hoekstra H, Kolacek S, Massar K, Micetic-Turk D, Papadopoulou A, de Sousa JS, Sandhu B, Szajewska H, Weizman Z, (2000). Lactobacillus GG administered in oral re-hydration solution to children with acute diarrhoea: a multi-center European trial. *J Pediatr Gastroenterol Nutr,* 30(1): 54–60, 2000 Jan.

13. Guarino A, Canani RB, Spagnuolo MI, Albano F, DiBenedetto L (1997). Oral bacterial therapy reduces the duration of symptoms and of visceral excretions in children with mild diarrhoea. *Journal of Paediatric Gastroenterology and Nutrition.* 25(5): 516–9, 1997 Nov.

14. Hirayama K, Rafter J (1999). The role of lactic acid bacteria in colon cancer prevention: mechanistic considerations. Antonie Van Leeuwenhoek, 76(1–4): 391–4, 1999 Jul–Nov.

15. Hoyos AB (1999). Reduced incidence of necrotizing enterocolitis associated with enteral administration of Lactobacillus acidophilus and Bifidobacterium infantis to neonates in intensive care unit. *Int J Infect Dis* 1999 Summer; 3(4): 197–202.

16. Hotta M, Sato Y, Iwata S et al. Clinical effects of Bifidobacterium

preparations on paediatric intractable diarrhoea. *Keio J Med*, 1987; 36: 298–314.

17. Kirjavainen PV, Apostolov E, Salminen SS, Isolauri E. 1999. New aspects of probiotics – a novel approach in the management of food allergy. (Review) (59refs). *Allergy*. 54(9): 909–15, 1999 Sep.

18. Krasnogolovez VN. Colonic dysbacteriosis. – M.: Medicina, 1989.

19. Lewis SJ, Freedman AR (1998). Review article: the use of biotherapeutic agents in the prevention and treatment of gastrointestinal disease. (Review) (144 refs). *Alimentary Pharmacology and Therapeutics*. 12(9): 807–22, 1998 Sep.

20. Lykova EA, Bondarenko VM, Sidorenko SV, Grishina ME, Murashova AD, Minaev VI, Rytikov FM, Korsunski AA (1999). Combined antibacterial and probiotic therapy of Helicobacter – associated disease in children (Russian). *Journal Microbiologii, Epidemiologii I Immunobiologii*. 1999 Mar–Apr; (2): 76–81.

21. Macfarlane GT, Cummings JH (1999). Probiotics and prebiotics: can regulating the activities of intestinal bacteria benefit health? (Review) (48 refs). *BMJ*. 1999 April; 318: 999–1003.

22. Metchnikov E. The Prolongation of Life. GP Putman's & Sons, New York, NY 1907.

23. Niedzielin D at al. A controlled, double-blind, randomised study on the efficacy of Lactobacillus plantarum 299V in patients with irritable bowel syndrome. *Eur J Gastoenterol Hepatol*, 2001 Oct; 13(10): 1143–7 Journal Code: B9X.

24. Nobaek S at al. Alteration of intestinal microflora is associated with reduction in abdominal bloating and pain in patients with irritable bowel syndrome. *Am J Gastroenterol*, 2000 May; 95(5): 1231–8 Journal Code: 3HE.

25. O'Sullivan MA, O'Morain CA. Bacterial supplementation in the irritable bowel syndrome. A randomised double-blind placebo-controlled crossover study. *Dig Liver Dis*, 2000 May; 32(4): 294–301 Journal Code: DQK.

26. Petrovskaja VG, Marko OP. Human microflora in norm and pathology. – M.: Medicina, 1976.

27. Rao CV, Sanders ME, Indranie C, Simi B, Reddy BS (1999). Prevention of colonic preneoplastic lesions by the probiotic Lactobacillus acidophilus NCFMTM in F344 rats. *International Journal of Oncology*. 14(5): 939–44, 1999 May.

28. Reddy BS, (1998). Prevention of colon cancer by pre- and probiotics: evidence from laboratory studies. *British Journal of Nutrition*, 80(4): S219–23 1998 Oct.

29. Reddy BS (1999). Possible mechanisms by which pro- and prebiotics influence colon carcinogenesis and tumour growth. *Journal of Nutrition*, 129(7 Suppl): 1478S–82S, 1999 Jul.

30. Roberfroid MB, Bornet F, Bouley C, Cummings JH (1995). Colonic microflora: nutrition and health. Summary and conclusions of an International Life Sciences Institute (ILSI) [Europe] workshop held in Barcelona, Spain. [Review] [33 refs]. Nutrition Reviews. 53(5): 127–30, 1995 May.

31. Rolfe RD. The role of probiotic cultures in the control of gastrointestinal health. *J Nutr*, 2000 Feb; 130(2S) Suppl: 396S–402S Journal Code: JEV.

32. Schwan A, Sjolin S, Trottestam U, Aronson B. Clostridium difficile enterocolitis cured by rectal infusion of normal faeces. *Scand J Infect Dis* 1984; 16: 211–215.

33. Shaw W. Biological Treatments for Autism and PDD. 2002. ISBN 0-9661238-0-6

34. Sullivan NM, Mills DC, Riemann HP, Arnon SS. Inhibitions of growth of Clostridium botulinum by intestinal microflora isolated from healthy infants. *Microbial Ecology in Health and Disease*, 1988; 1: 179–92.

35. Swedsinski A at al. Mucosal flora in inflammatory bowel disease. 2001. PMID: 11781279 PubMed.

36. Tabolin VA, Belmer SV, Gasilina TV, Muhina UG, Korneva TI. Rational therapy of intestinal dysbacteriosis in children. – M.: Medicina, 1998.

37. Tanaka R, Watamaba K, Takayama H et al. Effect of administration of Bifidobacterium preparation on antibiotic associated infantile protracted diarrhoea. Proceedings of V1 Riken symposium on the Intestinal flora. 1985; 43–64.

38. Voronin AA, Taranenko LA, Sidorenko SV. 1999. Treatment of intestinal dysbacteriosis in children with diabetes mellitus (Russian). *Antibiotiki I Khimoterapiia,* 1999, 44(3): 22–4.

39. Vorobiev AA, Nesvizski UV. (1997). Human microflora and immunity. Review.(Russian). *Sovremennie Problemi Allergologii, Klinicheskoi Immunologii Immunofarmacologii.* – M., 1997. c.137–141.

40. Vorobiev AA, Pak SG et al. (1998). Dysbacteriosis in children. A textbook for doctors and medical students. (Russian). M.: "KMK Lt.", 1998, ISBN 5-87317-049-5.

41. Venturi A, Gionchetti P, Rizzello F, Johansson R, Zucconi E, Brigidi P, Matteuzzi D, Campieri M (1999). Impact on the composition of the faecal flora by a new probiotic preparation: preliminary data on maintenance treatment of patients with ulcerative colitis. *Aliment Pharmacol Ther*, 13(8): 1103–8, 1999 Aug.

42. Vaughan EE, Millet B (1999). Probiotics in the new millennium (Revew/76 refs). *Nahrung.* 1999 Jun; 43(3): 148–53.

43. Wilson K, Moore L, Patel M, Permoad P. Suppression of potential

pathogens by a defined colonic microflora. *Microbial Ecology in Health and Disease.* 1988; 1: 237–43.

44. Yasui H, Shida K, Matsuzaki T, Yokokuta T (1999). Immunomodulatory function of lactic acid bacteria. (Review) (28 refs) Antonie van Leenwenhoek. 76(1–4): 38309, 1999 Jul–Nov.

Fats: the Good and the Bad (Part 2, Supplementation: Chapter 2) Cod liver oil (Part 2, Supplementation: Chapter 3)

1. Calabrese, Joseph R et al. Fish oils and bipolar disorder. *Archives of General Psychiatry,* Vol. 56, May 1999, pp. 413–14.
2. Conquer, Jilie A et al. Fatty acid analysis of blood plasma of patients with Alzheimer's disease, other types of dementia and cognitive impairment. *Lipids,* Vol. 35, December 2000, pp. 1305–12.
3. Denton M, Lacey R. Intensive farming and food processing: implications for polyunsaturated fats. *J Nutr Med* 1991; 2: 179–189.
4. Enig M. *Know your fats: the complete primer for understanding the nutrition of fats, oils and cholesterol.* Silver Spring: Bethseda Press, 2000.
5. Garrow JS, James WPT, Ralph A. Human nutrition and dietetics. 2000. 10th edition. Churchill Livingstone.
6. Hibbein, Joseph R. Fish consumption and major depression. *The Lancet,* Vol. 351, April 18, 1998, p. 1213.
7. Horrobin D. The madness of Adam and Eve. Bantam Press. ISBN 0 593 04649 8, 2001.
8. Joy, CB et al. Polyunsaturated fatty acid (fish or evening primrose oil) for schizophrenia. *The Cochrane Library,* Issue 4, 2000.
9. Kabara JJ. Antimicrobial agents derived from fatty acids. *Journal of the American Oil Chemists Society* 1984; 61: 397–403.
10. Laughame JDE et al. Fatty acids and schizophrenia. *Lipids,* Vol. 31, 1996, pp. S163–S65.
11. Puri B, Boyd H. 2004. The natural way to beat depression. Hodder & Stoughton.
12. Richardson A.J., et al. Red cell and plasma fatty acid changes accompanying symptom remission in a patient with schizophrenia treated with eicosapentaenoic acid. *European Neuropsychopharmacology,* Vol. 10, 2000, pp. 189–93.
13. Richardson AJ. Fatty acids in dyslexia, dyspraxia, ADHD and the autistic spectrum. *The Nutrition Practitioner,* Vol 3(3), 2001, pp. 18–24.
14. Severus W, Emanuel et al. Omega-3 fatty acids: the missing link? *Archives of General Psychiatry,* Vol 56, April 1999, pp. 380–81.
15. Sporn MB, Roberts AB, Goodman DS. The retinoids: biology, chemistry and medicine, 2nd edn. Raven Press, New York. 1994.
16. Tanskanen, Antti et al. Fish consumption, depression, and suicidality

in a general population. *Archives of General Psychiatry*, Vol. 58, May 2001, pp. 512–13.

17.   Udo Erasmus. Fats that heal, fats that kill. 1993. Alive books, Canada.

18.   World Health Organisation 1996. Indicators for assessing vitamin A deficiency and their application in monitoring and evaluating intervention programs. Micronutrient series 96–10. WHO, Geneva.

Digestive Enzymes (Part 2, Supplementation: Chapter 4)

1.   Augustyns K et al. The unique properties of dipeptidyl-peptidase IV (DPP IV / CD26) and the therapeutic potential of DPP IV inhibitors. *Curr Med Chem*, 1999 Apr; 6(4): 311–2

2.   Elgun S et al. Dipeptidyl peptidase IV and adenosine deaminase activity. Decrease in depression. *Psychoneuroendocrinology* 1999 Nov; 24(8): 823–32.

3.   Erdmann R. The amino revolution.1987. Century.

4.   Garrow JS, James WPT, Ralph A. Human nutrition and dietetics. 2000. 10th edition. Churchill Livingstone.

5.   Howell E. Food enzymes for health and longevity. 1986. Omangod Press.

6.   Horvath K et al. Improved social and language skills in patients with autistic spectrum disorders after secretin administration. *JAAMP* 9: 9–15, 1998.

7.   Sandler AD et al. Lack of benefit of a single dose of synthetic human secretin in the treatment of autism and pervasive developmental disorder. *N Engl J Med* 1999 Dec 9; 341(24): 1801–6.

8.   Santillo H. Food enzymes. The missing link to radiant health. 1993. Hohm Press.

9.   Seeley, Stephens, Tate. Anatomy and Physiology. 1992. Second edition. Mosby Year Book.

10.   The International Autism Research Centre. www.gnd.org

11.   Wolf M et al. Enzyme Therapy. 1972. Regent House, Los Angeles, CA.

Detoxification for People with GAPS (Part 2)

1.   Anthony H, Birtwistle S, Eaton K, Maberly J. Environmental Medicine in Clinical Practice. BSAENM Publications 1997.

2.   Bernard S et al. Autism: a novel form of mercury poisoning. *Med Hypothesis*, 2001 Apr; 56(4): 462–71.

3.   Coleman M et al. A review of epidemiological studies of the health effects of living near or working with electricity generation and transmission equipment. *Int J Epidemiol* 1988; 17: 1–13.

4.   Edelson SB, Cantor DS. Autism: xenobiotic influences. *Toxicol Health* 1998; 14(4): 553–563.
5.   Epstein SS. Unreasonable risk. How to avoid cancer from cosmetics and personal care products. 2001. Published by Environmental Toxicology, Chicago Illinois.
6.   Epstein SS. The politics of cancer, revisited. East Ridge Press, Fremont Centre, NY, 1998.
7.   Gerson C & Walker M. The Gerson Therapy. 2001.Twin Streams, Kensington Publishing Corporation.
8.   Kaplan S, Morris J. Kids at risk: chemicals in the environment come under scrutiny as the number of childhood learning problems soars. US News&World Report, June 19, 2000, p. 51.
9.   Kuhnert P et al. Comparison of mercury levels in maternal blood, foetal cord blood and placental tissues. *Am J Obstet Gynaecol* 1981; 139: 209–212.
10. McCandless J. Children with starving brains. A medical treatment guide for autism spectrum disorder. 2003. Bramble books.
11. McGinnis WR. Mercury and autistic gut disease. *Environmental Health perspectives* 109(7): A303–304 (2001).
12. Meyerowitz S. Juice fasting & detoxification. The fastest way to restore your health. 2002. Sproutman Publications.
13. Nielsen GD et al. Effects of industrial detergents on the barrier function of human skin. *Int. J Occup Med.* 6(2): 143–147, 2000.
14. Nylander M. Mercury in the pituitary glands of dentists. *Lancet* 1986; 1: 442.
15. Rogers S. 1990. Tired or toxic? A blueprint for health. Prestige Publishers.
16. Shaw W. Biological Treatments for Autism and PDD. 2002. ISBN 0-9661238-0-6.
17. Steinman D, Epstein SS. The safe shopper's bible. Macmillan, New York, 1995.
18. Stortebecker P. Mercury poisoning from dental amalgam through a direct nose brain transport. *Lancet* 1989; 339: 1207.
19. Wayland J, Laws E. Handbook of pesticide toxicology. San Diego: Academic Press, 1990.

Ear Infections and Glue Ear (Part 3: Chapter 1)

1.   Effective Health Care 1992, No 4. The treatment of persistent glue ear in children. Leeds. Univ of Leeds 1992.
2.   Crook W. The yeast connection. 1986. Vintage Books.
3.   Hagerman R, Falkenstein A. An association between recurrent otitis media in infancy and later hyperactivity. *Clinical Paediatrics*, Vol. 26, pp. 253–257, 1987.

4. Kontstantareas M, Homatidis S. Ear infections in autistic and normal children. *Journal of Autism and Developmental Disease*, Vol. 17, p. 585, 1987.

5. Nsouli TM et al. Role of food allergy in serious otitis media. *Ann Allergy* 1994: 73: 215–9.

6. Ostfeld E, Rubinstein E, Gazit E and Smetana Z, (1977). Effect of systemic antibiotics on the microbial flora of the external ear canal in hospitalised children. *Paediatrics* 60: 364–66.

7. Scadding GK et al. Glue ear guidelines. *Lancet*, 1993; 341: 57.

8. Seeley, Stephens, Tate. Anatomy and Physiology. 1992. Second edition. Mosby Year Book.

9. Shaw W. 2002. Biological treatments for autism and PDD. Self-published.

A Few Words about Education (Part 3: Chapter 6)

1. Barkley RA. Taking charge of ADHD – the complete, authoritative guide for parents. New York: Guilford Press, 1995.

2. Brooks R. The self-esteem teacher. Circle Pines, MN: American Guidance Service, 1991.

3. Donaldson M. Children's minds. Fontana, 1978.

4. Garber S, Garber M and Spizman R. Good behaviour – over 1,200 sensible solutions to your child's problems from birth to age 12. New York: St. Martin's Paperbacks, 1987.

5. Lovaas IO. Behavioural treatment and normal educational and intellectual functioning in young autistic children. *J Consulting and Clinical Psychology*, 1987, vol. 55, 1, 3–9.

6. Lovaas IO & Smith T. A comprehensive behavioural theory of autistic children: paradigm for research and treatment. 1989. *J Behav Ther & Exp Psych*. Vol 20, 1, pp. 17–29.

7. Lovaas IO. The development of a treatment-research project for developmentally disabled and autistic children. *Journal of Applied Behaviour Analysis*. 1993 Winter (4) 26, 617–630.

8. Lovaas OI. Teaching developmentally disabled children: The ME book. Austin: Pro-Ed. 1981.

9. McCarney S & Bauer A. The parent's guide: solutions to today's most common behaviour problems in the home. Columbia, MO: Hawthorne Educational Services, 1989.

10. Maurice C. Let me hear your voice. New York: Knopf. 1993.

11. Maurice C, Green H & Luce SC. Behavioural intervention for young children with autism. Austin: Pro-ed. 1996.

12. McEachin JJ, Smith T & Lovaas OI. Long-term outcome for children with autism who received early intensive behavioural treatment. *Am J Mental Retardation*. 1993, 97, 359–372.

13. Rief S & Heimburge J. How to reach and teach all students in the inclusive classroom. West Nyack, NY: The Center for Applied Research in Education, 1996.

14. Rief S. The ADD/ADHD checklist. An easy reference for parents and teachers. 1997. Prentice Hall Publishing.

15. Rhode G et al. The tough kid book (practical classroom management strategies). Longmont, CO: Sopris West, 1995.

16. Shure MB. Raising a thinking child. An Owl Book. Henry Holt and Company, Inc, 1995.

17. Stern J & Ben-Ami U. Many ways to learn – young people's guide to learning disabilities. New York: Magination Press, 1996.

18. Turecki S. The difficult child. New York: Bantam Books, 1989.

Index